It's Your Body:
A Woman's Guide to Gynecology

"An important book. Lauersen encourages women to abandon the traditional passivity of the patient and take a more active and effective role."

Helen S. Kaplan, M.D., Ph.D.,
Director, Human Sexuality Program,
New York Hospital—Cornell Medical Center

"Now is the time for getting to know your intimate self with this warm, sensitive knowledgeable physician as your guide."

Mildred Newman,
co-author of *How to Be Your Own Best Friend*

"Within the context of medical guides, Lauersen's book is impressive. He covers everything from abortions to orgasm in a manner that's unusually contemporary, sensible, sympathetic and detailed."

The New York Post

It's Your Body:
A Woman's Guide to Gynecology

by Niels Lauersen, M.D.,
and Steven Whitney

PLAYBOY PRESS
PAPERBACKS

CONTENTS

ACKNOWLEDGMENTS

There are many friends, colleagues, and patients who stimulated and encouraged us throughout the preparation of this book. To each and every one of them, we offer our gratitude.

The research, drafting, and critical analysis done by Kathleen H. Wilson, Jeffery Wood, and Craig Buck were invaluable in the completion of the manuscript. Our most profound thanks go to each of them. Without these three, this book would not be.

Others who helped immeasurably with research, verification, analysis, and drafting were Joel Surnow, Suzanne Grace, Mark Jacobsen, and Flansy Lewis.

The entire manuscript was typed by Lynn Scalla. The drafts, transcripts, and research notes were typed by Lori Leeds, Linda Elmore, Debbie Butler, Susan Donovan, Robin Fegley, Marsha Stein, Joann Froner, and Sue Janssen. Each of them also gave us insightful comments at every step.

The original art was done by Enrique Senis-Oliver, and the medical illustrations are the work of Pauline Thomas and Peter Ng. We also express our gratitude to Tom Saltarelli for photographic work and to Barry Cummings for photographic artwork.

So many others helped in so many ways, we can do little more than list them by way of saying thank you: Rob Morris, Janet Green, Phyllis Keitlen, Clair Sater, Allen Ralston, Harvey Rubin, Barbara Sater, Diana Davis, Jane Toonkel, Stafford Morgan, Tara Cole, Barbara Karpf, Laura Roth, David Schwartz, Vicki Till, Adrian Rothenberg, Steven Kriegsman, Tom Barad, and Cindy Boscowitz.

And a special thank you to Mel Sokolow, who saw the project through from beginning to end.

ILLUSTRATIONS

All drawings, graphs, diagrams, and photographs have been created solely for use in this book, except where noted by a credit line, and are the property of the authors.

NOTE

For the purpose of simplicity, the authors have chosen to designate the hypothetical gynecologists in this book with the male gender pronouns—he, his, him, etc. This gender rendering should not be viewed as a political or chauvinistic choice; rather as a means to greater clarification—making it easier to distinguish between the patient, who is always a *she,* and the doctor. It is true that more than 90% of all Ob.Gyn. specialists are men, but it is obvious to everyone that this field can only benefit by the increasing number of women who choose it for their profession. Hopefully, this future sexual balance in personnel will bring a greater closeness and understanding between doctors and patients.

INTRODUCTION

Today's woman is increasingly concerned with the well-being of her body. Consequently, she is determined to know more about her normal bodily functions and her medical care. The controversial effects of various drugs (such as the birth-control pill) and the epidemic proportions of certain illnesses (such as venereal disease) rightly concern every responsible woman. Too often, widespread media reports emphasize the more sensational aspects of medical findings, causing patients to be greatly confused by the apparently endless deluge of conflicting information. There is a need for practical and relevant information about a woman's body and the medical procedures relating to it. *It's Your Body* was written to fill that need.

We hope this book will help women realize the wonderfully complex functions of the female body. The normal functions are explained so that any abnormal functions that are symptoms of illness can be recognized in time to seek appropriate professional help. This should help inform and prepare a woman who does have an illness or malfunction become a partner in her own medical treatment.

However, our book was not written as a guide to self-treatment, but as a thorough encyclopedia of all aspects of a woman's life, from menarche to menopause, including a guide to sexual terminology and problems. The theory behind the book is simple: The best patient is an informed patient. We hope *It's Your Body* will help women understand their physicians' instructions and recommendations more completely. Through both its written words and its many illustrations, this book should lead women to a better understanding of a particular condition or a suggested treatment.

The data is the most recent available. For this reason, we hope our work leads women to the latest developments in the field of gynecology.

—NIELS H. LAUERSEN, M.D., NEW YORK
—STEVEN WHITNEY, LOS ANGELES

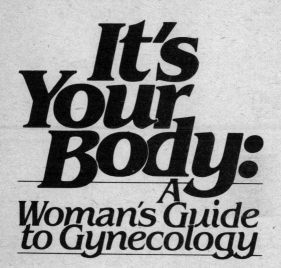

It's Your Body:
A Woman's Guide to Gynecology

chapter 1

SELF-EXAMINATION

GROWING UP AFRAID

A little four-year-old white boy is standing nude after taking a communal bath in his nursery school. He looks at the nude four-year-old black girl standing next to him. An expression of great puzzlement crosses his face as he continues staring at the black girl. Finally, he calls the teacher over to him and whispers in her ear. "Teacher, I didn't know there was such a big difference between white kids and black kids!"

A charming story, but, sadly, it is all too true. This statement and others like it are heard again and again at this age level, even between sisters and brothers. The reason is simple: a shocking lack of early education.

Most of us remember the time we first noticed the difference between penises and vaginas. Freud felt (and this is still a widely held opinion) that this was a traumatic event for little girls. His reasoning was this: Upon seeing a penis, the little girl was seized with jealousy and feelings of castration and inferiority.

> They notice the penis of a brother or playmate, strikingly visible and of large proportions, at once recognize it as the superior counterpart of their own small and inconspicuous organ, and from that time forward fall a victim to envy for the penis . . . She has seen it and knows that she is without it and wants to have it. [From *The Complete Psychological Works of Sigmund Freud,* The Hogarth Press.]

This statement, more than anything, seems to shed light on Freud's own phallocentricity. Today, "penis envy" has been called into question by many leading psychiatrists, who feel there is nothing superior or inferior in the way of genitalia; that everyone is equal. They feel Freud never considered the idea that little girls may have been jealous of the preferential treatment given to boys. The Victorian era was particularly repressive to women, and it is very possible that little girls of the time would have liked penises so that they, too, could have enjoyed the privileges bestowed on boys.

The girl who has enjoyed equal standing with boys and who has observed mutual respect between her parents should, upon viewing her first penis, notice merely that boys are different. If she has been allowed (mostly through example) to be proud of her body, she will probably be very happy with her streamlined build. Indeed, why should she envy the little boy his excess baggage?

Fortunately, there is a natural biological curiosity to discover and explore one's own body. A little girl discovers her opening and also discovers the pleasant sensation she derives from touching it. This pleasure is all too often offset by her parents'

Fig. 1–1: The reproductive organs in men and women have the same genetic origin. The sex of every child is determined at conception, but it cannot be discerned until the end of the eighth week after conception, or the tenth week after the mother's last menstrual period.

A small bud develops on the groin area of the fetus. If the child is to be a girl, this bud will form into the clitoris. Likewise, the bud will become a penis if the child is to be a boy. The tissue surrounding this bud folds back into the labia with girls, while it forms the scrotum in boys.

This tissue, which is called *genital tubercle,* begins to develop five weeks after conception, or seven weeks after the last menstrual period. This is shown in the top picture, where the genitalia is seen in the undifferentiated state. At this point, the bud appears as a phallus-like organ, but it is still too early to determine the sex of the fetus.

Ten weeks after conception, or twelve weeks after the last menstrual period, the development of *specific* sexual determination can be seen (see middle set of drawings), although a complete development of the penis or vulva does not occur until the fourth month (see lower set of drawings).

The illustration clearly demonstrates how the glands of the penis and the glands of the vulva both develop from the genital tubercle. The clitoral and penal foreskins are also developed from the same tissue in the undifferentiated state. The *labia minora* and the *raphe* (the tissue on the underside of the penis) are developed from the same tissue. Because of this, the *raphe,* like the *labia minora,* is extremely sensitive to touch.

THE DEVELOPMENT OF THE EXTERNAL SEXUAL ORGANS

UNDIFFERENTIATED

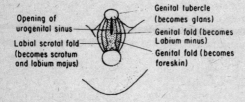

Opening of
urogenital sinus

Labial scrotal fold
(becomes scrotum
and labium majus)

Genital tubercle
(becomes glans)

Genital fold (becomes
Labium minus)

Genital fold (becomes
foreskin)

MALE

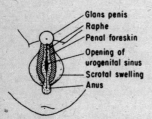

Glans penis
Raphe
Penal foreskin
Opening of
urogenital sinus
Scrotal swelling
Anus

FEMALE

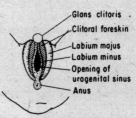

Glans clitoris
Clitoral foreskin
Labium majus
Labium minus
Opening of
urogenital sinus
Anus

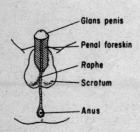

Glans penis
Penal foreskin
Raphe
Scrotum
Anus

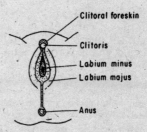

Clitoral foreskin
Clitoris
Labium minus
Labium majus
Anus

stern warnings not to play with anything "dirty" or of a sexual nature. This results in enormous anxiety and guilt concerning the exploration of her own body, an exploration that is the most natural urge of humanity.

Instead of having a knowledgeable feeling of comfort about their vaginas, then, little girls are caught in a complex mystery, and no one seems willing to explain what is going on. Girls hear old wives' tales and horror stories that fill them only with fear. They are told not to touch boys, not to bathe in the same water as boys, not to touch themselves, and not to ask questions. They grow up suspicious not only of men, but of themselves and their own sexuality.

Most girls, however, cannot resist the natural temptation to explore their own bodies. They go to the library to read about themselves and their vaginas. They even begin to probe the opening with their fingertips. Here they meet with trouble. As their fingers push against the hymen, they experience pain, which underlines the scare tactics used by their parents and grandparents. "Keep your fingers away from that, it is dangerous," they were told. And when they experience the pain on their own, those warnings seem warranted.

Of course, in recent years, attitudes toward sex education have become more liberal, and some of the stigma surrounding self-knowledge has been removed. Ironically, in many of the world's so-called primitive societies, the exchange of sex information between generations is considered an early responsibility of the tribe elders.

As liberalized as some segments of our society have become, the fact remains that *most* girls do not receive sufficient information. Confusion and mystery cloud the early years. When a girl gets her first menstrual period, the sudden appearance of blood is often a frightening, and sometimes a traumatic, experience.

It has been consistently shown in recent years that many—indeed, most—of the emotional traumas attached to adult sexual behavior have been caused by the refusal of parents to provide enough *correct* information to their children. In most cases, girls receive even less information than boys, so it follows that, as women, they must overcome even greater fears. Not surprisingly, many women come to regard the opposite sex with fear, suspicion, and confusion. And emotional friction between men and women serves no one.

The solutions are so simple.

First, there must be an open and honest communication between the girl and her parents. The differences between boys and girls should be examined, as should any other questions that arise in the girl's mind. Perhaps most important, every girl should be infused with the excitement and joy peculiar to becoming a woman.

Second, every girl should be given access to books which will help explain her budding sexuality. These books should show all the functions and relationships of the sexual organs. They should also provide clear illustrations, either drawings or photographs. (Be very careful in selecting the books you give to your daughter. Surprisingly, many of the new sex education books for children merely reflect the sexist attitudes of their authors. For example, there are many books that have no mention of the clitoris. Diagrams of the vaginal area *should* include graphic representation of the clitoris, followed by an explanation of its function.)

Third, girls should be given freedom to explore their own bodies without incurring the disapproval of their elders or their peers. Every child has a normal urge to explore her body, and this should be encouraged, not discouraged. As an adult, the more a woman knows about her body and its functions, the more she can appreciate the impulses constantly in motion within her. The more a woman knows about sex, the more she will be able to enjoy it.

EXPLORING YOUR VULVA

Many women mistakenly believe the vulva is itself an organ. They have heard their friends and physicians refer to it, and they have read books in which the word *vulva* is frequently used but never explained. The vulva, though, is not one specific organ. Instead, it is the name given the *entire outer area* of a woman's genital-urethral organs. The vulva comprises the *labia majora* (large lips), *labia minora* (small lips), the clitoris, the urethral opening, and the vaginal opening. The anus and the pubic hair are not, technically, considered part of the vulva, even though most discussions of the vulva inevitably mention them because of their close proximity to the vulva.

Mirrors

Throughout history, mirrors have been used to do more than can be described in this book. If ever there was an object whose development arose from insatiable curiosity, it is the mirror. From the beginning of time, men and women alike have enjoyed seeing their images reflected in a piece of glass. Unfortunately, in many minds, the mirror became to vanity what food was to gluttony; unfortunately, because the mirror is one of the world's most useful tools, and to confuse healthy curiosity with vanity is a sad mistake.

Unless you are a skilled contortionist, the mirror will be the most valuable tool at your disposal in examining your vulva. Certainly it will help you examine the outside region, but it will also, to a certain extent, allow you to look inside yourself.

Many physicians feel that mothers should use mirrors to show their daughters the exact location of the pelvic organs. Whether or not one subscribes to that theory, it must be admitted that a mirror, per se, is neither evil nor morally wrong. To

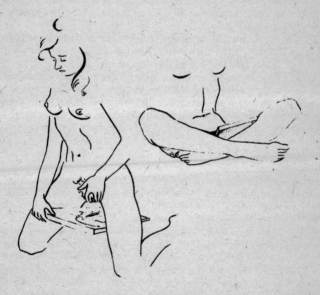

Fig. 1–2: Pictured here are two positions that are easy for most women to achieve in self-examination of the vulva.

At left, a woman is standing on her slightly separated knees with a mirror between her legs. This mirror is tilted, allowing the woman a clear view of her vulva through its reflection in the mirror. If the reflection is too dark, focus a beam of light against the vulval area.

At right, the self-examination is shown as it occurs in the lotus position. Here, the mirror is resting on the legs, giving you two free hands to spread the vulva apart, which will allow you to examine more specific portions of the vulva.

use a mirror to learn more about yourself and your body could hardly be considered harmful; indeed, it can and will do you a great deal of good.

Position

In using a mirror to examine your vulva, there are two easily attainable positions. You may either sit in the lotus position with your legs comfortably crossed, or you can simply kneel with your legs spread. In either position, you can lean backward or forward to reach the most comfortable state.

Regardless of which position you have chosen, place the mirror underneath you, between your legs. This will give you a relatively good view of the general area. To get a more specific view, though, you should use a flashlight, aiming it at the specific organs you wish to examine in detail. When you are doing this, you may also want to move the mirror closer to the specific organ you are examining.

Some women prefer using a mirror with some degree of magnification. This is certainly understandable, but it would probably be best to start with a mirror that will reflect the exact size of the organs. Once you have done that, though, you should feel free to use whatever sort of mirror you desire.

Labia Majora

Now that you are in a comfortable position and examining yourself with a mirror, the first organ to come to your attention will probably be the *labia majora*, or large lips. The *labia majora* contain deposits of fatty tissue and are covered with hair. As women get older, these lips become more flaccid and will contain less fatty tissue. In very old women, the large lips usually become just atrophic membranes, or shapeless pieces of skin.

These large lips may appear useless, but in fact they are extremely functional. The fat and the hair combine so that the large lips completely cover the vagina. In this way, no dirt or sweat can work its way into the vaginal opening. It might be said that the large lips are nature's contribution to preventive medicine. By protecting against dirt, the lips prevent a great deal of infection and disease.

Labia Minora

As the large lips are pulled aside, you will have a clear view of the *labia minora*, or small lips. These small lips are without hair, but they serve the same general purpose as the large lips—protection from dirt. They are the backup system, the secondary covering.

The small lips also play an important role in sexual activity. During any sort of sexually excited state, blood rushes to the small lips, filling and enlarging them in the same way blood causes an erection in the male penis. When a woman engages in intercourse, this sudden growth of the small lips creates a tighter grip around the penis, resulting in more pleasure for both parties. This enlargement also gives more cover to the vaginal opening, and so can help keep the sperm in the vagina after intercourse.

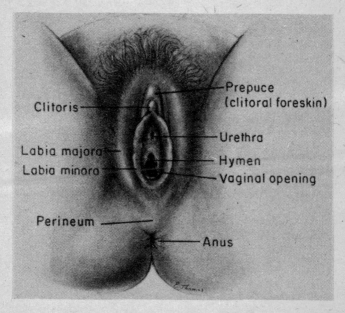

Fig. 1–3:   Above is a drawing of a vulva showing the normal anatomical relationship between the various parts of the vulva and the pubic hair and rectal opening (the anus). Every woman is slightly different and so is each vulva. Because of this, during self-examination, you shouldn't be disappointed if the anatomical parts of your vulva are not as easy to recognize as those in this drawing. The *labia majora* are here separated to allow a better view of the outer part of the vagina, locating the urethra and the hymen ring surrounding the vaginal opening.

During masturbation, the small lips are incredibly sensitive in their enlarged state. This, of course, should give greater physical pleasure.

The small lips are completely covered by the *labia majora* during early childhood, but as a girl becomes a woman, the small lips usually begin to protrude past the large lips to varying degrees. The small lips do, indeed, become larger for a variety of reasons.

First, the genetic factor undeniably influences the entire physical structure of each human being. Just as genes are responsible for the size and shape of the nose, they are equally responsible for the makeup of the *labia minora*. Some women will naturally have more pronounced *labia minora* than other women.

Second, extensive sexual activity, be it intercourse or masturbation, will also cause the *labia minora* to protrude beyond the large lips. Sexual activity stretches the *labia minora*, just as it stretches, to some extent, the penis. For example, women of African tribes usually have very pronounced *labia minora*, a fact sometimes attributed to the encouragement of early sex play in these tribes. Generally speaking, the more a woman masturbates or has intercourse, the larger her small lips become.

It follows that childbirth and abortion also stretch the small lips, though probably to a lesser extent, due to the relative infrequency of such events.

In rare cases, the *labia minora* might become so large that they cover the vagina to an extent that interferes with intercourse. If this happens, the excess skin can be surgically removed, restoring the *labia minora* to a more functional state.

The Clitoris

When one sees an early-developed fetus, it is impossible to determine whether it is a boy or a girl because the stemlike area in the pubic region could be either a clitoris or a penis. If it is a boy, this stem will grow into a penis; if it is a girl, the stem will open up into a vulva and vagina, with the clitoris remaining as what was the base of the early stem.

As you pull the large lips apart, the clitoris will be seen at the top of the inside folds where the large and small lips come together. The *prepuce,* or clitoral foreskin, is the name given to the additional folds which sit on the small lips at an angle and look like a triangular hat. The clitoris is directly in the middle of this small hat. In girls, the prepuce covers the clitoris very tightly, but it loosens its grip on the gland as the girl becomes a

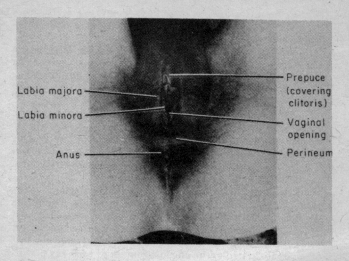

Labia majora

Labia minora

Anus

Prepuce
(covering
clitoris)

Vaginal
opening

Perineum

Fig. 1–4: Shown above is a photograph of the vulval area of a twenty-year-old woman. One can clearly see hair covering the *labia majora*. As in the majority of women, the clitoris is not completely visible and is covered by the *prepuce*, or clitoral foreskin. To see the clitoris, the prepuce must be pushed up. The *labia minora* are seen protruding between the *labia majora*. Notice also that the *labia minora* is without hair. The size of the *labia minora* varies from woman to woman. This difference can be traced partially to genetic factors and partially to sexual activity. The vaginal opening is visible between the *labia minora*. The area between the lower portion of the labia and the anus is called the *perineum*. Most women who have borne children will have scars in the area of the perineum. This scar is from the *episiotomy*—the cut made to enable the passage of the baby during delivery.

woman. If it does not loosen its hold, a portion of the prepuce can be removed, a process akin to circumcision.

When you get the head of the clitoris between your fingers, you can feel it as a small mass and that is what it is—a small mass, or a gland.

When you play with the clitoris, you will find that, like a penis, it is an extremely sensitive area, and it will become stiffer and larger with manipulation. By extensive clitoral play, you will usually bring on an orgasm.

It is important to bring on this sensation by self-manipulation, and you should train yourself to do it for two major reasons. First, it will enable you to recognize an orgasm when you have one, and second, the more these organs are trained to reflexive action, the easier it becomes to have an orgasm.

Unfortunately, the clitoris is in a rather inconvenient position for intercourse. It is, sexually speaking, too high up in the vulvar region. When the penis enters the vagina, it will not usually rub against the clitoris. The lack of stimulation to the clitoris is, perhaps, the main problem in intercourse. Because of this, it is often necessary for either a woman or her partner to stimulate her clitoris during intercourse.

Orgasm is not caused merely by clitoral sensation, but by the nerves of the entire, sensitized vulvar area. Each woman must explore and manipulate each organ to find out which one is the most sensitized and most likely to bring orgasm.

The clitoris becomes larger with extensive masturbation or manipulation. The size of the clitoris is also genetically factored. Some women have larger clitorises than others. But the size of the clitoris has no influence on the facility to reach orgasm. What is influential is the training and learning of the reflexes of the nerve endings.

SEEING INSIDE

The Hymen

When looking inside the *labia minora*, it is usually a good idea to insert a finger into the vaginal opening, using the finger to stretch the opening to allow a better view. About half an inch inside the vaginal opening, you will see a small membrane or rudiment of a membrane. This is the *hymen*. The hymen is usually broken after the first intercourse, but fragments of it exist throughout a woman's life. When it is broken, the hymen looks like small pieces of flesh sitting along the half-inch circumference of the vaginal wall. Occasionally, the hymen lingers as a long piece of flesh, and this can be surgically removed if it is bothersome.

Some women are born with extremely small hymens. These women will have little problem or pain upon first intercourse, and sometimes the hymen does not even rip.

Other women are born with hymens almost completely closed. Sometimes the hymen is so tight it is almost impossible to penetrate during intercourse. In such an event, the hymen might have to be opened by surgery *(hymenectomy)*. In most cases, though, patience and a slowly induced finger can break

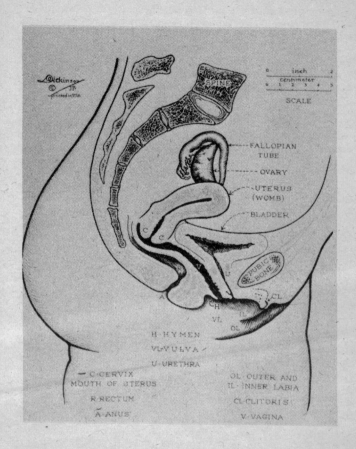

Fig. 1–5: This picture shows the relationship in position and size of the pelvic organs in a standing woman. The uterus in this drawing is in the *anteverted,* or front, position. It should also be clear that the vagina is not a hole, but a collapsed space directed backward and connected to the uterus by the cervix at an almost right angle. Notice that the clitoris is located at least an inch from the opening of the vagina. For this reason, during normal intercourse, no direct rubbing of the clitoris takes place. (Dickinson Anatomical Chart—reproduced by permission of Educational Department, TAMPAX Incorporated, Lake Success, New York.)

the closed hymen, even one that will not allow the penetration of a penis. With some women, an emotionally or physically traumatic event will open the hymen.

Of course, the hymen can open during horseback riding, or bicycling, or even because of a simple fall. In cultures where virginity is prized above all else in brides, many a tragic horseback ride has been confessed in many a bedroom.

The Vagina

If you have not yet had intercourse, it might be impossible to explore deeper into yourself with a mirror and a light. The hymen might obstruct a clear view.

On the other hand, even if you have had intercourse, it might still be difficult for you to see into the vagina. The reason is simple. Although many people (women included) think of the vagina as a sort of hole, it is, in fact, a *collapsed space surrounded by muscle*. Some physicians and women prefer the term *muscle tube* in describing the vagina.

Being comprised of muscle, the vagina is controllable. You can train yourself to contract and/or expand these muscles. The effect is obvious—it increases sexual pleasure. During intercourse, a woman tightens the muscles around the penis, giving not only the man, but herself as well, more sensation, since more friction is created between the penis and the vaginal walls.

Under certain physical and/or psychological situations, the muscles of the vagina will tighten to the degree where it becomes difficult for the man to pull out. This can, of course, be desirable if planned and controlled, but if it is an accidental reflex, the woman must train herself to relax and train her muscles to respond to her desires. If this happens and the woman has not yet learned to relax, nature still compensates. At the moment of orgasm, the upper part of the vagina balloons out, almost like a silent explosion, after which the muscle tension naturally decreases and the man is able to withdraw.

Vaginismus is a more serious problem. Again, for either physical or psychological reasons, this condition occurs when the muscles of the vagina tighten so much that nothing, much less an erect penis, can enter the space. This problem will be explored fully later in this book.

The length of the vagina has been the topic of discussions ranging from the *Kama Sutra* to the locker room. Just as men and women believe many myths concerning the length of a penis, they are apt to be just as silly about the length of a vagina. In general, black women have longer, deeper vaginas than their

white European counterparts. However, unless a woman has
hang-ups about this, the length of the vagina has no bearing on
either productivity or enjoyment.

Most surface abnormalities in the vagina, like warts or discharges, will be seen through the mirror. With discharges, it is
very important to note the coloring. This can aid in the diagnosis of an infection. Venereal warts, brought on by a sexual
virus, are in the back part of the vagina and drain out with a
discharge. The warts sometimes spread all the way down to the
rectal opening.

If you see either warts or discharges, or any other abnormalities that worry you, see your physician.

The Cervix

By sitting down on your heels or by standing up with one leg
on a chair or toilet seat, you can merely bend down and insert
your index finger or middle finger into the vagina. As you push
your finger deeply into the vagina, you will feel something like
the tip of your nose. This is the *cervix*. It is a hard area with a
small depression in the middle at the top of the vagina.

The cervix serves as a valve between the vagina and the
uterus (which lies behind the cervix), and the small depression
that you feel with your finger is the tiny hole through which
sperm enter the uterus, blood flows from the uterus during
menstruation, and babies come during birth.

The area around the cervix on the vaginal side is called the
fornix, and it not only surrounds the cervix but serves as the
outer, protective wall of the uterus.

The uterus will not be accessible to you during a self-
examination, so it will be dealt with in a later chapter. However,
the interaction of the uterus, the cervix, and the vagina can be
partially explained here.

During intercourse, the penis may push hard against the cervix, hitting the uterus and throwing it higher up inside you.
Certainly this will be more frequent when you are in the
superior position, because the muscles push down on the bladder, shortening the vagina. You should not worry about this,
unless, of course, there is unusual pain during or after sex. If
you have an intrauterine device, your partner may think he is
hitting the IUD and he might complain. Although this is possible, it is much more likely that he is, instead, pushing against
the cervix.

In some positions, the uterus is tilted into an abnormal position, and this may cause some pain. This depends on the length

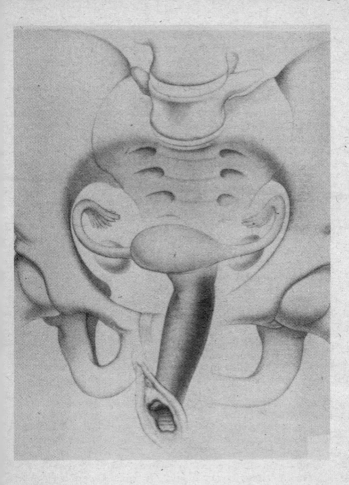

Fig. 1–6: A frontal view of the female reproductive organs, showing their relation in size and position to the pelvic bones. The vulva and the vaginal opening are clear. The muscular tube of the vagina is pointed to the back and the cervix can just be seen in the upper portion of the vagina. The uterus is tilted forward, anteverted in the normal position, and the fallopian tubes lead away from the uterus toward the egg-shaped ovaries. (Reproduced by permission of Ortho Pharmaceutical Corporation, Raritan, New Jersey.)

of the vagina, and may be avoided by knowing that the vagina achieves different lengths in different positions. You may feel how this happens by moving from one position to another by yourself with your finger in the vagina. You will notice how the vagina expands and contracts as you move. This is, of course, an interaction with the uterus, which is pushing against or away from the top of the vagina. Because of this tendency, the knee-chest position is a favorite of many women, especially those with shorter vaginas. In the knee-chest position, the vagina is stretched to its greatest extent, usually allowing the greatest degree of pleasure.

Obviously, when examining the vagina and the cervix with your fingers, if you feel a lump or something that you think is irregular, you should ask your physician about it. In fact, if you have any questions concerning any part of your self-examination, you should not hesitate to bring it up with your gynecologist.

With your finger, you will probably be able to palpate, or touch, the cervix. If you have an IUD, this palpation is particularly important (see chapter 9), but even if you don't have an IUD, it is useful to be able to judge the depth and the breadth of your vagina by such a palpation.

EXTRA TEXTURES

Usually considered a part of the vulva are the anus (rectal opening) and the pubic hair. In fact, they are separate from the vulva, but their close proximity makes it convenient to examine them at the same time as you are exploring your vulva.

Pubic Hair

The hair covering the *mons pubis* is another dirt-collecting agency, protecting the orifice below. It also absorbs a great deal of sweat.

Pubic hair should generally be in a triangle, the top of which is usually a fairly straight line. Orientals generally have less pubic hair, and do not necessarily have a straight upper line. In Blacks and white European women, however, if the upper line of the pubic hair moves in a triangular direction toward the navel, it usually indicates a higher than average presence of male hormones in the system. If this is true, the hair itself will also be of the male hormone type, and there will probably be more hair on the legs, arms, and even perhaps on the face.

Possessing more male hormones in no way affects your femininity or your womanhood. It is probably just a genetic happenstance. But if you recognize this tendency, you should be aware that it is often associated with a condition known as polycystic ovaries, or Stein-Leventhal disease, discussed in chapter 14. This condition can be evaluated by your physician, and he should be able to answer any questions you have.

The Anus (Rectal Opening)

Approximately one or two fingers'-breadth below the lower end of the vagina, you will see the anus, or the opening to the rectum. This is usually a very tight area, but if you engage in frequent anal intercourse, it will appear more relaxed. Also, the area around the rectal opening is usually very smooth, but after childbirth there might be external hemorrhoids, which are seen as pieces of flesh sitting on the outside.

Any lumps, warts, or other irregularities that you see around the rectum should be reported to your doctor, who can check them out. If these irregularities are not serious (such as prickly heat), be sure you can recognize them the next time around. It will save you needless, but normal, worry.

chapter 2

HOW TO CHOOSE A GYNECOLOGIST

Many women have more trouble finding a good gynecologist than Stanley had tracking down Livingstone. Some women, trying to avoid the dilemma of a search altogether, give the matter little thought. They quickly settle either on someone in the neighborhood or become loyal, if dissatisfied, patients of their mother's gynecologist. Other women realize they must shop around to find a doctor they like, just as they must shop around for any good buy. The trouble here is that many of these women are insecure about judging doctors (it is something they have been taught by society not to do), or they are not sure they could recognize a good gynecologist if they saw one.

The easiest way to begin this search is by eliminating certain doctors who don't fulfill even the simple basics of the profession.

If a gynecologist is cold or unsympathetic, he probably won't be able to support your emotional needs. If the physician is rushed during your first examination, or if he is terribly disorganized, you will probably have to look elsewhere. You want a gynecologist who doesn't resent the time spent with patients, and you want one organized at least to the point that it is your file he's reading when he's with you. For most women, unusually high fees are another basic that sends them elsewhere. It must always be remembered that high fees do not necessarily guarantee good medicine.

These are basics that everyone knows. Still, they must be

repeated time and again. Unfortunately, even these do not provide sufficient information for choosing a gynecologist who is right for you.

This book cannot offer a definitive list of competent gynecologists, but it can give you some basic guidelines for finding a good one. In following these guidelines, you must be as tough and as critical as you would be in any other area of your life. It is a very important *personal* decision, but it is also a hard *business* decision; you are paying money and you should get the very best value for your dollar.

Although you must find a physician with complete technical competence, he must also fit your specific psychological and emotional needs. The human element is very important—a technically superb gynecologist may be right for your neighbor's emotional needs, but wrong for yours. It is essential to find a doctor with whom you can relate easily. Such a doctor will make you feel as comfortable as possible and will gain, as well as earn, your trust and confidence.

After all, you and your doctor are engaged in the healing process. To accomplish this, you will be working closely together. If there is little or no rapport between the two of you, the healing process will suffer.

Of course, you should have alternatives from which to choose. To settle on the first doctor you hear mentioned would be unfair to both you and the physician. Neither should you rely solely on the advice of family or friends. A doctor who is good for your mother, your sister, or your best friend still may not be good for you.

If you are a young woman and your mother's doctor is older, as is often the case, his opinions about birth control or his knowledge of the latest techniques may not be compatible with your needs. His practice, in this case, would probably consist mostly of older women, contemporaries of your mother, whose problems, illnesses, and emotional needs would be different from those a younger woman would have.

Usually younger women want a doctor closer to their own age, not only for his more recent medical training, but also because it may be easier to relate personally to someone more contemporary. Such a physician will also be able to tend the younger woman throughout her lifetime, just as her mother's doctor tended her for years.

Some younger women are concerned also that their mother's doctor might, as a gesture of innocent friendship, tell the mother more about the daughter than the daughter wishes her to know. Whether this is classified as spying or as motherly concern, the problem is avoided by finding your own doctor.

HOW TO FIND A GOOD DOCTOR

The selection process begins by seeking advice from trusted friends. As different doctors are discussed, you should discover how long your friend has been seeing the gynecologist she has recommended. A woman who has seen a doctor for years is undoubtedly more qualified to judge than a woman who has been seeing one for only six months.

You should also find out the recommended doctor's opinions on such matters as abortion, birth control, estrogen therapy, or any other topic which concerns you. Regardless of a physician's skill, most women prefer gynecologists to share at least some of their beliefs. Again, get the name of more than one doctor—you may have to visit quite a few before finding one who is compatible with your beliefs.

If you have moved to a new town or if your friends fail to supply you with satisfactory choices, you might get the information you need from the nearest good hospital, preferably one associated with a medical school. The chief resident of the hospital should be able to help, as should a hospital administrator or any other knowledgeable staff worker. Such a person should give you three or four names to consider. This can be particularly valuable when you are seeking a second opinion.

You may wish to visit a nearby hospital to seek advice. Nurses and interns, both of whom work closely with a number of doctors, can often give well-grounded opinions about the better doctors on the staff. Better yet, interns and nurses often are not caught up in the medical game of protecting other doctors.

A local Planned Parenthood chapter or the county medical society can usually provide the names of a number of well-qualified gynecologists in the area.

If you are specifically looking for a woman gynecologist, you should contact the American Medical Women's Association in your area for their recommendations. Be advised, though, that as a medical association, they cannot recommend one doctor over another; they can only supply a list of women gynecologists, from which you will have to do further study. In many areas, the National Organization of Women (NOW) can refer you to a women's health organization.

Certainly one of the most common methods of choosing a gynecologist is to ask your own internist or family doctor, if you have one, particularly if you are pleased with him. Good doctors tend to associate with other good doctors, and should be an excellent source of referrals.

HOW TO EXAMINE YOUR GYNECOLOGIST

After you have the names of several recommended gynecologists, you will want to find out more about them for yourself. You may be justifiably concerned about not having the medical background to decide which doctor is most qualified for your needs. The average person is not expected to have medical training, but there are still some simple ways to evaluate a doctor.

Start by looking up the doctors who interest you in the *Directory of Medical Specialists,* available in medical libraries, many public libraries, and at local county medical society offices. The directory lists a physician's birthdate, medical school, and the hospital where he took his residency. This information is a good point of departure. An older physician may be more traditional in his outlook and perhaps less involved with the latest ideas or techniques. Perhaps a younger doctor's practice may not be as large, allowing him more time per patient.

Although medical schools are not all alike, they all provide a basic standard of education. Because of this, the medical school a particular doctor attended is not, by itself, grounds for determining a doctor's qualifications. More important is where the physician took his residency, because this is the institution where he received training in his specialty. Hospitals or medical centers associated with medical schools are usually the best places to serve a residency. These are teaching hospitals, in which doctors become familiar with a greater variety of cases and conditions than is possible at smaller or nonteaching hospitals. A residency lasts a long time, generally three to five years. A longer residency training usually produces a more qualified physician, so you should take special note of the length of residency. Taking residency at a good hospital associated with a medical school generally indicates a high-quality physician.

There are other factors you may wish to consider. If a woman favors abortion, for example, and she notices that a doctor was trained in a Catholic medical school or hospital, she would probably do better to find someone else. This is not merely a philosophical problem, but can be one of practical experience as well. As Catholic hospitals perform very few abortions, the doctors trained there are not nearly as experienced in this procedure.

The directory also provides a physician's hospital affiliation.

Good hospitals are your best assurance of quality medical care, and a doctor's ability is strongly indicated by which hospital has appointed him to its staff. The best physicians are usually affiliated with the best hospitals, and the best hospitals are those associated with medical schools. Remember, this is the hospital where you, as a patient, may be admitted, so it bears serious consideration. The hospital reflects the care you may receive, as well as the doctor's standing within his profession.

Another important consideration that is sometimes overlooked by the general public is that of a physician's board certification. Board certification indicates a true specialist in a particular field; in this case, gynecology. To become board certified, a doctor must train in residency for three to five years and pass several difficult examinations in his specialty. These examinations have a failure rate of nearly 40 percent. Passing these boards indicates a doctor of top professional standing in his specialty. The doctors who complete these requirements are known as board certified, while physicians completing all but the final examination are board eligible, which is almost as significant. Studies have shown that specialists holding board certification provide a significantly higher standard of medical care. A doctor may call himself a specialist even without passing these boards, so it is your responsibility to examine this fine point. Whenever possible, especially if you have a complex problem, you should seek a doctor who is board certified. This information is available from the *Directory of Medical Specialists,* local medical societies, and some libraries. You might even ask the gynecologist or his secretary in which specialty he holds certification.

After you have checked out a number of physicians and narrowed your list on the basis of their qualifications, you should call their offices and compare fees. A polite question to the secretary about the doctor's fee for your initial visit and examination is completely proper, and you should not hesitate to ask. It makes no sense to pay one physician significantly more for the same services provided by another, equally qualified, physician.

It is also an excellent idea to talk with the gynecologist and discuss your personal needs. This is a good way to determine if the two of you are emotionally and philosophically compatible. If he is too busy to talk to you or fails to return your call, he probably is not the man for you. You may have a particular problem (infertility, for example), with which you want special help. Doctors often have subspecialties within their specialties.

In this case, you would want to consult a gynecologist whose subspecialty is infertility.

Contrary to popular myth, studies have shown that doctors who are members of group practices usually provide a better standard of care than single or "solo" doctors. The environment of several doctors consulting and checking one another's results naturally keeps doctors at peak performance.

THE GYNECOLOGIST AS PRIMARY PHYSICIAN

The changing life-styles of women have led to changes in the role of the gynecologist. More women than ever before see their gynecologists for problems unrelated to the reproductive organs. In many cases, the gynecologist has replaced the family doctor or general practitioner as the primary physician. Consequently, it is likely that you will see your gynecologist for many reasons, and he should perform routine checks for high blood pressure, diabetes, and similar illnesses.

There is a faction of the American College of Obstetricians and Gynecologists which feels a gynecologist should be educated in the fields of gynecology, obstetrics, family planning and abortion, endocrinology (the study of glands, such as the thyroid or pituitary), and surgery. He should have widespread education in medicine and medical diseases, so he can serve as a primary physician, able both to treat a woman for minor illness and to make knowledgeable referrals to specialists in more serious cases. Gynecologists themselves are accepting this new responsibility of becoming the primary physician.

As with any physician, you certainly should not wait for an emergency to try to locate a gynecologist. This is especially true if he is to serve as your primary physician. Find yourself a doctor *now*, when you can think slowly and logically. Do not wait until you are under the stress and emotion of an emergency, when you must take whomever you can get.

A MAN OR WOMAN GYNECOLOGIST?

While most women realize the necessity of gynecological examinations, it is, nonetheless, an uncomfortable experience. Some women are uneasy because the examining physician is male; others are reassured by that very fact. Many women seek women gynecologists, feeling they are better able to relate to a woman doctor, while others feel no need to do so. This is perhaps the single most personal decision you must make in finding a gynecologist who is right for you.

Medicine is dominated in this country by men, and there are far more male gynecologists than female. In fact, only about 6 percent of American gynecologists are women. Still, this does not indicate any difference in ability based on sex. Given the same training, men and women should be of equally high caliber. In Russia, for example, nearly 65 percent of all physicians are women. It is probably the traditional American sex bias that is responsible for the small percentage of women in medicine, as well as the feeling that women doctors are somehow inferior to their male counterparts. There is certainly no room in the medical profession for such opinions, nor for jealousy between men and women gynecologists.

As a matter of practical consideration, however, men have been given greater opportunities, especially in the past, to receive medical training. Residency programs have provided many more men than women with opportunities for advanced work. It stands to reason that more advanced training produces better physicians. So, while many women are excellent physicians, others have not been afforded the opportunities for equal training, especially in surgery and other complex specialties.

Gynecology is a relatively new field. Many of the older gynecologists were general practitioners, or perhaps surgeons, who went into gynecology. Their training in advanced or developing fields, such as endocrinology, may not be the latest, be they male or female. You may find some older female gynecologists with a strong antimale bias, or older males with strong feelings on what is proper conduct for a woman. While each physician certainly has an individual identity, points like these should be considered when you are personally evaluating a gynecologist.

Some women feel they can more easily identify with a female gynecologist, and this transference of identity eases their fears and apprehensions during examinations. Or you may simply feel more comfortable being examined by a woman. Perhaps it is easier for you to relate to a younger, woman gynecologist, finding you have a lot in common socially and philosophically. If you think you would best relate to a woman of your own generation, then you should find such a doctor. Conversely, many women believe they can be more honest with a doctor of the opposite sex. They are more at ease asking questions and more comfortable during the examinations, sometimes to the point where they do not even wish to have a woman nurse in the room during the examination.

What is really being discussed is the association between you and your physician. If you are looking for a young woman doctor whom you can treat as a friend as well as a physician, then find one. If you feel more comfortable with a male, that's fine, too, and you will have a few more to choose from. You are seeking an honest, open, and therapeutic relationship with your gynecologist, so consult whichever sex best helps you fulfill this relationship.

GAMES NOT TO PLAY

By now, you should be able to identify a physician who is highly qualified. There are, however, several popular but ill-conceived notions about what makes a good doctor. This folklore has absolutely nothing to do with the quality of medical care. For example, many people are concerned with the social status of a physician or the status of his patients. A wealthy society doctor with patients of high social standing certainly indicates a high fee, but says little about the caliber of the physician. It is easy to see how such a notion developed, but it is equally clear that there are better considerations for choosing a gynecologist than simply "all the best people use him." The same can be said for doctors in exclusive neighborhoods or for those who charge significantly higher fees. It is entirely possible in the case of a specialist or an exceptional physician that high fees are indeed appropriate, but fees *themselves* say nothing about the quality of care. The quality of a physician is determined by his education and expertise, not his fee. Doctors in the most exclusive neighborhoods with higher office rents must pass these high rents on to the patients. You are paying for medical care, not a classy address, and should act accordingly.

You should not be greatly influenced by the size of a doctor's practice. A large practice is no guarantee of a fine physician. Perhaps the physician does not refer enough patients to other doctors, or maybe he has not solved the problems of his own patients. Also, consider that while a younger doctor may be equally skilled, it normally takes several years to establish a sizable practice. It can be to your advantage to catch a new doctor when he is young and eager, and you may receive less hurried and more personal care. Then, of course, you will find the physician who cannot possibly see you for at least a month. Usually even the best specialist can see you within two weeks. If you have to wait much longer, perhaps the physician already has more patients than he can handle, or perhaps he plays a lot

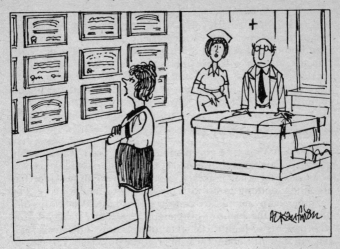

"No wonder you don't know what's wrong with me. You spent half your life in school!"

Fig. 2–1: Reproduced by permission of the artist, Al Kaufman, and *Ob. Gyn. News*, Rockville, Maryland.

of golf. Either way, a long wait for an appointment, unless it is for something quite specialized, tells you nothing about the caliber of the physician. The same can be said for a gynecologist who consistently keeps you waiting for long periods in his office for your appointment. Maybe he feels you have nothing better to do with your time or thinks you really enjoy reading those health magazines all afternoon. Occasional delays and reasonable waits are to be expected, but there seems no logical reason why you should select a gynecologist who schedules too many patients in too short a time, unless you enjoy being examined by an overworked physician.

THE DOCTOR'S PERSONAL SIDE

Besides seeking someone who is medically well qualified, you are also looking for a physician with whom you can establish a personal relationship. It is important for your medical care that you be able to communicate easily with your gynecologist, and to do so, you must have a comfortable relationship with the physician. Each woman naturally seeks a different psychological and emotional relationship with her gynecologist. To accommodate the patient, a gynecologist must often fulfill somewhat different roles for different patients. Some women prefer a gynecologist who is somewhat paternalistic, who acts like a reassuring father. Other women wish to keep the relationship on a strictly matter-of-fact basis, or perhaps even prefer a gynecologist who is aloof and more of an adviser. Gynecologists are usually aware of their patients' varying psychological needs and try to act accordingly. It is most important that the two of you are satisfied with the nature of your relationship.

You certainly should expect the gynecologist to treat you personally and to sympathize with your problems and concerns. Being rushed through a doctor's office makes any woman feel slighted, as well as indicating the physician's lack of personal concern. There are any number of qualified physicians, and you need not tolerate being tossed about by a gynecologist who is consistently too busy.

Women should not allow their gynecologists to hide behind the mystique and prestige of the medical world. Physicians who adopt rigidly medical postures or who frequently confuse you with endless medical jargon may be intentionally building a

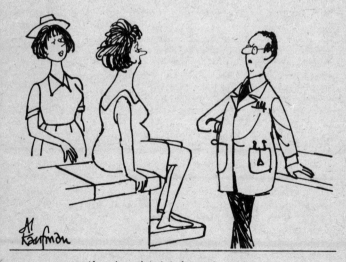

*'I can't explain it in laymen's terms.
I don't know any laymen's terms.'*

Fig. 2–2: Reproduced by permission of the artist, Al Kaufman, and *Ob. Gyn. News,* Rockville, Maryland.

barrier between you, the lowly patient, and him, the seer of science. This mystique makes it all the more difficult to communicate with him and to establish a comfortable relationship. Gynecology has made many advances in recent years, but a doctor who insists on acting like a mystical and inscrutable Merlin is ignoring the fact that he is treating intelligent women who want hard talk, not a Latin lesson.

As a patient, you should not tolerate a doctor who treats you in a condescending manner, shields you from reality, or assumes you cannot make your own decisions. The discussions between the two of you should be open and honest. You have the right to expect a physician to take time to answer your questions thoughtfully and sympathetically. You want somebody who understands your concerns and answers your questions in plain English. It is not difficult for a physician to explain a problem or procedure to you in language that you can understand, and it certainly helps your peace of mind to know exactly what is happening. A physician who constantly answers your questions with, "Don't worry, it will be all right," or, "Why don't you just leave that to me," is not giving you the consideration you deserve. He is violating your right to know, and shows little respect for your concern and intelligence. Physicians should not regard questions, if they are properly put, as challenges to their medical authority or ability. Similarly, a gynecologist who asks you many questions may be indicating his genuine concern with your problems. This give and take is beneficial to a close association between you and your doctor.

GYNECOLOGY IS A MUTUAL EFFORT

The past decade has seen women take more active responsibility for their own lives. This affects the relationship many women expect to have with their gynecologists. Women are rightly demanding greater participation in medical decisions which affect them. They seek doctors willing to present alternative solutions to medical problems and to allow women to be part of the medical team. This gives you the chance to offer your informed consent to the treatments prescribed by the gynecologist. There is increasing resentment of physicians who prescribe a treatment more or less by decree, rather than giving the woman herself several alternative solutions. This is especially true in areas such as birth control, in which some methods are more suited to you than others. Rather than telling a woman what she will be using for birth control, the understanding gynecologist describes several methods and their respective advantages, allowing the woman to participate in the selection of the method most suited to her own life-style. This gives you more active control over your medical and sexual life. The gynecologist is your *partner*, not an omnipotent medical seer. As a team in active partnership, you can proceed for your mutual benefit.

If you are partners, a doctor cannot simply tell you what to do. You want a doctor to inform you of your options and state a medical opinion. To remain independent, however, you cannot allow the gynecologist to impose his morality or opinions upon you. As often as is possible, a doctor should be a neutral observer, giving you the opinions and information necessary for both of you to reach decisions. There are obviously times when a doctor must not remain neutral, and he would be negligent of his medical responsibilities if he did not insist on a specific course of action. This, however, is a matter of medical expertise, and not a decision based on personal moral codes. If, after informed discussion, you disagree with your doctor's course of treatment, by all means seek a second opinion from another physician.

What we must realize is that gynecologists are, or should be, healers. They are not philosophers or moral leaders. Gynecologists have no business deciding the moral or sexual standards of their patients. A doctor has no right to deny you the ability to make judgments which affect your life.

If you are an unmarried woman who wishes some manner of birth control, you should expect a doctor to give it to you without a lecture, snide remarks, or other opinions that have nothing to do with medicine. Your life and sexual activity is your own business, and you should not be subjected to a lecture by a physician with ideas on how you should be living.

Abortions are now legal throughout the United States. There are, however, certain doctors, clinics, or hospitals which still refuse to perform abortions. An individual doctor has the right to refuse to perform abortions, according to his own ethical convictions, but such a doctor should refer you to a physician who does perform this procedure. In the case of hospitals or clinics, especially those supported with public funds, the right to refuse abortions is, at this time, an open question. Although abortions are legal, there are areas of the country in which certain individuals opposed to them are powerful enough to prevent physicians otherwise willing to perform abortions from doing so. It is unfortunate that women are made to feel that they are seeking a disgraceful or illegal solution to a common problem. If a physician does not wish to perform an abortion, a woman needing one should seek another doctor.

A gynecologist's personal morality can also cost you money. Encouraging you to have more children or to have children sooner than you planned can simultaneously increase the doctor's income. You should not be pushed into anything a doctor feels is good for you because it fits his personal wishes.

Treating the "Total" Person

A good gynecologist understands the complex emotional nature of his patients. When a woman is feeling anxious, insecure, or suffering from emotional strain, these feelings are often manifested in her pelvic organs, causing physical dysfunctions or so-called psychosomatic illnesses. Many physical illnesses do, indeed, derive from emotional stress, so a doctor must treat the mind as diligently as he treats the body.

The gynecologist must consider your background, desires, physical capacities, and life-style, and place these into proper perspective for both of you. The doctor should assist you in feeling comfortable about yourself and should help you live happily with who and what you are. Feeling good about who you are and comfortable about your life as a woman is the most important aspect in maintaining good emotional and physical health. The good gynecologist brings all these factors together.

Your Duty as a Patient

The more you know about the nature of your body or your illness, the more you are able to help yourself. Seek information. Ask questions. Get to understand what the doctor is doing with your body. Don't hesitate to speak up when there is something you don't understand. Offer the gynecologist the best information you can about your condition. The more accurately you describe your symptoms and their occurrence, the better they can be treated. Your physician needs feedback, and hiding conditions or symptoms makes the doctor's work more difficult.

At the same time, be human and do not hesitate to express your emotions honestly. In order to treat the *total* person, a doctor must know what you are thinking and feeling; you cannot expect him to rely on guesswork.

Whenever possible, see that the doctor gives you a choice in the course of your treatment. Do not hesitate to ask for alternative methods for dealing with problems, and have confidence in your ability to help make these decisions. The more knowledge you have, the better decision you can make. In addition, refuse to be bullied or intimidated into something you do not want. Remember, if you have any doubts about a course of treatment, seek a second opinion.

If you believe the relationship between you and your gynecologist is no longer beneficial to you, have the confidence to leave him. An antitherapeutic relationship does no good. The sooner you realize this, the sooner you will seek more satisfactory care.

You must look for mutual participation, a situation in which you and your doctor work together for your good health. By selecting a well-qualified gynecologist—one who meets your emotional and philosophical needs—and by upholding your responsibilities as a patient, you can achieve good health care.

THE GREATEST BARGAIN ON EARTH

If you have any doubts about the value of becoming an active participant in your health care, you should think twice about your priorities. The average American spends more money each year on the purchase and maintenance of automobiles than on health care. This same American spends countless hours, days, and weeks looking for the best buy or the best repair shop. Prices, standard equipment, warranties—everything about a car is usually carefully researched before purchase.

Yet the topic of discussion here is not your car—it's your life. Is there anything more important to you? If you ask hard questions and have high standards when buying a car, shouldn't you have even harder questions and higher standards when dealing with your life? If you refuse to buy a car that doesn't meet the standards you set, don't you think you should refuse to see a gynecologist who does not meet your standards? Remember, when you choose a doctor, you are selecting someone who might one day be the difference between your life and your death.

Isn't that worth a little work on your part?

chapter 3

THE PELVIC EXAMINATION

Two women are talking quietly in a department-store cafeteria. The second woman has been summoned by the first, and tension fills the air.

ANN: Susan, something happened the other day that has been bothering me.

SUSAN: What is it?

ANN: It's . . . it's . . . it's damn embarrassing, that's what it is.

SUSAN: That's all right. What is it?

ANN (is silent for a moment, then makes an inner decision to tell all): Susan, how long does it take to do a pelvic examination?

SUSAN: Why? Is something wrong?

ANN: I don't know. I went to my family doctor yesterday and it took him forty-five minutes to complete the pelvic exam!

A Broadway play? Hardly. But the dialogue is representative of a real-life drama that is played every day somewhere in the world. Unfortunately, it has too many repeat performances. The exact question may not be the same, but the questions, doubts, and fears surrounding the pelvic examination affect almost every woman.

Until recently, it was the rare patient who had any idea at all what her gynecologist was doing during her pelvic exam. Even today, the majority of women have no notion whatsoever about what is going on inside them.

Part of the blame, of course, must be placed with doctors. Sadly, many physicians feel that any explanation of procedure would only confuse their patients and open the door to what these physicians would consider needless questions. The correct method, particularly during a woman's first pelvic examination, is clearly and patiently to explain the whats and whys of every step of the pelvic exam. A physician who does not have the time to explain these things may also not have the time to perform the examination correctly.

On the other hand, women must take some of the responsibility. Unlike a surgical procedure, where the patient is anesthetized, a pelvic examination is a two-way street. A woman who is completely ignorant of her own body certainly will not be able to ask the right questions during the pelvic exam, nor will she be relaxed, and an anxiety-ridden patient makes the pelvic exam much more difficult.

What are the right questions? Simply, those that relieve your worries and help you toward understanding the procedure.

And why should you be relaxed? After all, doctors are paid, and some are paid very well, to perform the procedure no matter what your condition. First of all, a woman who is relaxed responds much better than one who is tense. That in itself is a good reason for relaxation. Second, the pelvic organs are extremely difficult to outline when the patient is abnormally tense.

One of the most difficult tasks for medical students is merely to understand the location and shape of the pelvic organs. The pictures and drawings in medical textbooks are not adequate substitutes for the real thing, and since each patient exhibits individual differences, it is only upon the examination of the actual pelvic organs that understanding dawns. Even then, it is no easy task to determine the exact location of the organs. If a woman exhibits extreme tension, these organs become almost indistinguishable and a good examination is hard to accomplish.

Obviously, communication is of prime importance during the pelvic examination. A relaxed patient and a relaxed but alert physician can go a long way to remedy the mistakes of the past.

THE PRELIMINARIES

Communication is one of the oldest, yet still one of the best, tools of medicine. For that reason, your first visit to any gynecologist should begin with a complete medical history. Ideally, this should be conducted with your doctor, but many times the exigencies of a medical practice dictate that the nurse review the patient's history. In either case, you as a patient should be totally honest in giving information. You should also consider the method used by your interviewer, whether it is the doctor or the nurse. If the interviewer makes you feel uncomfortable at this stage, the discomfort often increases as the examination progresses to more personal aspects.

The gynecologist's medical history will pay specific attention to your menstrual record—the onset of your first period, its regularity or irregularity, and the duration and quantity of blood flow. Another important factor to discuss is how much pain, if any, you experience, and its direct or indirect relationship to your period.

During the history, you must be *totally honest* about yourself and your medical history. Your doctor knows how embarrassing certain disorders, infections, or diseases are. But your doctor will not be embarrassed nor in any way judge you (aside from medical judgments) because of your history.

It is important to stress here that if your doctor does make any moral or personal judgments, or makes any disparaging remarks about your present condition or history, this physician will probably not be suitable for you. Doctors are medical practitioners, not philosophers or moralists. If you are seeking moral, religious, or philosophical guidance, you would be better advised to find counsel in a church, in a university ethics department, or with a good friend. Your doctor's task is to understand you and your world, and any doctor who refuses to offer that understanding will very likely be a destructive influence on your general mental and emotional health. Since there is great interaction between physical and mental or emotional health, finding a physician who understands this interaction, and who understands you, is vitally important.

As vulnerable as telling your medical history makes you feel, it is necessary. Your doctor cannot be blamed or held responsible if he or she makes the wrong decision when it is based on an incorrect history. More than that, if a serious condition does develop, you want to know that your physician's decisions are based on correct information.

There are many women who have qualms about relating their medical histories. These qualms run so deeply that these women will not be likely to reverse themselves just by reading here that they should be honest. Still, a good physician should be able to recognize this problem and should be able to help. A big part of any gynecologist's job is to make the patient feel at ease. Commonly called the bedside manner, this quality should be apparent in the office as well as in the sickroom.

If you have made the appointment with some specific questions in mind, the time to ask them is during the history or the first part of the examination. In that way, if your doctor does not have an immediate answer, he will at least know what is troubling you and be able to check it during the actual examination. Many women make an appointment with several questions in mind and then forget those questions when they get to the office. This is a human foible—none of us has a perfect memory—yet it is annoying for the patient as well as the doctor. For this reason, you should write down in advance all the questions you want to ask your doctor and take the list with you to your appointment.

It is likely that questions will arise during your examination, and you should feel free to ask them when they arise. It is also important to remember the name of any pills or medication you are or have been taking prior to your examination. A drug of any sort will influence or alter your chemistry, and the doctor has to know what it is to make a proper diagnosis. Here, again, you should write down the name of any medication of this sort and bring it with you to the doctor's office. Or you may want to bring in the bottle itself. Describing the pills will not provide sufficient information; either bring the medication with you or have its complete, exact name.

So relax, be honest, and come prepared with questions and information. If you do that, any doctor will turn somersaults to treat you—although he will still send you a bill. About that, nothing can be done.

The Physician's Observations

While taking the patient's history, the doctor should observe the patient's entire appearance. The patient's color is important; so, too, is the mental state of the patient. These things should tell a well-trained observer a lot about the patient—whether she is nervous, happy, unhappy, tense, or depressed. This type of observation often helps the physician reach the final diagnosis which enables him to give the patient the best treatment.

This initial observation will also tell the physician the most simple aspects of the patient's general health—whether she appears too fat or too thin and, further, if she looks tired or healthy. If the patient is extremely pale, she might be anemic, which, in turn, might account for all her health problems. If the patient is yellowish, it may indicate jaundice secondary to liver damage, or it might be that the woman just eats too many carrots. It might even be due to genetic coloring.

From these examples and many more, it is easy to see that the initial observation is very important in ferreting out a woman's health problems. Appearance is always a good indicator, and the physician follows these indicators like a detective tracking down a bad guy. In this case, the bad guy is any abnormality that affects your health.

The gynecologist who finds any medical problem outside his special domain should refer you to the proper specialist. The gynecologist should, of course, explain to you exactly why he is referring you to another doctor.

Medical Checks

Since a gynecologist is often considered the primary physician to attend a woman, it is now a commonly accepted practice for this doctor to care for the woman's entire health. Because of this, your doctor should probably perform a complete physical examination on each visit. This includes a breast and pelvic examination; a blood-pressure check; examination of the head and neck, heart and lungs, and abdominal and pelvic organs. The gynecologist should further check the patient's weight and encourage diet if the weight is outside normal limits. A urinalysis should be performed, and if the patient complains of extreme fatigue, a blood count should be taken. In short, a total examination.

Preparations for the Pelvic Examination

After the history has been taken, your gynecologist should instruct you to empty your bladder. Although a urinalysis will be taken on the specimen during your examination, there is another important reason for this procedure. When the bladder is full, it pushes the uterus backward. This makes the pelvic examination more difficult both for you and your doctor.

The urinalysis is a test for sugar and protein. If there are traces of sugar in the urine, it might indicate that you are developing diabetes. If any protein is present, it might indicate kidney damage or malfunction. If either of these checks is positive, it will, of course, be further investigated.

At the same time as you are collecting the urine sample, you will be asked to undress completely for your examination. Many women are uptight about this, but it is necessary. No one can perform an honest and good examination through clothing, and as uneasy as it might make you, you should realize that when you are asked to undress completely, it only means that the physician intends to examine you thoroughly.

Regardless of the need to undress, though, you should be given a private room in which to undress or, at the very least, a curtain or screen behind which you may disrobe. You should also be given a loose gown to wear during the examination so the doctor is able to examine specific parts of your body without exposing your whole body.

If the gynecologist does not have a special gown for you to wear during your examination, you should be properly draped by sheets. Usually two sheets are used, one to cover the body and one to cover the legs.

Unfortunately, some physicians have abused women by not having them dressed in gowns or draped in any fashion. The reasons are numerous and are better dealt with in a separate book. Suffice it to say that if your doctor examines you while you are completely nude, you are well within your rights to object. If this happens, and if the doctor does not pay any attention to your objection, you have the right to end the examination at this point. Indeed, you probably should, for this treatment of you by the doctor will probably create tension and thus will not be conducive to a good examination. Apart from the issue of decency, this is totally unprofessional behavior on the part of the physician. Many women have gone along with this sort of treatment in the past, mostly because of the indoctrinated social training we all receive about the doctor-patient relationship. But the patient is also a consumer engaging the services of a professional, and if those services make you feel bad or uncomfortable, you should probably find a doctor more in tune with your personal preferences.

Once you have given your urine sample and been gowned or draped, the nurse or the doctor will probably take your blood pressure before you rest on the table. Since most people live their day-to-day lives on their feet—walking, running, and so forth—the blood pressure should also be taken in that normal state. If the test is taken while you are lying down, it will not accurately reflect the blood pressure that you normally have; it will only reflect the pressure at rest.

Your weight will be taken at this point, and your urine will be checked. In that way, the doctor will begin the actual physical examination with these tests completed and, therefore, with a better idea of your general health.

The doctor is now ready to begin the physical part of the examination.

THE PHYSICAL EXAMINATION

Now that the preliminary work has been done and you are gowned or draped, your physician will probably ask you to get on the table. Although this table should be relatively comfortable, you shouldn't expect it to rival your favorite chaise lounge, unless your favorite lounge comes equipped with stirrups. Still, the table should not be a torture rack.

Since your gynecologist should be sensitive to the vulnerabilities inherent in any examination, he will begin his general and well-established check of all organs with an area commonly overlooked—the skin. The covering of your body is just as much an organ as any other and, accordingly, your doctor should examine it thoroughly for any major abnormalities. If any are found, you should be referred to a specialist, but actually, starting with the skin is a doctor's method of psychologically easing you into the sensitive areas of the examination.

It must be stressed that any doctor who goes immediately to the pelvic examination is probably insensitive to your feelings. There are no concrete medical arguments against starting in the pelvic region; rather it is an issue of human understanding. A doctor without compassion and sensitivity is a little like a lawyer with no sense of justice—they might both be good technicians, but it would be difficult to call them complete professionals. Certainly compassion and sensitivity are not salable commodities—no more than is justice—but you as a consumer *have a choice.* You can choose any gynecologist you wish, and you may choose one for whatever qualities you desire in your physician. Most women want the human touch added to the technical proficiency, and they should get it.

The physician will next probably look at your hair and examine your entire head, checking the condition of your hair and whether there is any change in it, either in structure or in amount. Loss of hair might indicate a hormonal imbalance or malnutrition, or it could simply be caused by a lack of vitamins such as vitamin B complex. A decrease in thyroid-hormone production could also cause this condition, and if the doctor suspects this, it should be checked by a blood test to determine the blood-thyroid concentration (a PBI or a T_4 test).

Your eyes should be examined to see if they have a normal appearance. Protruding eyes usually indicate a thyroid gland condition in which too much thyroid hormone is produced. The mucosal coloring underneath the eyelids should also be checked. If the mucous membrane is extremely pale, the patient is usually anemic.

If you complain of "buzzing," the doctor will examine your ears for obstruction and discharge. Naturally, if a serious abnormality is found, the gynecologist will refer you to a specialist.

Your nose will also be checked for any obstruction to the nasal passages; bleeding or abnormal discharge should be investigated.

The doctor will examine the condition of your teeth, gums, and tongue. If there is any unusual bleeding, that should also be noted. The doctor will also examine your throat for the size and condition of your tonsils and/or pharynx.

Next, the doctor will examine your neck for enlarged lymph glands indicating infection, in which case the nodes will be very tender. In rare cases, enlarged lymph glands might also indicate a malignant blood disease such as leukemia or Hodgkin's disease.

The thyroid gland is located in the middle of the neck and is formed like an H, with the bar of the H located one to two fingers beneath the Adam's apple. The gland's arms are located on each side of the bar of the H. This gland produces thyroid hormones, which are extremely important for metabolism. One common function of the thyroid is regulation of weight. If you have a low thyroid function, you might have a slow metabolic rate and will tend to be fat even with minimal food intake. On the other hand, if your thyroid is overactive, your metabolic rate will be high and you will be constantly hungry and able to eat without gaining weight. If that sounds too good to be true, it is; people with overactive thyroids also tend to feel hot and sweaty most of the time, whereas people with slow thyroid functions tend toward fatigue and are extremely sensitive to cold.

The thyroid gland is also closely associated with ovulation pattern. Since the gonadotrophic hormones, produced by the pituitary and regulating the ovarian function, are influenced by the thyroid hormones, a slow or fast thyroid function might interfere with ovulation through interaction with the pituitary hormone.

The thyroid gland can be checked by a blood test to examine the blood content of the thyroid hormone, or it can be checked by a basal metabolism test. This blood test has to be taken on an empty stomach, since food intake containing high amounts of iodine can upset the real values. Infertility (the inability to conceive) has often been corrected just by giving small amounts of thyroid medication to the patient with a slow thyroid function.

Enlargement of the thyroid gland can occur from many causes. It might be due to an overproduction of thyroid hormone by the glands, or it could be caused by a tumor or cancer of the thyroid gland. Of course, there can always be a simple explanation as well. Insufficient iodine intake will cause enlargement of the thyroid gland. This causes the thyroid to enlarge in order to increase the production of thyroid hormone to keep pace with need. This condition is called *goiter (struma)* and is corrected by increasing iodine intake or by adding thyroid hormones to the diet. Goiter is more common than you might imagine and is the reason that many cities and towns add iodine to their drinking water. If you live in an area with an uncontrolled water supply, an iodine supplement may be needed.

The physician should next examine the heart and lungs. This is done by listening, either through a stethoscope (*auscultation*), or through percussion (palpation or knocking on the area with fingers). The breathing sounds of the lungs will change when conditions such as asthma, bronchitis, or pneumonia are present. Excessive cigarette smoking will also change the breathing sounds. If the physician finds any suspicious symptoms, he might want to send you for a chest X-ray or to a lung specialist.

The heart is examined for size. Normally, the higher your blood pressure, the bigger your heart is. The doctor will also listen to the heart to detect any murmur or other abnormality that might warrant an electrocardiogram (ECG) or a referral to a heart specialist.

The breast examination is the next step in the procedure. Remarkably, this is a relatively new aspect included in your visit to the gynecologist. Just a few years ago, the breast examination was often overlooked: The general practitioner felt the gynecologist should do it, while the gynecologist felt the general practitioner should do it. However, it is now firmly entrenched as a part of the gynecological examination, again because the gynecologist is becoming the primary physician for many women.

The breasts are examined individually. First, each breast is checked for abnormalities in configurations and skin coloring. Cancer, for instance, is often shown by abnormal skin coloring in the area where it is developing, and the skin will often pull down a bit in that area.

Thereafter, the physician should feel each breast with both hands to be sure it is freely mobile to all sides. At the same time, obvious lumps will be felt.

During the breast examination, the physician mentally divides each breast into four quadrants—upper outer, lower outer, upper inner, and lower inner. Generally speaking, the breast is divided in this fashion by intersecting two invisible straight lines at ninety-degree angles, the center of the intersection being at the nipple. Each quadrant is examined by the gynecologist, both visually and by touch, for extra masses or any other irregularities.

In the middle of each breast is the nipple, and behind the nipple is the milk gland. During the menstrual cycle, the milk gland will be influenced by hormonal changes, commonly resulting in cystic enlargement of part of the milk gland or enlargement and tenderness of the entire milk gland. The physician will thoroughly check the breast for any abnormalities.

If there are any suspicious lumps in either breast, a biopsy might be needed. This, of course, is usually performed by a surgeon and is not considered part of the gynecologist's routine procedure, even though it is often done by the gynecologist. Before a biopsy is done, though, if a suspicious mass is found, the gynecologist should send you for an X-ray examination of the breast by mammography or xeroradiography, or by thermography. The thermographic examination picks up abnormal heat patterns in the breast. Since a carcinogenic lesion will be more virulent, it will also vary in color from the rest of the breast on a thermographic X-ray (see Chapter 18 on Breast Examination).

After the examination of each breast, the corresponding axilla (armpit) is carefully examined. This is to check for cancer metastasis, since the lymph nodes in the axilla are the first place the cancer will spread. Each axilla should be explored carefully.

If there are any suspicious abnormalities of the breasts up to this point, your gynecologist should have you sit on the edge of the table with the lower part of your legs dangling over the side. The physician will then reexamine your breasts from this perspective. Your hands should first be at your side, then placed behind your neck to reexamine the axilla.

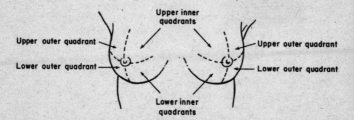

Fig. 3–1: While conducting a breast examination, the physician mentally divides each breast into four parts, or quadrants. The above illustration describes the area of the quadrants. By doing this, a physician can more easily diagnose the location of any mass and also can more easily monitor such a mass on subsequent examinations.

Following the breast examination, the physician will examine the abdominal region to make sure there are no visible abdominal masses or lesions protruding from the abdominal cavity. The doctor will also ascertain if there are any abnormalities of the skin in this region. The abdomen should then be systematically palpated for abnormalities. The area underneath the right rib cage will be explored for any possible enlargements or abnormalities of the liver. The physician usually should not be able to feel the liver's edge. This is important, since if you do have an enlargement of the liver, a tumor, or even hepatitis, you should not use birth-control pills. As soon as the doctor has finished exploring the right side of the rib cage, you should raise your hands above your head so the left side under the rib cage is exposed. This permits the doctor to ensure that the spleen is not enlarged. This is done both by touch and by sound; as the doctor palpates the area, he naturally feels any abnormality. Percussion, the sound which occurs when a physician knocks on a finger placed on the skin, will be high if there is no mass and low if there is a mass present.

At this point, the doctor will examine the right and left flanks for pain or possible enlargement of the kidneys. If either is present, it may indicate tumors or infections in that area. Again, palpation and auscultation are employed. In this case, auscultation equates with listening through a stethoscope to the sound of the peristalsis of the intestines, a sound which changes if there are any intestinal obstructions or abdominal infections present. Although you need not know the normal sound of the peristalsis of the intestines, it might make you more comfortable just to know what your doctor is doing.

The physician should next examine your pubic hair. The hairline should be almost straight, although this is somewhat dependent on race. If, however, the hairline is triangular moving toward the naval, this may indicate a higher concentration of male hormones than is usual. This in itself is not dangerous, and you certainly should not worry if your hairline is not straight. However, a high concentration of male hormones is sometimes a symptom of ovarian tumors or, more commonly, of a condition called ovarian polycystic disease (also called the Stein-Leventhal syndrome).

The doctor next examines the lower portion of your abdomen by feeling just above the symphysis (the major pubic bone just beneath the hairline). The gynecologist will be able to feel your uterus and will be able to ascertain if there are any tumors present or if there is a pregnancy beyond the three-month stage.

The groin should be checked for lymph node enlargement at this time. If you have any history of infection on your legs, toes, or in the vulval area, the infection will have spread to the lymph nodes. It might be useful to think of the lymph nodes as soldiers that fight infections. They catch all the bacteria and either kill them or stop them from spreading to other parts of your body. If it weren't for the lymph nodes, many bacteria would spread throughout your body each time you had an infection, and sepsis infection in the blood would be the result. Luckily, the lymph nodes create a sort of immunity as you grow older. By the time you are an adult, you will have had many infections of different types, and the lymph nodes created to fight the bacteria of these infections have increased in number. These lymph nodes give the body more time to fight the infection, but as they increase, you will be able to feel them in your groin. Tenderness in the lymph nodes indicates an active infection, either in your vulval area or in your legs and/or feet. This condition should be checked. On the other hand, an enlarged lymph node that is not tender merely indicates that you have had a past infection. Of course, if there is a marked increase in the size of the lymph nodes, it should be examined, since most cases of leukemia and some other diseases start in the lymph nodes. In these cases, a biopsy might be the best procedure to follow, especially since cancer also spreads through the lymph nodes. The physical examination, although it seems complicated, need only take a few minutes.

THE PELVIC EXAMINATION

Up to this point, you will usually have been in the supine position (flat on your back) on the examining table. Now it is time to get into the gynecological position. This is one that makes many women nervous, mostly because of misconceptions and exaggerated horror stories. It should not, though, be an uncomfortable situation if you are seeing a gentle and competent physician who cares enough to put you at your ease. Some women find it embarrassing, but the internal examination should be seen strictly as a necessary medical process and not as a procedure to embarrass you. It is the only way to examine you internally and to obtain a Pap smear. Because of this, you should try to relax as much as possible.

In the gynecological position, your legs are spread and your knees are bent as you lie flat on your back. In most examining rooms, the doctor will have a table equipped with stirrups, and you will be asked to place your feet or knees in these to control your position. It is important that your hips are all the way down at the edge of the table. This insures that the doctor can work very close to the area under examination. The physician stands or sits between your legs, facing the vulva.

Before the internal pelvic examination is started, the gynecologist should be sure that the sheet or drape is covering you completely so that only the vulval area is visible. This makes the examination much less embarrassing for you.

However, if you are interested in observing the procedure, feel free to remove the sheet. Many women feel that watching the doctor's moves lessens the fear of the unknown. Familiarizing yourself with the pelvic examination should also remove the notion of the doctor being in control of your body.

Many people wonder if the internal pelvic examination is a sensual or sexual experience. Suspicions that the doctor performing the examination relates to the patient sexually worry many, and some husbands and boyfriends even wonder if their partners enjoy the examination. It should therefore be stated that even though the pelvic examination should not be an unpleasant experience, neither should it titillate or excite. It is a medical examination—a piece of work that has to be done thoroughly and carefully. If you receive any hints that your doctor is deriving anything but scientific pleasure from your examination, you will obviously feel a little uncomfortable. Again, if this happens, do find another physician.

Sitting or standing between your legs, the gynecologist points a light at the vulvar area. The surface examination includes almost exactly what you can examine yourself with your own light and mirror. The doctor will inspect the entire vulvar area, checking the pubic hair first for lice and growth. He will then see if there are any profuse discharges from the vagina or if there are any obvious lesions or growths such as venereal warts, syphilitic lesions, herpes sores, or abscesses in the area. The physician should then inspect the clitoris and the *labia majora*, spreading the large lips and looking for any lesions or tumors. At the same time, the doctor will usually insert a finger into the vagina and palpate the two Bartholin's glands that are located in the lower aspect of the vagina. These are the glands that produce hormonal secretion to the vagina, and sometimes the ducts leading to these glands will be clogged due to infection. Although most often a gonorrheal infection partially causes this condition, any type of mixed infection can clog these ducts. If they are clogged, the doctor will feel an enlargement on each side.

If you ever feel what seems to be a lump between your legs or in the lower aspect of your vagina reaching toward the rectum, it is probably a Bartholin duct cyst. It might become inflamed and may cause an abscess. This is an extremely painful situation and usually warrants an operation to correct it. If, though, there is an enlargement not accompanied by pain, it will sometimes disappear just with the use of sitz baths and/or with local treatment advised by the gynecologist, which may clear the Bartholin's ducts and drain the cyst.

Immediately inside the vulva underneath the clitoris is the urethra, the short channel from the bladder that drains the urine. The physician will look to see if any glands, cysts, or other abnormalities surround the urethra. Because urine will sometimes dribble down into the labia, it is not uncommon to have a slight irritation in this area.

The Speculum

For some women, the internal examination is a frightening experience. There might be logical reasons for this, but still, these fears can be corrected by a gentle and competent physi-

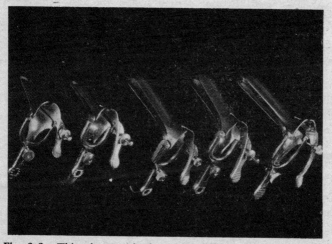

Fig. 3–2: This photograph shows the different sizes of vaginal specula. While the following photograph shows just the different size of the blades, this one shows how the two blades on each speculum open and close by pushing on the handle.

cian. Most of the fears involve the speculum, an instrument which the gynecologist inserts into your vagina.

Part of the fear surrounding the speculum comes from a careless, and mistaken, nickname the instrument has received. Many women actually call the speculum *clamps,* and the image this word provokes is indeed frightening. To correct this, your gynecologist might give you a quick explanation of the speculum, telling you that it doesn't clamp anything. Just the reverse is true—it opens the vagina so the doctor can get a clear view of the inside. The insertion of the speculum should not be painful, though admittedly it might be a little uncomfortable.

The most common complaint in this area is the temperature of the speculum. Many women will swear their doctors keep the speculums in a block of ice, and, indeed, too many physicians thoughtlessly keep these instruments in cold places, though few actually freeze them in ice. In winter, drafts or a lack of heating in the examining room can result in a cold speculum. Women are right to complain—there are few things in life worse than an ice-cold speculum entering your vagina.

The solution here is simple, and up to the gynecologist. Either the speculum should be kept in a heated cabinet (readily available in the medical marketplace), or the doctor should be careful to place the instrument where it will remain warm. The doctor might hold the instrument under hot water or even heat the instrument with his hand before using. As a consumer, you should insist on a warm speculum. Remember, if your gynecologist is so inconsiderate as to insert a cold speculum, this same physician might also be insensitive to you in other important areas as well.

The problem of pain associated with the speculum is more complex. The patient should be as relaxed as possible, especially since any tension just increases the possibility of pain. A woman who is anxious might make sudden, jerking movements, causing pressure when the speculum is in her vagina. Her muscles will also tighten and perhaps even clamp around the tool. All of this causes pain, and the only remedy is relaxation. That, of course, is easier said than done, but the woman in this situation should ask herself why she is so anxious. If it is because she does not trust her doctor, perhaps she should switch doctors. If it is a more general fear associated either with all doctors or with anything having to do with medicine or penetration of her body, she should certainly try to resolve the conflict by discussing it with her doctor.

The doctor, too, can cause the pain, and for many reasons. Primarily, the doctor might be too rough during the examina-

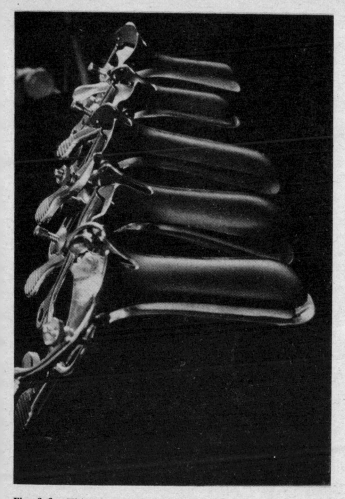

Fig. 3–3: This photograph shows the different sizes of vaginal specula, also referred to by laypeople as clamps. The speculum is available in various sizes, from the small "virgin" type with very small blades to very large speculae to be used for women who have borne several children. The physician should perform a cursory examination of your vaginal opening before inserting the instrument to determine which size is right for you.

tion, and this is certain to cause discomfort. Supposedly some very progressive medical schools have instituted a policy where every male student is placed in stirrups while a strange woman doctor enters the room, squeezes his testicles, then leaves without saying a word. Although this is perhaps an extreme example, if it teaches these young men to be more sensitive to their patients, it has probably helped some women. One would hope that extreme teaching methods such as this would not be needed to make young doctors more sensitive to women, but that sensitivity, especially when it comes to handling the speculum, is necessary.

If you do experience pain on the insertion of the speculum, it might also be caused by the doctor using the wrong size instrument on you. Speculums are available in different sizes, and if the gynecologist inserts one that is too big, it will cause pain. If it is your first visit to a particular gynecologist, the doctor may have to discover what size instrument should be used. Although this is sometimes an uncomfortable process, it should never be excessively painful. A physician should always use a very small instrument if you are a virgin or have only infrequent intercourse. If, however, you have regular intercourse, the doctor will probably use a medium-sized speculum and then increase or decrease the size of the instrument until finding the appropriate one for you. In this manner, an oversized speculum is avoided. Once the right speculum is found, you should ask what size it is for future reference; remembering the size will save testing if you switch doctors.

Once you know the size speculum you should use, don't lie about it. Many women feel that it is more ladylike to have the smallest speculum, and they even insist their doctors use this. In such a situation, the doctor has difficulty performing the examination. Certain prostitutes insist on a small speculum to minimize their sexual activity, and thus prevent the physician from performing an adequate examination.

If your gynecologist is using the right size speculum but is using it too roughly, ask him to be more gentle. If your physician is offended by this, you should look for a gentler doctor. However, before taking this step, be sure it is the gynecologist's rough handling of the instrument and not your anxiety that is causing the pain.

The gynecologist should place a finger on the lower part of the vagina before inserting the speculum. The finger should be pressed gently down so the speculum, inserted sideways, can slide into the vagina on the top of the finger. This prevents the instrument from scratching any part of the vagina. The speculum should be moved slowly into the depth of the vagina, then turned to the right position and opened, again slowly. This avoids pinching any part of the interior. When the physician opens the speculum, it should be opened only to the point where the doctor has a good, clear view of the cervix and the mucosa of the vagina. Opening the speculum any more than this is needless, and sometimes causes pain as the speculum presses against the vaginal wall.

When the speculum is inside you, there might be some occasional pain, but it should not be excessive or anything but occasional.

THE INTERNAL EXAMINATION

After the speculum has been inserted, the doctor will check the wall of the vagina to be sure it is the right color. If everything is in order, the vaginal wall will be pink and clean. If, though, there is any type of discharge, the physician will notice its color. In several cases, the color of the discharge indicates exactly what type of infection is present.

Often, there is a cheeselike discharge, which indicates a *Monilia* infection. If *Monilia* is present, the patient will usually come into the office complaining of a discharge and some type of burning sensation.

If a discharge is greenish yellow, it usually points to a *Trichomonas* infection. If this is suspected, the gynecologist will swab the vaginal wall, smear the discharge on a glass plate, mix it with a saline drop, and examine it under a microscope. If it is present, the doctor will see the *Trichomonas* organism, with two or three small tails, on the slide. This organism is extremely mobile and will move constantly on the slide. There are other methods of determining *Trichomonas*, but this is the most common.

A gonorrheal infection will usually show up as a profuse yellowish discharge originating from the opening of the cervix. If gonorrhea is suspected, a culture should be taken and sent to the lab for immediate examination. The gonorrheal bacteria is very sensitive, so if this specimen is not examined immediately, it will be of no use whatever (this is often the case in offices that are not close enough to laboratories). Once the specimen has reached the lab safely, it usually takes about two days for the bacteria to grow on the culture medium before the bacteria can be diagnosed. Even if the bacteria is not gonorrheal in nature, this method will produce the correct diagnosis.

The gynecologist will next inspect the cervix and the area around it. As you noticed in your self-examination, the cervix feels like the tip of your nose and is in the very back of the vagina. As the physician looks at the cervix, there is a small hole in the center of it, which is the passageway to the uterus.

Occasionally there will be an irritation on the edge of the cervix, which is called *cervicitis*. One cause of cervicitis is a chronic inflammatory reaction, particularly common during pregnancy. When a woman is pregnant, the blood supply to the cervix changes. This in turn increases the probability of irritation and infection to the mouth of the womb. Most often this manifests itself as a sore or an erosion, and is called cervicitis.

Another cause of cervicitis is too high a concentration of the female hormone, estrogen. This most often occurs in women on the high-estrogen birth-control pill. Again, this concentration of estrogen causes an increased blood supply to the cervix, resulting in more breakage and infection in the cervical area.

There are many ways to treat cervicitis. If the birth-control pill is the cause, it would be wise to place the woman on another type of pill with less estrogen. In some cases, antibiotics alone will clear up the infection. Sometimes the doctor will coagulate the cervix with silver nitrate. These treatments clear up most minor cases, but if the infection persists, electrocauterization or cryosurgery might be the solution. Although most women are familiar with the technique of cauterization, cryosurgery (wherein the area around the cervix is frozen) is a relatively new procedure which has been found effective in the treatment of chronic cervicitis.

If you have an IUD (intrauterine device), the gynecologist should see the tail of it. The body of the IUD should not be visible, but the visibility of the tail will enable your gynecologist to determine if the IUD is in the right location (see diagram).

At this point, the physician will obtain a Pap smear (more completely, a Papanicolaou smear). This test consists of swabbing cells shed from the vaginal pool and the cervix, and examining them for any abnormalities. For this reason, you should not douche for at least twenty-four hours prior to an internal examination (even though we are brought up to be clean before going to a doctor, douching might, in this instance, wash away and, therefore, cover up the trace to an accurate diagnosis. You should still wash the outside of your vulva before an examination). With the Pap smear, three samples are taken—one from the vaginal pool, one from the inside of the cervical canal (the *endocervix*), and one from the area immediately surrounding the mouth of the cervix. All three samples are placed on a slide and sprayed with a special solution to fix the cells so their contents will not be altered in the transport to the lab. In the lab, the samples will be treated with a special Papanicolaou stain or

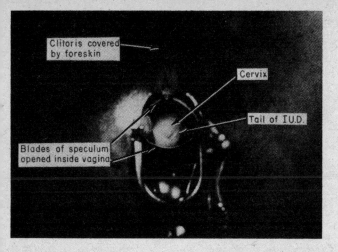

Fig. 3–4: This photograph shows what a doctor sees through a medium-size speculum inserted into the vagina. The cervix is clearly visualized at the end of the vagina. The tail of an IUD is seen protruding through the cervical mouth. The body of the IUD cannot, and should not, be seen, since it is positioned inside the uterine cavity. If a part of the IUD body *could* be seen, it would indicate that the IUD was not in the correct position.

color and then examined for cell content. The lab physician will be able to detect if the cells are normal or abnormal. If there is a malignancy pending, it will be spotted early and treated properly. Along with aiding in the early detection of cancer, the Pap smears can also be examined to ascertain the estrogen index and can detect other infections of the cervix, including *Trichomonas.*

Following the examination of the vagina and the cervix, the doctor will withdraw the speculum. Reversing the process of entry, the gynecologist closes the speculum, turns it on its side, and slowly removes it from the vagina. Again, this avoids any pinching of the vaginal wall.

The Bimanual Examination

The physician will next conduct a bimanual pelvic examination. It is important for this part of the examination (of the uterus, the fallopian tubes, and the ovaries) that you have emptied your bladder and that you are not constipated. If you appear at the gynecologist's office on a day when you are constipated, the doctor might send you home with a few enemas and ask you to come back another day. There is a good reason for this.

It is very easy to confuse a mass or a cyst with an ordinary fecal mass. Don't forget that the intestines are right next to the ovaries and the pelvic organs. Any sort of lump will come under suspicion, and it is not the doctor's fault if you had a large meal the night before. If, though, your pelvic organs are easily palpated, constipation may not cause a problem. In this case, the physician might have to insert a finger in your rectum to examine you thoroughly.

The bimanual examination begins when the gynecologist slides one or two fingers (with jelly) into the vagina. If you are a virgin or if your vagina is inordinately tight, only one finger should be inserted. This is a procedure to examine you, not hurt you; however, it is again important that you are relaxed. If you are tense, the examination will be infinitely more difficult. If you are worried about the fingers entering your vagina, you should think of the logic of the situation. Certainly your physician's finger will be smaller than your sex partner's penis. If your vagina can receive an erect penis, it will be able to withstand the penetration of your physician's fingers, even though the sensation will be less pleasurable.

With his finger(s) inside your vagina, the doctor puts the finger on the cervix and slowly moves it. The doctor will then place his other hand on your abdomen. As he presses slowly on your abdomen, he slowly rotates your uterus by pushing the cervix from the inside. This helps determine the position and size of your uterus.

The most frequent position of the uterus is forward, or anteverted. Occasionally the uterus will be in a posterior, or retroverted position, or even in what is called the midposition. Many women are frightened if the uterus is not in the forward position, and this is reinforced by many ignorant or dishonest physicians. The "tilted uterus" syndrome is one of the most destructive myths of gynecology. In the earlier part of the century, it was the source of many needless surgical operations. The belief then was that a woman with a tilted uterus could not have a baby, so an operation was performed to rotate the uterus into the "correct"—that is, forward—position. This was all nonsense. The position of the uterus is determined by genes. If your mother had a retroverted uterus, the chances are you will also have one. But your mother gave birth to you, and you can

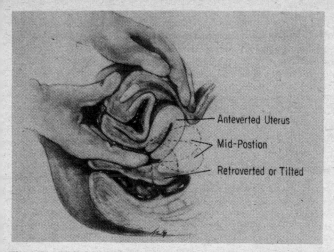

Fig. 3–5: This drawing shows how a physician examines the location and size of the uterus. The doctor here has inserted two fingers into the vagina against the cervix. The other hand is placed on the abdomen. The gynecologist then slowly pushes the cervix with his fingers, forcing the uterus up against the abdomen. This enables him to palpate the uterus. By rotating the cervix, the doctor can get an approximation of the size and location of the uterus. He will also be able to determine most abnormalities of the uterus.

The uterus in this illustration is in the anteverted, or front, position. This is not only the most common position, but also the one most accessible to the doctor, particularly in thinner patients.

The broken lines show the two other possible uterine positions—the mid-position and the retroverted, or tilted, position. As can be discerned, the physician will need to push much harder against the abdomen to get an exact description of either of these two positions. With a retroverted uterus, the physician often must insert a finger into the rectum, the canal lying just beneath the vagina in this picture, to diagnose any abnormality in a tilted uterus.

certainly have children, all other factors being equal. Unfortunately, the operation on the tilted uterus provided these doctors with a good source of income, and today, even though we know better, there are still many operations of this type performed.

It cannot be overstated: *The position of your uterus does not make any difference to your health or to your ability to have children.*

This does not mean you shouldn't know the position of your uterus. This knowledge sometimes eases an examination. As the doctor is rotating the uterus, he should tell you exactly what he is doing and the position of your uterus. If your uterus is in the posterior position, the examination will be a bit more difficult, but that is only because the uterus will be more inaccessible to the gynecologist.

The physician outlines the uterus while holding it, and should let you know what he is feeling. If there are any abnormalities, such as fibroid tumors, the doctor should outline them and tell you their exact size. It is extremely important to explain these things to the patient, because when she is examined the next time, she will know if the tumor has grown. To a certain extent, and surely with women who jump from one gynecologist to another, women have to monitor their own health to make sure the correct treatment and attention is given to each infection or abnormality. With tumors, it is important that women know the approximate size of each tumor, for it is the patients who will have to monitor any growth in the tumor, especially if they have changed physicians.

In rare instances, when an IUD has penetrated the walls of the uterus, it may cause a problem. In this case, nature has its own remedy. The *omentum* is a fatty membrane which hangs from the upper portion of the colon like a curtain. If there is a localized infection in the abdomen, the omentum encapsulates the infection, almost like glue, preventing its spread. When this occurs with an IUD, the omentum will cover the penetrated part of the IUD. Of course, this will sometimes result in the omentum sticking to the area which the IUD has penetrated. This, in turn, causes a pelvic adhesion, which decreases the mobility of your uterus. In such a case, there can be pain when the gynecologist is rotating your uterus. It is important here that you are not stoical, telling the doctor that something does not hurt when it does. The most common symptom of many infections and abnormalities is pain. If you do not complain, the doctor may very well bypass the area.

If there is pain when the physician moves your uterus and it cannot be connected to an IUD or some other foreign object, an infection or disease should be suspected. Every movement and pain is important in diagnosis, and you the patient cannot afford to forget this.

With his fingers still in your vagina, the physician will move his free hand to either side of your abdomen and try to find the area of the fallopian tubes. These tubes are normally slightly tender when squeezed, but if there is *extreme* tenderness or pain when the doctor touches them, it may indicate an infection. If the tubes are enlarged with a mass, it might be due to an *ectopic* (or tubal) pregnancy, a tubal abscess, or a tumor.

Even though the ovary is usually just the size of the end of your tongue, a good physician will be able to outline it for you while moving up from the fallopian tubes. If a patient is obese, it will be difficult to outline each ovary, but the gynecologist should still be able to feel any uncommon masses.

When the physician squeezes an ovary from the inside and out, it will hurt, just as when one squeezes a man's testicles. That is because there are more nerves in this area.

This process is repeated on both the right and left sides, outlining the fallopian tubes, then the ovaries. If your uterus is in the retroverted, or posterior, position, it will probably be more difficult for the physician to find the tubes and he will necessarily have to press a little harder. At the same time, the doctor should engage in an almost constant flow of conversation, telling you exactly what he is feeling and why.

Following the examination of your uterus (including the tubes and ovaries), the physician withdraws his hand from your vagina. It is at this point that some gynecologists insert a finger into the rectum to be sure there is no abnormality behind the uterus. This is not always done. Some physicians feel that if the pelvic examination has been done on a slim and relaxed patient, they need not put a finger in the rectum unless they suspect an abnormality there. If you are overweight and/or uptight, though, you will probably be subjected to a rectal examination. But—take heart—it lasts only a few seconds.

That completes the pelvic examination. The rest of your appointment should deal with what the gynecologist has found and with any questions, general or specific, that you may have concerning your examination. The doctor may schedule various tests for you, and should tell you the exact reasons for such tests. If the doctor does not explain adequately, ask.

Do Some Women Achieve Orgasm during the Pelvic Examination?

Word of mouth has it that some women really look forward to their pelvic examinations, supposedly because they get a kick when the gynecologist is holding the uterus between his hands. This has to be a very rare response, but then some people are turned on by plum pudding.

The vast majority of women do not come anywhere close to orgasm during the pelvic examination. Of course, during the insertion of a speculum, the vagina will, in many cases, balloon up just as it does during orgasm. This creates a feeling of well-being, but it is no more erotic than a licensed masseur working a kink out of your neck.

Without a doubt, what turns most women on is when the gynecologist tells them they are perfectly all right and that they need not come back until their next physical.

Do Some Gynecologists Achieve Orgasm during the Pelvic Examination?

No. If so, change gynecologists.

A gynecologist does not look at your sexual organs as anything but medical organs or scientific problems. When something is wrong, the doctor has a problem and is looking for a solution. Being human, it pleases a gynecologist when he solves a problem, but the pleasure is ego-gratifying, not libidinous.

Certainly there are horror stories of gynecologists or general practitioners who love to look at nude women. One story told of a doctor who asked his patient to stand nude on one leg while he looked at her for about half an hour. Another patient recently reported an unethical incident which occurred while she was vacationing in a New York hotel. Feeling ill, she visited the hotel physician, a distinguished-looking older man. She was asked to undress in his lavish office while he went elsewhere to make a phone call. After she disrobed, the woman realized there were no sheets or gowns to cover her. When the doctor reappeared, she was standing in a corner of the office, shivering. The doctor asked her to parade back and forth in front of him while he observed her movement. He then asked her to sit on the examining table, where he interviewed her and performed a lengthy examination. He spent an excessive amount of time examining her breasts and conducting the internal examination. By this time, the patient suspected the doctor's professionalism. While she was still in the stirrups, he told her he had diagnosed the problem. Leaving the room, the doctor announced he would return in a few minutes to start treatment. When the doctor returned, he was completely nude. Moving to the table and positioning himself between her legs, he told her she needed "an internal massage." Panic set in, and the woman jumped off the table, grabbed her clothes, and ran from the office. Because she was not an American citizen, and was therefore unfamiliar with the country's laws, she did not report the incident until recently. By then, it was too late. The doctor had left the hotel and the charges made by the woman would not hold up after the enormous lapse of time.

This type of behavior belongs in the massage parlors, not the gynecological examining room, and physicians of this type should be barred from practice. Both as a consumer and as a patient, it is important that you report any behavior that you feel is unprofessional on the part of your doctor.

Do Women Make Advances to Their Gynecologists during the Pelvic Exam?

This is a question many husbands and boyfriends ask, or want to ask. The answer is a qualified no.

Generally speaking, women do not make advances to their doctors, especially during the examination. Interestingly enough, it has been found that women who do play up to the gynecologist during the internal examination are usually frigid. There are many reasons why these women might release their desires only during the pelvic examination, but that is better dealt with in a book on psychological disorders.

Suffice it to say that those are extremely rare cases.

How Long Does a Pelvic Examination Take?

The internal exam takes no more than two to five minutes. If it takes longer, the doctor should tell you exactly what he is doing and why he is taking the extra time.

HOW MUCH SHOULD I KNOW ABOUT MY GYNECOLOGICAL HEALTH?

Everything you can. And your gynecologist should be patient and understanding. There should always be an open and honest communication between doctor and patient. If you have trouble understanding something, the doctor should perhaps implement his explanation with a simple drawing to help you understand.

If the gynecologist has to tell you bad news, it should be broken slowly. It should also be explained *in full*. In such a case, the gynecologist should be sure you leave the office knowing exactly what is wrong. Fear does not help any patient on the road to recovery.

chapter 4

THE STORK AND OTHER MYTHS

Since the creation of humankind, conception has been one of life's greatest mysteries. Amazingly, it has only been in the last two centuries that facts concerning the reproductive process have been scientifically proven. In the countless centuries before this understanding of conception, many myths compensated for the lack of knowledge. Even now, a surprising number of people still cling to these stories about where babies come from.

Human beings were aware at a very early stage that there existed some mysterious connection between the menstrual period and conception. These people realized that pregnant women did not bleed. Unfortunately, this connection was misread. Bleeding was associated with sickness and the lack of bleeding was associated with good health. Obviously, then, the normal, healthy state for women seemed to be one in which they did not bleed. Therefore, it followed that woman's natural state was pregnancy.

The ancient Hindus believed there were three essential components needed for the formation of a baby. First, the father provided white semen, which formed the bones, the brains, and the whites of the eyes. Second, the mother provided the red semen, which produced the skin, the hair, and the iris of the eye. It was left to God to provide the expressions of the face, sight, hearing, speech, and movement.

Another belief concerning the mystery of conception was offered by the Koran. A man was created from "a choice extract" of clay, then placed as semen in "a sure place." The semen was created in a clot of blood, and the clotted blood was formed into flesh. In simple language, humans were clots of various seeds developed into coagulated blood.

Very often the power of conception was linked to animals and birds. Since these beliefs dealt in more metaphorical terms, many of them passed into legend and folklore, where the answers they provided satisfied many people for ages.

Usually these legends concerned beings possessed with supernatural powers and the birds that surrounded and protected them. Ancient Hindus and Egyptians thought the ibis (a cranelike bird) brought children. Young couples would accordingly offer prayers to flocks of these blessed birds. The crane and the butterfly served this purpose in Japan, while early Mexicans honored the red spoonbill.

It was left to ancestral Teutons to develop the most lasting myth of all. This ancient people believed the stork brought children to young married couples, and the familiar picture of a stork flying to its destination carrying a small infant has remained with us to this day. Teutons also believed that to prevent any additions to an already large family, they had only to keep the stork away. When this proved an unsuccessful method of contraception, it gave rise to the theory that the stork flew only in the dark and that babies were born in the hours of darkness.

Belief in the stork was widespread—people in England, the Scandinavian countries, and Germany, as well as in great portions of eastern and western Europe, gave credence to the story. Some of the details of the stork myth were confusing and even contradictory. For instance, it was believed that the stork flew to a hot climate, usually thought to be Egypt, for the winter, and then returned in the spring. Obviously, some babies were born in the winter, and this fact would not support the stork legend.

Yet there might have been a cyclical variation in the nature of those people that could explain this apparent fallacy. At that time, the majority of children were conceived in the late summer. Early explanations reasoned that winters were long and people were more tired. Later researchers found that the energy given off by summer heat was greater than in winter and this caused increased fertility. Since a late-summer conception would result in spring birth, most babies were, indeed, born in the spring, when the stork supposedly returned.

Belief in the stork was strong. A new family would build a stork house on the roof in the hope that they would be given many children. The first children in the family were given the task of luring the stork to the house by placing sugar on the windowsills. Modern-day Scandinavian postcards still commemorate this tradition.

In present-day cultures where the legend of the stork continues, it does so as a children's fairy tale. The stork as a bird is seen as a figure of joy—unthreatening and sometimes even graciously silly. It is a comfortable image for children, and actually not harmful—as long as the truth is eventually told to the children.

Another basically Scandinavian legend concerned the spirit child who lived in lakes, streams, springs, and in the fruits of trees. If a woman happened to bathe in the waters or eat a fruit that was inhabited by a spirit child, she would become pregnant. This myth had its origins in primitive tribes who believed that all children came from the spirit world. These early tribes made no connection between sexual intercourse and pregnancy. The reproductive power of semen was completely unknown.

People in Papua were closer to the actualities of conception. Although ignorant Papuans thought pregnancy was caused by bathing in streams inhabited by eels, an enlightened minority believed the seminal fluid ejaculated by men was the prime force of reproduction. The actual flesh and blood of the child was believed to have been formed by an accumulation of semen. It followed that pregnancy could occur only after repeated intercourse. This gave Papuans a socially based motivation for frequent and lively intercourse, so it naturally became a popular belief.

At the same time, many primitive tribes held to the theory of the wandering-room child, a creature who crawled in and out of a woman's mouth in the shape of a toad while she slept. When it was outside the woman's body, this toad-child would eat and drink, then return to the woman.

In approximately 400 B.C., Hippocrates (generally considered the founder of the medical profession) formulated his own theory of conception. This ancient Greek physician felt that pregnancy was caused by combining male and female semen. When conception occurred, menstrual blood flowed into the uterus daily, not monthly. This accumulation of menstrual blood formed the flesh of the new child. Hippocrates believed that ovaries, like testicles, produced semen—a controversial tenet since it stated that a child owed its genetic heritage as much to the mother as to the father. Hippocrates was convinced that a child's resemblance to either or both parents was due to the semen from both. He believed semen was a representative *extract* of the whole body.

One of Hippocrates' most vocal critics was Aristotle, an early chauvinist who strongly opposed all theories implying that women contributed seeds of any kind to the embryo. Aristotle had observed that a woman could become pregnant while remaining absolutely passive (without orgasm). Exactly how Aristotle observed this phenomenon is not known, but he felt it proved that women made no genetic contributions. After all, men were active during sex while women could be completely passive (at least, one supposes, in Aristotle's case), so it was obvious that men contributed the vital elements to the child. Aristotle granted that the menstrual flow was important to creation, but only as a nutrient to the embryo. He also drew a parallel between menstruation in women and animals in heat. Aristotle felt that the dynamic principles—thought, morality, feelings, and so forth—were transmitted only by the male semen. "The mother of what is called a child is no parent," wrote Aristotle, "but only a nurse to the young life that is sown in her. The parent is the male—she is only a stranger, a friend whose fate bears the plant, preserving it until it is put forth."

Aristotle's thinking in this matter was not as original as some of his other, and philosophically sounder, tenets. The early Egyptians believed fathers alone were responsible for lineage, while mothers provided only nourishment to the fetus. This corresponded with a widespread belief in the old world that a woman's body was nothing more than a farmland in which men planted their seeds. If the farmland (woman) was watered and treated properly, it would reward the farmer (man) with a wonderful harvest. This belief can be seen clearly by examining the war practices of the time. Male prisoners were usually killed, while women survived because there was no fear that they could contribute children in the future of the defeated race.

One point on which almost all Greeks agreed, and one that was even taught in medical schools of the time, was that boys developed in the womb much faster than girls because the male fetus occupied the right, and warmer, side of the womb.

Many feel the Greeks had the most advanced culture of their time. That might have been true, especially in their regard for philosophy and humanism. Yet in the matter of conception and childbirth, their knowledge was meager and inaccurate.

One of the problems during ancient times in understanding the woman's role in conception was the invisibility of the uterus. Being an internal organ, the uterus was misunderstood in size, shape, and function. As far back as the Ebers Papyrus, the uterus was regarded as an animal with an independent life. Its form varied—sometimes it was shaped like a tortoise, other times like a newt, and frequently it took the shape of a crocodile. Abdominal palpations and vaginal inspections were sometimes undertaken just to determine the temporary location of the uterus and its temporary animal form.

In the second century, Arateus also thought the womb resembled an animal because it moved about freely. It was Arateus' postulate that the womb moved toward certain odors and away from others. Some of his generation agreed, and Galen even tried to prove that women played some role, even if a small one, in conception. Although Galen could not reconcile the fact that no woman ever conceived by herself, he still clung faithfully to his belief that women had something to do with baby making.

The idea that men are the sole creators is a ploy used in most patriarchal societies. A patriarchal culture, by definition, oppresses women. All too often the oppression reaches the point of denying women their most obvious attribute: the amazing ability to procreate. It is natural for the oppressor to fear the capabilities of the class it subjugates. In the case of patriarchy, man's fear of woman eventually gave rise to the spiteful, damaging myths concerning her body.

Myths and ignorance on the subject reigned for the next thousand years. There were many variations on the theme, but it was generally accepted that only men had any active reproductive power.

In 1520, Paracelsus theorized conception as involving putrefaction. He began a series of futile experiments with this decaying process in the hope that the tests would provide answers to genetic diseases or birth defects. Although a few manuscripts before the tenth century had mentioned the concept of female eggs, it was only in the age of Paracelsus that chemical methods were applied to the ideology.

Fallopius examined the ovaries and vesicles in search of seminal elements. He found none, so agreed with the historical concept of woman's inferior role in conception. A sidelight of this failed exploration was the discovery of the tubes on either side of the ovaries. These were later named fallopian tubes.

In 1621, Fabricus arrived at a new theory of conception. He organized animals into two categories. In the first were those spontaneously produced from eggs. The second category included animals produced internally by mothers and formed from seminal fluid.

In 1676, a medical student named Ham discovered sperm by

examining it through Antony van Leeuwenhoek's invention—a tool called the microscope. Leeuwenhoek was Ham's mentor, so it was his honor to present the discovery to the Royal Society of London.

Leeuwenhoek knew this would be an extremely controversial discovery. Not only did it go against the prevailing knowledge of the time, the entire subject was considered offensive to polite society. He made every effort to convince the Royal Society that the semen in which the sperm was discovered was not gotten by any immoral means, such as masturbation. In his paper to the court, Leeuwenhoek wrote:

> What I here describe was not obtained by any sinful contrivance on my part, but the observations were made upon the excess with which Nature provided me in my conjugal relations. And if your Lordship should consider such matters either disgusting, or likely to seem offensive to the learned, I earnestly beg they be regarded as private, and either published or suppressed, as your Lordship's judgment dictates.

Leeuwenhoek's discovery was published in 1677, but his contemporary colleagues fought firmly against it. They thought these sperm to be only "animalcules"—parasites that were totally unrelated to fertility.

The discovery of sperm ranks among the great discoveries of natural science, but, as can be seen, it was not widely accepted at the time. The more popular belief was purely preposterous. Using Leeuwenhoek's microscope, most scientists claimed they saw minute forms of men with arms, hands, and legs swimming around in the semen. Some microscopists said they saw a figure of a miniature horse riding through the semen taken from a stallion. Animals with long ears were likewise seen in donkey semen. This belief was widely held through the middle of the eighteenth century. Many medical books and pamphlets included drawings showing little men living inside sperm. The masses took this as microscopic proof that the male semen was the sculptor, the menstrual blood was the block of clay, and the fetus was manufactured from this reproductive combination. This phenomenon of miniature men floating in semen illustrated that seventeenth-century scientists were as ignorant in their own way as primitive tribes had been thousands of years before. And at least primitive tribes made their conclusions without benefit of the microscope!

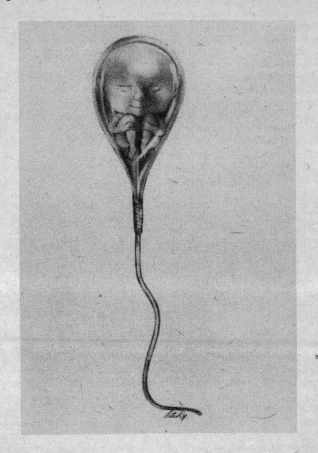

Fig. 4–1: 1976 was the tricentennial of the discovery of the sperm. When it was discovered, though, the sperm was completely misunderstood. Above is an artist's rendition of the human sperm as it was thought to be upon its discovery. Although microscopists never actually *saw* little men in sperm, they believed all new life originated in the male sperm, which they thought contained microscopic entities with all the characteristics necessary to develop into human beings. Women played no role in creation, and the uterus was believed merely to house the growth of the new individual encased in the male sperm.

Almost a hundred years passed before the next vital break-through. In 1775, an Italian biologist named Lazarro Spallan-zani performed an unusual experiment. From waxed fabric, Spallanzani fashioned tiny pairs of "trousers" which he put on male frogs. These frogs then mated with female frogs, but the male semen was caught and encased by the trousers. When the females failed to conceive, Spallanzani knew he was onto some-thing. He then collected semen from other male frogs in the same manner and mixed the semen with female eggs. The eggs became fertilized and Spallanzani should have been able to link the sperm to conception. Sadly, he did not. Instead, he felt that some vague element in the seminal fluid was the agent respon-sible for conception.

It was Dr. T. Barrie who finally made the important step in 1843, when he discovered the cellular origin of the sperm-egg union. From that date forward, scientists and medical people have been in agreement concerning the roles the male sperm and the female egg play in conception.

Each person is formed by genetic factors passed on through the mother and father. The sperm is the medium by which chromosomes from the father are taken and joined to the mother's egg, which carries her half of the chromosomes. This union of sperm and egg forms the fetus and, ultimately, the individual.

A spermatozoon is 0.002 inches long. Appearing almost like a microscopic snake, it has a small, oval head and a long, whiplike tail. It would take three billion sperm to fill a thimble. In every ejaculation, a healthy man releases approximately three hundred million active sperm. This high number of sperm is apparently necessary for the journey to the egg, a journey which few sperm survive. Along the way, half the sperm enter the wrong oviduct. Others are stranded in folds and crannies in the oviducts that trap sperm, preventing their contact with the egg. The opposing current which carries the egg down to the sperm also evacuates many sperm traveling upward to the egg. Many sperm die before they swim the distance—about a foot—to the egg. Sperm swim at the rate of about three inches per hour. All in all, only about one hundred of the original three hundred million survive. Even then, ovulation must be occur-ring for conception to take place.

From the time of Barrie's discovery, science did not ade-quately explain conception to lay people. For years, the masses continued their beliefs in myths and stories. Even while the correct information was readily available, ignorance on the subject remained widespread. Some old stories even acquired new twists to help them bridge the gap into the modern world.

The stork was one of the birds to survive the leap from the age of ignorance to the age of neglect. In many countries, when a woman was about to give birth, she would leave home to go either to a hospital or to stay with a midwife. If this woman already had children, they were rarely told the real reason their mother was gone. They were usually told only that their mother would be gone for a few weeks and, in the meantime, the stork would come and give them a new baby. When the mother returned to the family, she might still look pregnant to the children because her abdominal muscles would be stretched and her uterus would be hypertrophic, or enlarged. Since their mother looked about the same as when she left, the children actually believed the stork had brought their new brother or sister.

Today, of course, the mother does not leave home for weeks on end, but that is a relatively new treatment. It was recently found that the long bed rest given to women after childbirth was a common cause of phlebitis and related syndromes. Nowadays, the mother is released from the hospital as soon as possible. This has drastically reduced the occurrence of phlebitis due to long bed rest. Modern childbirth methods have also made it difficult for the illusion of the stork to survive in the minds of the mother's other children.

The problem of educating children on the subject of conception today is different. Science knows how conception occurs, and so, generally speaking, do the masses. Yet most people are still embarrassed about the sexual aspects of conception and are either too shy or too uncomfortable to explain it to their children. A modern-day child may believe in the stork for a while, but by the time the child is about to reach puberty, the stork no longer seems logical and the child must look for other answers. If parents do not provide the correct facts, the variety of theories children receive concerning conception is truly astonishing.

Some children are told that babies come from semen, which at least starts with the right premise. But then they are told that the semen is spread out and as soon as the sun's rays touch it, it turns into a child and the semen flows into the mother, where it grows and is finally born.

In the midwestern United States, children sometimes learn that a woman has three vaginas leading to three different uteri. As a man enters a woman, he lodges in one of the three locations. The mother's egg is supposedly in only one of the three uteri, and if the man enters the vagina leading to the uterus containing the egg, the woman will get pregnant. This Russian roulette sort of theory lends a hidden excitement and danger to sex for early teenagers, and perhaps that is the reason this myth has not died.

Of course, modern society encourages complete sexual education. Although this is to be praised, we must be careful not to go overboard in a backlash of past ignorance. A child's psychological attitude toward sex and conception is vitally important, and it is just as vital that the child is given correct information in a comfortable and natural way. Society must not force-feed sex education to three-year-old children; they may not want it, and further, they may not be able to cope with it.

Teaching children about sex and conception should perhaps be handled in the same way children are taught the three Rs—gradually. As each new step is easily and comfortably consumed by the child, another new facet of sex can be explained. This can be done in a variety of ways, such as parental talks, picture books, and even showing parallels in the animal world.

Whatever method is chosen, it should not be one that will shock, upset, or disgust the child. Recently, a well-known psychiatrist told of his ultramodern method of educating his daughter. When the child was eight years old, this man encouraged her to watch him have sex with his wife. The child could not absorb this because the man's wife was, of course, *her mother*, and her image of her mother did not coincide with this behavior. Eventually, the girl would have come to know her mother as a sexual being, but in this case, the experiment was too much, too soon. The child was traumatized and she is now in a psychiatric institution.

If there is a lesson to be learned from the stork, perhaps it is that the idea of conception and childbirth is one that is best related to children in a spirit of love and gentleness. Now is the time for loving, caring, and gentle parents to replace this giant white bird, who so lovingly served children and their parents for so many generations, with the truth, told gently and gradually. No woman can afford not to do this.

chapter 5

THE REPRODUCTIVE CYCLE

LEVITICUS 15

19 And if a woman have an issue, and her issue in her flesh be blood, she shall be put apart seven days: and whosoever toucheth her shall be unclean until the evening.
24 And if any man lie with her at all, and her flowers be upon him, he shall be unclean seven days, and all the bed whereon he lieth shall be unclean.
28 But if she be cleansed of her issue, then she shall number to herself seven days, and after she shall be clean.
29 And on the eighth day she shall take unto her two turtles, or two pigeons, and bring them unto the priest, to the door of the tabernacle of the congregation.
30 And the priest shall offer the one for a sin offering, and the other for a burnt offering; and the priest shall make an atonement for her before the Lord for the issue of her uncleanness.

THE CURSE—A BLESSING IN DISGUISE

If you have ever wondered why the aura of shame surrounds menstruation, look to your Bible. Although most patriarchal cultures have antifemale myths, we can blame Leviticus for our Judeo-Christian menstrual hang-ups. These few lines sufficiently capture the essence of male fear concerning the menses.

The purpose here is to dispel the image of the "unclean woman." Menstruation is a healthy function. Contrary to biblical belief, menstruation is a cleansing process, whereby the uterus prepares itself for the next ovulation.

There have been more nicknames and euphemisms concerning the menstrual period than perhaps any other female function. So much so that the word *menstruation* is hardly even in the everyday vocabulary of many women, who prefer even in these modern times to refer to their monthly bleeding process as a "period." For other women, a period is still only something that ends a sentence, and these women might refer to this quite normal phenomenon as "the curse." Women known for discretion smile sweetly and announce to co-workers that "my good friend is visiting." Others—usually teenage American girls—whisper to schoolmates that "Mary just fell off the roof!" Very rarely does a woman announce the onset of a menstrual condition with anything but embarrassment or irritation.

Men don't help at all in this area. In fact, quite possibly, men are more insensitive to the monthly bleeding pattern than to any other facet of a woman's physical condition. They crudely tell their friends that their wives or girl friends are "on the rag" or "riding the cotton pony," obvious references to sanitary napkins and tampons.

The reasons behind this subterfuge are many but simple. More frightening stories and descriptions have been associated with menstruation than with any other physiological aspect of a woman's life. Like stories concerning conception and contraception, myths and misconceptions on the topic vary from one culture to another. Most patriarchal societies exhibit misogynist tendencies regarding menstruation, while matriarchal cultures reverse the trend.

Thousands of years ago it was thought that the menstrual period was a sign of fertility. Ancient peoples connected the event to the bleeding in animals that aroused sexual excitement. Some cultures even thought menstruation heralded a two- or three-day time in which women were to be fertilized. Now, of course, we realize they were wrong and, conversely, that if there is any time of the month that is less fertile than others, it is during a woman's monthly bleeding.

Ancient cultures naturally observed that this bleeding occurred approximately once a month. Ironically, the Romans gave it the name *mens*, not a sexual designation, but rather a word that translates as *monthly.*

No connection was made in the Greek culture between menstruation and childbearing. Birth was considered a gift from God that happened once every couple of years. Strangely enough, the connection made was between breast-feeding and childbirth. The ancients thought that women would not become pregnant while they were breast-feeding, so the gift of God was thought to be given only to women not breast-feeding a child. Many women, therefore, breast-fed their children much longer than was necessary in the hope they would not become pregnant again.

This fairly common belief enslaved women in a perpetual state of pregnancy or breast-feeding. Since menstruation did not occur in either state, most women did not have regular periods. Therefore when bleeding occurred, it was looked upon as a sign of abnormality. Because of this, every time a woman started to bleed, it was thought she was sick inside or was bleeding from internal scars or sores caused by childbirth or disease. When she conceived again, or stopped bleeding, she was considered healthy. It was a vicious circle, made more tragic by the fact that women of the past often died during childbirth at a young age because of anemia or other diseases which attacked them while they were in weakened states of health.

Another reason women were constantly pregnant was the low rate of survival among their children. In those days, medicine knew few cures for the diseases that ravaged populations. Babies were extremely susceptible to major illnesses, diseases, and viruses. Only a few of the strongest could survive before the advent of modern medicine.

This was an era in which there was no knowledge of the menstrual cycle—a time when it was known merely that intercourse had some vague, but unclear, connection to conception. The belief that men dominated the reproductive cycle was universally accepted, so menstruation was ignored for many centuries.

A true understanding of the menstrual cycle and an exact comprehension of the pattern of ovulation and its relationship to the menstrual period was not discovered until 1930. At that time, two physicians—one Austrian, one Japanese—arrived independently at the same conclusions concerning ovulation. These men established that ovulation occurs approximately twelve to sixteen days prior to each menstrual period. That discovery, coupled with the knowledge of the full twenty-eight-day menstrual cycle, made it possible to determine almost positively the exact days of fertility. The most immediate effect of this discovery was the creation of the "safe period" of intercourse—the time just before, during, and after the menstrual period when a woman could have sex without worry of pregnancy.

Of course, this new "safe period" was completely opposite to prior beliefs. For centuries, the period was associated with animals in heat and was, therefore, considered the proper time for reproduction. At the same time, many women who had sex during the previously regarded safe period when they were not bleeding found themselves pregnant. Now we know that the bleeding function is not only reproductive but sanitary, and that it cleans the internal organs, washing away dead and dying cells with monthly regularity.

Even today, misconceptions about menstrual bleeding run rampant. There are even twentieth-century subcultures which encourage the belief that menstrual bleeding is a sign of unhealthiness.

For a long time, the Jewish heritage, and in particular the Orthodox sects, demanded that a woman be taken from her home during her period because she was considered dirty. These women would be locked up until their bleeding stopped; then they would be washed and their vaginas fumigated before they were considered clean enough to reenter their families and society. This type of irrational belief only traumatized women and gave vent to no true understanding of what it was to be a woman.

Other, more matriarchal cultures taught women that their periods cleansed them. Even so, there were many misconceptions. As recently as twenty years ago, American women were told by many doctors not to bathe or swim during their periods and to get plenty of bed rest. This would indicate that these physicians thought bleeding was akin to the flu or common cold, something which required medical attention. Although the period was considered beneficial to a woman's overall health, the stigma attached to it was difficult to shake.

With the personal and political choices being made by women today to have fewer or no children, the menstrual period is more and more being viewed not as a curse but as a blessing. For women who do not use any form of birth control, and even for those who do, the period signals one more month in which they have not gotten pregnant.

WHAT IS MENSTRUATION?

Stated simply, the uterus is an organ which is under the influence of hormones and which is constantly undergoing changes throughout the monthly cycle. The *endometrium* (the lining of the uterus) increases in thickness throughout the monthly cycle by becoming thicker and more vascular (increas-

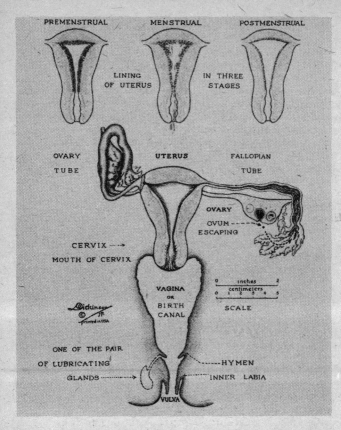

Fig. 5–1: The lower part of this picture is a cross-section of the vagina, the cervix, and the uterus that approximates the relationship of the ovaries and the fallopian tubes to the uterus.

On the right is a further cross-section of an ovary and a fallopian tube. Shown is an egg (ovum) escaping from the ovary and in the process of being caught by the end of the fallopian tube.

At the top is a cross-section of a uterus and *endometrium* (the lining of the uterus) during the premenstrual, menstrual, and post-menstrual phases. Each month, the *endometrium* accumulates a mass of vascular tissue. This prepares the uterus for conception. If conception does not occur, the egg disintegrates and the *endometrium* is expelled via the menstrual flow. (Dickinson Anatomical Chart—reproduced by permission of Educational Department, TAMPAX Incorporated, Lake Success, New York.)

ing the blood supply). This readies the uterus for conception, but if conception does not occur, the build-up of the endometrium is essentially wasted. To enable the process to begin for the next month, the build-up of wasted cells in the lining of the uterus must be cleared away. The menstrual blood is the medium by which these waste matters are disposed of, washing them away from the uterus through the cervix and vagina. The blood removes the dead cells from the uterine lining, but it does not clean the lining. The cleaning is accomplished by the endocrine function, in which the hormonal changes are activated and deactivated. It is this endocrine function which affects the entire body, another reason women often feel better immediately following their periods.

Because it is the endocrine function which actually cleans the uterus, the amount of blood flow during the period has no connection to the amount of cleaning accomplished. Some women mistakenly feel that if they have a heavy blood flow, they are cleaner than women who experience a light flow. This is untrue. The amount of flow may affect the speed by which the uterine lining is cleaned, but not the extent of cleaning itself.

Some women express concern that menstrual blood is also evacuating cells which are beneficial to good health. This is a natural and somewhat logical worry, but a needless one all the same. Menstrual periods merely indicate a loss of the *unused* and *unnecessary* lining of the uterus. Nothing that is essential to good health is removed by menstrual blood.

The interaction of these two functions—the removal of the dead cells by the blood and the cleaning of the uterus/uterine lining by the endocrine function—is the *total sanitary process* of menstrual bleeding.

Physical and Emotional Changes during the Menstrual Cycle

The physical and emotional ups and downs most women experience during the menstrual cycle cannot and should not be overlooked. Most of them are caused by the hormonal changes every woman endures during her cycle. The basic body temperature rises. The levels of progesterone and estrogen are also higher just prior to the period.

One physical manifestation of this hormonal change occurs because the hormones bind salt, and the salt, in turn, binds water. Because of this, many women retain water and feel bloated immediately prior to menstruation. This bloated condition makes many women feel worse and many physicians prescribe diuretics to ease the malady. Other doctors tell their patients simply to avoid excessive salt intake, particularly before their periods. The decrease in salt content in the body will likewise cause a decrease in water retention. Acne and nausea also commonly occur prior to or during menstruation.

These physical disturbances accompany and/or cause emotional upset, such as depression. But depressions can also occur without these physical manifestations and are quite common. Studies have shown that more women commit suicide just prior to their menstrual periods than at any other time.

Depression has been a justifiable motivation for women thinking of their periods as a curse, but now something can be done even about this. It has recently been discovered that there is an increased need for vitamin B6 immediately prior to menstruation. Since women on birth-control pills (which contain higher than normal hormone levels) were also found to require an increased amount of B6, the need is probably a result of the similarly increased hormone levels prior to menstruation.

The lack of B6 has been associated with some premenstrual depressions, and many women have found relief from these depressions by consuming increased amounts of B6 at that time. An advantage of B6 is that it often clears up acne, which is also associated with a lack of B6.

It is therefore recommended that women suffering from premenstrual depression and/or acne should take a multivitamin containing high amounts of vitamin B6. Special multivitamins with B6 have been suggested by researchers for use in connection with oral contraceptives. These same multivitamins are ideal for the prevention of depression and acne. One can also take a vitamin B complex, as long as it contains a high amount of B6.

If vitamin therapy is the solution to your menstrual ills, you will probably find the exact intake for your particular problem on your own or in conjunction with your doctor. In most cases, one multiple vitamin per day is taken throughout the menstrual cycle, and if acne or depression is severe, the vitamin intake is usually doubled or tripled just prior to menstruation.

Although hormonal changes certainly account for some or most of the depressions, research has shown that even these depressions can be caused psychosomatically. For instance, a woman who has been fed frightening stories about her period will dread its onset. Even though her hormonal changes alone would not lead to a depressed state, she psychologically braces herself for the period by sublimating her fear. This fear grows subconsciously and the effect, if not the cause, is the same: depression. This is one very obvious proof of the harm done by menstrual myths, and it should be reason enough on its own for seeking to destroy those myths.

During menstrual bleeding, a woman will lose iron from her body. It is disadvantageous to have a heavy flow, since more iron is lost. If you feel weak or tired after a particularly heavy menstrual flow, the cause may be an iron deficiency. In such a case, you will have to replace the loss with vitamins and iron pills to keep your hemoglobin level up. This should make you feel much healthier. Of course, if you have been placed on some type of hormone pill that prevents iron loss, you should feel consistently energetic.

Manipulators

The few women who abuse their periods should not be overlooked, either. These are women who try to reinforce the myth that a woman's period is a terrible thing to endure and who manipulate people around them by exaggerated displays of suffering. These women get out of dates, business meetings, or gym classes at school on the excuse that their periods are having a devastating effect on their health. Some of these women don't consciously want to manipulate, but just want a little sympathy, and this, sadly, is one of the few ways they can get it. Other women will use their periods to punish their sex partners subtly, saying they can't have sex during their periods. And the small offenders are those women who use their periods to indulge in activities they don't normally support, like smoking or drinking.

In the long view, women who abuse their periods might be getting back at the society which has, from the beginning, perverted the concept of menstruation.

What Happens after Menstruation?

After their periods, women should feel better, both physically and psychologically. Not only have they disposed of uterine waste; the hormonal levels which were high prior to their periods have returned to normal. This causes a lower progesterone and estrogen level. They also dehydrate and lose some of the water they had retained. This would make anyone feel better.

THE FIRST MENSTRUATION—MENARCHE

Because of incorrect histories and scare stories concerning the menstrual cycle, a mother's explanation about the process to her daughter is extremely important. Before the child has her first menstruation, her mother should tell her to expect menstrual bleeding and should explain the entire process to her in a reassuring and positive manner.

If the child is not told, one day she will start bleeding and, not knowing what is happening, she will probably think something is terribly wrong with her internally. The resulting psychological trauma could very well follow her the rest of her life.

Most children begin menstruating at age eleven, twelve, or thirteen. The time of the *menarche* (first menses) varies, of course, and two girls who are otherwise almost totally alike may experience their first bleeding three or four years apart.

However, if a girl starts to menstruate very early, say before ten years of age, she should be seen by a physician, since certain types of hormone-producing tumors could be located either in the adrenal glands or in the ovaries. These tumors sometimes cause early menstruation, and that very menstruation is a signal of the tumors.

Likewise, if a girl does not menstruate until very late, say fifteen, she should also be seen by a physician, since there may be some sort of organic malfunction which is responsible for the late menstruation.

These variations in onset of the first menstrual period may also be due to very simple causes. Genetics is one factor: If a mother menstruated at a late age, her daughter will probably show that same tendency. Variations might also be caused by different nutritional intakes or by psychological strain. It is important to realize that the menstrual period is part of a very delicate process, and almost any upset might delay or speed its onset.

THE MENSTRUAL CYCLE AND IRREGULARITIES

The regular pattern of the menstrual period varies from woman to woman. The majority of women have their periods approximately every twenty-eight days, but other women exhibit irregular patterns of ovulation. When a woman has an extreme weight gain or loss, this likely is reflected in her menstrual cycle and the cycle probably becomes irregular.

It is now known that the menstrual period is closely associated with the hormones LH (luteinizing hormone) and FSH (follicle-stimulating hormone), both of which are secreted from the pituitary gland in the brain. LH and FSH are further influenced by hormones released by the hypothalamus, which is, in turn, influenced strongly by a woman's psychological and emotional state. Because of this, if a woman enters a time of extreme stress (and the definition of extreme stress also varies from woman to woman), *amenorrhea* (a stoppage of the bleeding pattern) will result. It is important for women to know that their menstrual periods are affected by emotional conditions and/or stress. Armed with this knowledge, women might find it easier to cope with stressful situations and their resultant menstrual irregularities.

Certain other medical conditions can cause irregular menstrual bleeding. Polycystic ovaries, which is a cystic enlargement of the ovaries, can cause irregular bleeding. Many other diseases and infections can cause menstrual irregularity, but each abnormal menstrual malfunction should be evaluated individually to find the cause.

Hormonal Changes during the Menstrual Cycle

During the menstrual cycle, there is a close relationship between the pituitary hormones (FSH and LH) and the ovarian hormones (estrogen and progesterone). These hormones are responsible for ovulation as well as for the cyclical change of the endometrium (the lining of the uterus).

Immediately after menstruation, there is an increased discharge of FSH from the pituitary, which stimulates the follicles in both ovaries. *Follicles* are cells in the ovaries that might develop into eggs. As the follicles start to increase in size, their production of estrogen also increases. For unknown reasons, each month one follicle will surpass the growth of the other follicles and develop into a Graafian follicle, which produces the egg for that particular month. In the case of unidentical multiple births, several Graafian follicles produce several eggs for the month. At present, there is no rigid pattern that can be discerned in ovulation, so it cannot be determined if a woman has one or many Graafian follicles in her ovaries at any given time, or in which ovary ovulation might occur.

The increased amounts of estrogen produced immediately prior to ovulation have a feedback to the pituitary, resulting in a decrease in FSH production and a surge in LH production. This will result in ovulation.

After the egg is released from the Graafian follicle (the

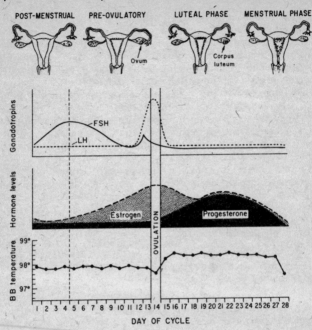

Fig. 5-2: This graph illustrates the close relationship between the brain hormones (gonadotrophins), the ovarian hormones (estrogen and progesterone), and their influence on ovulation, the menstrual period, and the Basal Body Temperature (BBT).

At the top of the illustration, one ovum is seen developed in the preovulatory phase. Note also that the end of the fallopian tube is reaching down toward the ovum to ensure that the tube will catch the ovum during ovulation.

As illustrated, the BBT, which has been steady during the first two phases, usually drops 0.1° to 0.2° at ovulation.

After ovulation, the graafian follicle containing the ovum of the month changes into a special cellular unit called the corpus luteum, shown here in the luteal phase. It should also be observed that the end of the fallopian tube here releases its grip on the ovary.

process of ovulation), the Graafian follicle changes into a *corpus luteum* (yellow body). The cells in the corpus luteum then produce progesterone. Progesterone is a Latin name; *pro* means "for" and *gesterone* means "gestation," therefore *progesterone* means "for gestation." In medical circles, it is also

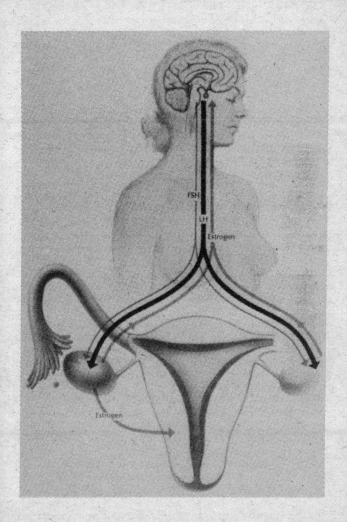

Fig. 5–3: The interaction of the pituitary, the ovary and the uterus during ovulation caused by the secretion and stimulation of LH, FSH, and estrogen. An egg has been released by the woman's right ovary and is about to be picked up from the fimbriated end of the fallopian tube. (Reproduced by permission of the Ortho Corporation, Raritan, New Jersey.)

called the hormone of the mother, since it helps maintain pregnancy. Progesterone is an ovarian hormone that is partially responsible for the changes in the endometrium and for the change in basal body temperature (BBT). The BBT is the temperature obtained in the morning immediately after a person awakens and before any active movement. This temperature is approximately 97.5 degrees for the two weeks after menstruation, with a slight decrease at the time of ovulation; a one-degree increase occurs thereafter, to approximately 98.5 degrees, from the time of ovulation to the time of menstruation.

If conception does not occur, the corpus luteum disintegrates immediately prior to menstruation. This results in a steep drop in the amount of progesterone and in the BBT approximately a day before menstruation.

SEX AND MENSTRUATION

All manner of scare stories have been told to women about the terrible consequences of intercourse during the menstrual period. Like many stories told for shock value, several of these tales start with one fact and then travel into the realm of total fantasy.

It is true that during menstruation the uterus is open and pumping waste through the cervix. Consequently, as the penis goes into the vagina during menstruation, it will push bacteria from the penis into the uterus. If this bacteria is harmful or the kind that spreads easily, such as venereal bacteria, it will probably spread infection or disease. Because of this, it might be wise to have the man use a condom if you have intercourse, at least during the first couple of days of your period, or when the flow is heaviest. As the blood flow decreases to a minimal amount, the uterus will usually be almost closed again and it will not be dangerous to have condom-free sex. This is the one and only danger of sex during menstruation, assuming all other factors are equal, and any other scare stories should not be believed.

Several men have been told that if they have intercourse during a woman's period, and the woman uses the superior position, blood will run into the penis and cause damage. This is patently ridiculous and has no basis in fact. In fact, the origin of this fear is an acceptance of the misogynist myths society has foolishly embraced for such a long time. If you cannot convince your male sex partner of the silliness of this myth, let him use a condom if he wants. He will probably worry less and therefore be free to give you more sexual satisfaction. If this doesn't work, you might be better off finding a less neurotic bed partner.

If you find that a heavy flow reduces the amount of friction you need during sex, you can temporarily halt the flow by inserting a diaphragm. If your partner is particularly neurotic about the presence of blood, you can douche to remove the last traces. Douching should *not* be done if you are using a diaphragm for contraceptive purposes, as the contraceptive jelly will be washed away.

Remember, the presence of menstrual blood is a sign of health. A woman need never be self-conscious about her period during sex. If there is a psychological problem here, it is probably the result of believing the male-originated myths about menstruation.

Sexual Stimulation during Menstruation

A majority of women describe an increased sexual desire during their menstrual periods, particularly in the last few days of bleeding. This is not abnormal, because the blood acts as an aphrodisiac by stimulating, or tickling, the sexual organs of the woman. This aphrodisiac effect of menstruation is usually highest in the last few days of the period, when the flow is light and there is no association with painful menstrual cramps.

Some women feel an increased sexual desire immediately prior to the period, a phenomenon probably due to an increased sensitivity in the nervous system.

As mentioned before, intercourse is not harmful at these times. To the contrary, it might even help relieve the tensions built up at this time.

IS MENSTRUATION NECESSARY?

In recent years, several physicians have investigated the menstrual pattern in an attempt to determine whether or not the period is a necessary or desirable part of a woman's life. The newer birth-control pills, especially the low-estrogen-containing contraceptives, usually retard the stimulation of the uterus or the lining of the uterus which causes the tissue build-up responsible for menstrual bleeding. Therefore, with this type of pill, women experience very little menstrual bleeding.

If it is ever proven that menstrual bleeding is, indeed, unnecessary or harmful, many women will rebel against the proof since they feel their periods are an inherent part of being a woman. If and when this comes to be, a program of wide reeducation may be necessary. Certainly the presence or absence of a single function in a woman has little bearing on her womanliness. Women who have hysterectomies or mastectomies are no less womanly than other women, and this logic would carry through to menstrual bleeding.

Obviously, many women benefit from the low-estrogen contraceptive pills. Women who experience too much bleeding early in life, causing a huge loss of iron, or women who have *dysmenorrhea* (extremely painful menstruation), find many of their physical problems lessened by use of these pills. It is important to teach women that this treatment will not harm them in any way. The glands which produce menstrual blood are not damaged or altered, just put in a state of rest as a natural function of this type of birth-control pill. Some of the new birth-control pills lessen bleeding; others stop it altogether, causing complete amenorrhea (cessation of menstruation).

What is vitally important is that the physician completely explain to each woman what she can anticipate with each type of pill. If you are on a birth-control pill containing a lower level of hormone, you will have very little menstrual bleeding. If you are placed on the minipill, you might have regular bleeding in the beginning and then later on have almost no menstrual bleeding. If you are on the newly researched antigonadotrophic hormones such as Danazol, you might have no bleeding whatsoever.

Studies in England have shown there may be an important link between the menstrual cycle and breast cancer in women. Researchers there found that older women who had little menstrual bleeding when they were younger because they were constantly pregnant or were breast-feeding had a significantly lower incidence of breast cancer than the general female population. These test results have sparked concern among physicians and have given new support to the birth-control pill. The results show that the cyclical changes of menstruation, where the breasts change size month after month, might possibly cause cancer. If this is borne out by further research, women might be better off being placed on ovulation-suppressing birth-control pills.

DO MEN HAVE A TEMPERATURE CYCLE SIMILAR TO WOMEN?

Recent investigation indicates that men appear to have a temperature cycle synchronous with the temperature changes of the women with whom they are living. This is interesting, since men do not undergo any significant fluctuations in hormone levels such as women do during their menstrual cycles.

Factors that influence a partner's cycle can, however, secondarily affect the other's cycle. In reported findings, the male cycle ran from seventeen to thirty-five days, which fairly closely coincides with a woman's cycle. Men *seem* to have behavioral changes occurring in the same rhythmic fashion as women.

A typical male pattern shows temperature drop in the middle of the month, near or at the same time as his female partner has the ovulatory mid-cycle temperature drop. A man's temperature then rises to a high level, also compatible with the one occurring in women after ovulation.

A major difference shown in the survey was that a man's temperature usually dropped approximately a week after his female partner's ovulation, where a woman's temperature remains high for approximately two weeks after ovulation.

The type of hormone changes or causes of this male temperature cycle are unknown. It was found, however, that when partners were not in cyclic temperature harmony, there appeared to be more strain and difficulty in the relationship.

OVULATION

Ovulation occurs only once a month, approximately fourteen days before a menstrual period. Even women with irregular bleeding patterns ovulate two weeks before their next period. The egg is released from only one ovary at a time, and there is no way to predict which ovary will release the egg at any given time. Women who have had one ovary surgically removed will still ovulate regularly from the remaining one.

The first day of menstrual bleeding is called *day 1* of the menstrual cycle. The bleeding is accompanied by a decrease in estrogen and progesterone, a hormonal change that might create a tendency toward mild diarrhea, and creates a water and weight loss, making the woman feel lighter and healthier.

During the first five days of the cycle, the decreased estrogen results in a release of follicle-stimulating hormone (FSH) from the pituitary gland. The FSH stimulates the follicles in the ovaries. This matures several of the stored eggs, and as they grow, they produce estrogen.

The estrogen stimulates the growth of the endometrium (the lining of the uterus). The mucous plug of the cervix becomes thinner and more slippery, ready to aid the sperm in their travel through the cervix. During this part of the cycle, one of the still undeveloped follicles (the mass of cells containing the almost-mature egg) begins to outgrow the others, becoming the Graafian follicle that produces the egg of the month. As the Graafian follicle grows to the surface of the ovary, preparing to expel the egg, the fallopian tube on the same side reaches down around the ovary to catch the egg. The increasing estrogen level starts to block the FSH from the pituitary.

As ovulation nears, the Graafian follicle has a higher amount of *prostaglandins* (fatty acids present in many tissues), which cause the ovary to contract and expel the egg. As this happens, the ovary turns to the side close to the fimbriated, or fringed, end of the fallopian tube, which, like a hand with fingers, grasps the egg and its surrounding protoplasm (egg white).

In the fallopian tube, the egg travels slowly toward the uterus, propelled by fine, fingerlike *fimbria*. The ruptured Graafian follicle becomes a corpus luteum, or yellow body, and begins to produce progesterone and estrogen to stimulate the uterine lining to become thicker and spongy. This is accompanied by an increase in basal body temperature (BBT). The temperature decreases slightly at ovulation, while increasing one degree to about 98.5 degrees the two weeks after ovulation.

If conception does occur, the corpus luteum does not disintegrate. This causes a persistently high level of progesterone and the BBT remains about 98.5 degrees. This is the first proof of pregnancy.

CAN A WOMAN TELL WHEN SHE OVULATES?

Ovulation occurs two weeks prior to each menstrual period, but since many women are not sure when their next period will take place, it can be difficult to determine the exact time of ovulation. By taking the basal body temperature for a few months, a woman can get an approximate idea of when ovulation takes place. This, however, is only possible if she has a regular cycle. The temperature usually decreases slightly on the day of ovulation and increases sharply on the day following ovulation.

Some women state that they know exactly when they ovulate because they feel several changes in their bodies. Many women experience mild pain or backache at the time of ovulation. Other women even experience severe pain (called *Mittelschmerz*). Several women say that around the time of ovulation they feel more sexually aroused and erotically stimulated. This is actually a known phenomenon among animals in heat on the day of ovulation.

STAGES OF OVULATION AND FERTILIZATION

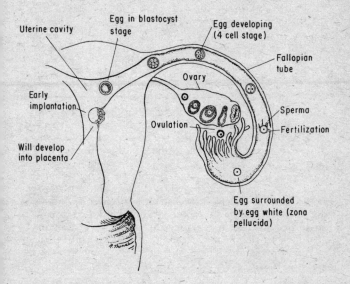

Fig. 5–4: This schematic drawing shows the various stages involved in ovulation and fertilization. In the ovary, the development of an egg into first a follicle, then a Graafian follicle, followed by expulsion of the egg, ovulation, and remaining corpus luteum can be seen. The fimbriated end of the fallopian tube reaches toward the ovary; the egg passes into the fallopian tube. In the tube, the passage of the egg toward the uterus is assisted by the motion of small, hairlike projections called *cilia,* and is nourished during this time by the egg white, the *zona pellucida* that surrounds the egg. Fertilization, the conjunction of the egg with sperm, usually takes place in the mid-portion of the fallopian tube. As it continues its journey toward the uterus, the fertilized egg, called a *zygote,* begins to divide first into two cells, then into four, and then, by geometric progression, into a hollow ball consisting of many cells, called a *blastocyst.* In the blastocyst stage, the fertilized egg enters the uterine cavity and implants in the uterine wall. At the site of implantation, blood vessels develop which provide blood to the developing placenta, the source of nourishment to the fetus. It usually takes an egg 3 to 5 days to make the journey from the ovary to the uterus. If the egg is fertilized and this journey is interrupted due to some fallopian-tube abnormality, the blastocyst might implant in the fallopian tube, resulting in an *ectopic,* or tubal, pregnancy. The egg and sperm in this illustration are not drawn to scale.

The environment of the secretion within the vagina is generally acidic, but this secretion becomes slightly alkaline at the time of ovulation. By measuring the acidity in the vagina, a woman can get an indication of when ovulation occurs. The acid-base balance is checked by using a special test paper.

It has recently been discovered that the activity of the enzyme called *alkaline phosphatase* decreases significantly at the time of ovulation. A self-examination of the amount of alkaline phosphatase in the cervical mucus might provide a practical method for determining the time of ovulation. Such a test is still not commercially available.

The cervical mucus changes throughout the menstrual cycle. The mucus is thick and scant immediately after the menstrual period. As ovulation approaches, the amount of cervical mucus increases from ten to a hundred times and becomes clear and slippery. This is called *the wet period.* Many women easily feel this change, which can be used as another sign of ovulation approaching. When the estrogen level peaks and ovulation occurs, the cervical mucus has reached its maximum change. A new device the size of a tampon is being developed in laboratories in Boston. This device, called an Ovutimer, is designed to read the direct change in the cervical mucus and thus indicate the time of ovulation. The device may be commercially available in the future.

MITTELSCHMERZ—INTERMENSTRUAL PAIN

Intermenstrual pain, or *Mittelschmerz,* usually occurs at the time of ovulation. Normally, ovulation causes no pain, or sometimes just a dull cramping. Occasionally, ovulation is combined with such severe pain that a woman cannot walk and is confined to bed. Often a physician is seen because the woman might easily think she has appendicitis or a pelvic infection. *Mittelschmerz* can occasionally be associated with vaginal bleeding. This sometimes scares women, although it is a normal physiological happening. The pain is probably due to intra-abdominal bleeding from the ovulation site. This causes a reaction from the peritoneum in the abdomen, which results in pain from the nerve endings. The vaginal bleeding which occurs is usually due to spillage of hormone, mostly estrogen hormone. The spillage of this hormone can cause a change in the body's mechanism and can alter the contraction pattern of the uterus. Some of the endometrial lining of the uterus is then shed, resulting in bleeding. The pain usually disappears in a few days. There is no treatment save bed rest with a heating pad. The bleeding is usually slight and self-limiting. The bleeding site usually heals and no other problem occurs. However, if pain continues, one should see a physician.

CONCEPTION

Conception occurs when the sperm fertilizes the egg in the fallopian tube. This happens between one and three days after ovulation. The egg remains in the fallopian tube for about four or five days before moving into the uterus.

The round egg cell is the largest single human cell, yet it is smaller than a single dot. The sperm cell is considerably smaller. Though shaped like a comma, it would take about 2,500 sperm cells to cover a comma. In fact, all the sperm required to repopulate the earth would be no larger than an aspirin tablet. Sperm have tails, which they use to propel them-

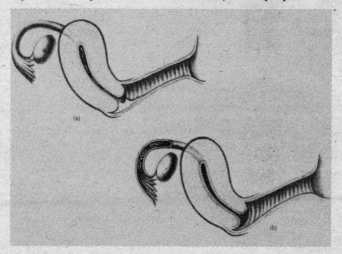

Fig. 5–5: The vagina, uterus, fallopian tubes and ovaries in cross-section, with the approximate angles of these pelvic organs in a woman lying on her back. In picture (a), the ejaculate is lying close to the cervix and sperm have begun their migration through the uterus toward the fallopian tubes. The egg is about to be expelled from the ovary and caught by the fimbriated end of the fallopian tube. In picture (b), the egg and sperm meet in the mid-portion of the fallopian tube, the most common place for proper fertilization. (Reproduced by permission of the Ortho Pharmaceutical Corporation, Raritan, New Jersey.)

selves, much as fish use their tailfins. They move quickly, reaching the fallopian tubes eight to ten minutes after being ejaculated into the vagina.

A fertilized egg implants in the uterine wall six to seven days after ovulation, or approximately three weeks after the last menstrual period. It unites with the blood vessels inside the uterus, and a human being begins to develop. The spongy uterine wall in which the egg lodges becomes the placenta, providing the developing fetus with nourishment.

The exact mechanism enabling the sperm to penetrate the egg shell is unknown, but hormones in the head of the sperm probably effect the fertilization. Though approximately two million sperm cells are present in a normal ejaculation, only one penetrates the egg during conception. If fertilization of the egg does not occur, the egg disintegrates and is slowly expelled from the uterus.

Fertility drugs containing LH and FSH in abnormally high doses overstimulate the follicles, and several eggs may be released as a result. This can result in multiple birth if several eggs are fertilized.

How Can a Woman Tell if She Is Pregnant?

The first sign of pregnancy is usually a missed period. If you miss a period, you should take your basal body temperature (BBT) every morning to confirm or deny any suspicions of pregnancy. If you are pregnant, your BBT does not drop; it remains elevated around 98.5 degrees. A routine urine test for pregnancy will probably not be positive until two weeks after the missed period.

A new and more sophisticated urine test which has been recently developed can detect a pregnancy within two weeks of conception. That test, known as a *radioimmunoassay* (RIA), is expensive, time-consuming, and available only in major medical centers.

The most widely used pregnancy test, called the *slide test*, is cheap, fast, easy to perform, and available in many doctors' offices. But it is not usually accurate until after the first month of pregnancy.

At the Cornell Medical Center, a new blood test has been developed but its use is still limited. It can occasionally diagnose pregnancy even before a missed period. This test is a so-called *receptor assay*, which detects very small levels of human chorionic gonadotrophin (HCG). HCG is a hormone manufactured by the placenta, the organ which nourishes the fetus. If a woman is pregnant, HCG is in her blood and urine. The level of HCG will be so small in the beginning of a pregnancy, however, that it cannot be detected by the available, routine pregnancy tests. This new test enables a woman to know if she is pregnant at the earliest possible date, an important consideration whether she is interested in abortion or in establishing a healthy environment for the fetus.

There has been a recent proliferation of over-the-counter home pregnancy kits which are based on the detection of HCG in the urine, but their ability to detect very early pregnancy is still being tested. The kits range from $9 to $15.

A physical examination by a gynecologist should reveal some blueness of the cervix and a slightly enlarged uterus if you are pregnant. The cervix should also be soft and pliable (positive Hegar's sign), the breasts should swell, the areolas around the nipples should become darker, and the blood vessels in the breast become much more visible. Morning sickness frequently occurs.

Pregnancy Care

As soon as a woman suspects that she is pregnant, she should contact her physician to confirm the diagnosis of pregnancy. If she wishes to bear a child, a proper diet should be started, she should avoid any drugs, and proper antenatal care should be instituted. If there is any abnormal bleeding or pain during this very early part of the pregnancy, a physician should be immediately contacted. Full information on pregnancy and childbirth is beyond the scope of this book, which deals strictly with gynecological rather than obstetrical matters. There are, though, several excellent books on obstetrics available.

Egg Cells

All potential egg cells, or follicles, are present at birth in women. Thus, every month, the egg that descends into the fallopian tubes at ovulation is as old as the woman. When a woman reaches forty, the eggs begin to feel their age. Occasionally, the genetic mechanism suffers, causing possible birth defects or miscarriage. Modern medicine has developed certain tests to analyze the amniotic fluid around the fetus and determine whether the chromosomes are normal. Obstetricians are particularly worried about the possibility of delivering a child with Down's syndrome (sometimes called mongolism), which happens much more frequently in women over the age of forty. Today, women at that age can safely carry a child if the pregnancy is carefully monitored by an obstetrician associated with a modern medical center. To be on the safe side, these women should undergo amniocentesis when they are between sixteen to eighteen weeks pregnant to exclude mongolism or other genetic abnormalities.

Men do not have this problem because sperm is freshly produced. Even if the man does not ejaculate, old sperm cells are automatically expelled.

CAN YOU CHOOSE YOUR CHILD'S SEX?

Much has been written lately about various techniques used to preselect the sex of a child. To date, however, only one method has been proven successful—a method which raises a serious ethical question.

Around the sixteenth to eighteenth week of pregnancy, it is possible to insert a needle into a woman's abdomen, withdrawing some of the amniotic fluid that surrounds the fetus. Laboratory tests can then determine the sex of the fetus. If the fetus is not the desired sex, an abortion can be performed. The moral questions in this type of sex determination are obvious, and the test should be performed only in very special cases, such as when there is the possibility of hemophilia, which is a sex related disease.

History of Predicting Sex

The Berol Papyrus, written around 1350 B.C., described a method by which both pregnancy could be ascertained and the fetal sex predicted with the aid of urine taken from the potential mother. Barley and wheat in two bags were moistened daily with the urine. If the barley germinated, a girl would be born; if the wheat germinated, a boy. If no germination occurred, the woman was not pregnant.

Doctor Manger, who presumed that estrogen in the urine stimulated the germination of barley but had the opposite effect on wheat, repeated the experiments in 1933 and reported a correct prediction in 80 percent of the cases. Other physicians, however, were unable to find any correlation between the content of estrogens or gonadotrophins in the maternal blood and the sex of the fetus. Nevertheless, pregnancy serum, like urine, does contain one or more substances which stimulate the growth of certain plants.

According to the Egyptian papyri, the sex of the unborn child was also indicated by the color of the mother's face. A pregnant woman whose face had a greenish hue could be sure of giving birth to a boy. The Hippocratic school, on the other hand, taught that a woman with child, if it were to be a boy, had a good color. If she was carrying a girl, her facial color would be poor. Aristotle held that females were on a lower developmental level than males; consequently, a male fetus made more demands on the mother than a female fetus, needing greater body warmth and better circulation.

The sex of the fetus has also been thought to be an influence on the mother's disposition, a male fetus making her cheerful (Arabian), happy (Indian), and untroubled (Jewish).

Similarly, some people believed that a woman's desires reflected those of the sex she was carrying, and that her dreams were equally telling. In India, she dreams about men's food if she is carrying a boy. In Russia, dreams of knives or clubs are associated with boys, whereas dreams about spring or parties signify the arrival of a girl. In Japan during the tenth century, Temba taught that women desiring boys should concentrate on male pursuits, such as hunting. Until recently, it was a Japanese myth that if the husband called to his wife while she was on her way to the toilet, causing her to turn suddenly to the left, the outcome of the pregnancy would be a girl.

Modern Suggestions for Sex Determination

Many gynecologists prescribe programs of timing and douching to determine sex. Unfortunately, these programs have not been proven effective. Some programs even contradict other programs.

One of the most popular methods of sex preselection was developed by Dr. Landrum B. Shettles. Dr. Shettles created two programs—one to produce boys, one to produce girls—which patient couples are to follow with strict adherence. If a couple wants a girl, Dr. Shettles suggests the following procedure:

1. No intercourse for two to three days before ovulation.
2. Since a lower sperm count may increase the couple's chance of conceiving a girl, they should engage in intercourse freely before the two or three days prior to ovulation.
3. Precede intercourse with an acid douche of two tablespoons vinegar to one quart water.
4. The woman should avoid orgasm, since it increases alkaline vaginal secretion.
5. The missionary (male superior) position should be used so the sperm can be deposited at the mouth of the cervix.
6. Penetration should be shallow at the time of male orgasm.

For a boy, the procedure is different:

1. Intercourse should be timed as closely as possible to the time of ovulation.
2. To ensure the highest possible sperm count, intercourse should be avoided from the beginning of the menstrual cycle until the first day of ovulation.
3. Precede intercourse with a douche of two tablespoons baking soda to one quart water.
4. The woman's orgasm should be encouraged simultaneously or before the man's.
5. Vaginal penetration should be from the rear position, in order to deposit the sperm at the entrance of the womb where the secretions are alkaline.
6. Penetration should be deep at the time of the male orgasm.

This program is questioned by many reputable gynecologists. On the other hand, Dr. Shettles claims an 85 percent success rate. (David M. Rorvik with Landrum B. Shettles, M.D.; *Your Baby's Sex: Now You Can Choose;* Dodd, Mead, Inc.; 1970.)

Whether or not Dr. Shettles's program is effective, research in this area is accelerating. Even skeptics admit that the days of clearly proven sexual predetermination are not far off.

What Is the Theory behind Sex Preselection?

The *female sperm,* which carries an X chromosome, is larger than the *male sperm,* which carries the Y chromosome. The male sperm seem to move faster because they are smaller. If intercourse occurs at the time of ovulation, the fastest-moving sperm supposedly reach the egg before the slow-moving sperm. Therefore, there is a better chance of pregnancy with a male fetus if intercourse occurs at the time of ovulation.

The acidity in the vagina is highest several days prior to ovulation. The larger female sperm has a greater chance of surviving in this environment than the male sperm. Intercourse several days prior to ovulation should give a higher probability for a female baby.

It is true that vaginal secretions become increasingly alkaline during a female orgasm. This milieu might be better for the Y chromosomes. However, these changes are so sudden that they may have no influence on the sex.

Recent reports indicate that the X and Y chromosomes can be separated by centrifugation, and artificial insemination can be performed using either female or male sperm. Whether this will ever be a clinically available technique of preselecting a child is unknown.

If You Had the Choice, Which Sex Would You Choose?

Research on sex preference has shown that there is an overall preference for a male child as the first-born child. Eighty percent of the couples interviewed preferred a girl as the second born.

This might be very unhealthy, since it tends to separate the sexes even more. It has been theorized that first-born children of either sex are more ambitious, creative, achievement oriented, self-controlled, serious, and adult oriented. They are also more likely to attend college and to achieve eminence. This is all characteristic of masculine sex-role stereotypes.

Second-born children of either sex have been described as cheerful, easygoing, talkative, popular, practical, likely to seek help, and nervous. These characteristics supposedly resemble female stereotypes.

If exact sex preselection were possible and a majority of couples chose boys as the first born and girls as the second born, this could create even greater dissimilarity between the sexes and further the sexist stereotypes that are so destructive for us all. Perhaps, though, because of the recent examination of sexist values, more couples in the future will choose to a have girl as their first child.

PROBLEMS ASSOCIATED WITH THE MENSTRUAL CYCLE

Premenstrual Tension

Premenstrual tension usually occurs three to five days before menstruation, coinciding with the time during the menstrual cycle when the amount of ovarian hormones, estrogen and progesterone, is at its highest level. One of the most characteristic symptoms is water retention, usually between two to five pounds. This occurs because the hormones bind sodium chloride, and sodium retains excess fluid. Water retention gives a bloated, uncomfortable feeling, and might be responsible for headaches, dull aching or heaviness in the abdomen, and backaches. The high estrogen and progesterone levels give a general feeling of malaise, tiredness, and lethargy. Hormone levels are also responsible for nausea, breast enlargement, and pain.

Some women become more irritable, tense, or depressed during this period. Many women also develop acne. This is the time during the menstrual cycle when a woman may have a tendency to be more nervous and irritable. Statistics show that the highest suicide rate for women occurs during the premenstrual period, and that women experience more emotional and nervous breakdowns at this time. The swelling of the pelvic organs and/or pelvic congestion can affect the bowels, resulting in constipation and the bloating or swelling of the stomach.

Premenstrual tension is clearly associated with the increased hormone levels immediately prior to menstruation. Some women have described the same symptoms when they initially start taking birth-control pills, particularly a birth-control pill with a high estrogen level. Researchers have found that women who suffer from premenstrual tension produce too much estrogen compared to progesterone.

It is not the hormone levels alone that determine the degree of symptoms, since many women never experience any premenstrual difficulties. Premenstrual tension depends to a great extent on a woman's mental state. If a woman is well, happy, and in good physical shape, she might have no or very few complaints. However, if a woman is anxious, nervous, and run-down, she will be more affected by premenstrual hormone changes and could develop severe symptoms.

Recent studies show that women who suffer severe premenstrual tension are more likely to react poorly to stressful situations and are more prone to psychosomatic illnesses.

Treatment of Premenstrual Tension

Most women suffer from sodium retention. The elimination of excess water by reducing one's salt intake or by adhering to a no-salt diet is recommended one week prior to menstruation. It is also necessary to drink a large amount of water to wash out the excessive waste products in the blood stream. If this is not sufficient, diuretics should be prescribed.

Recent discoveries show that there is an increased need for vitamin B6 prior to menstruation, since the lack of B6 has been associated with premenstrual depression and acne. Women suffering premenstrual symptoms should increase their intake of vitamin B6 or take a multivitamin containing a high amount of B6 prior to menstruation.

Women who have a high estrogen level but a relatively low progesterone level have found relief when they take progesterone tablets prior to menstruation. Some women have found relief when on low-estrogen birth-control pills, while others have found that this precipitated the symptoms.

There have been suggestions that spasmodic and congestive discomforts are due to calcium loss. If that is the case, extra calcium intake in tablet form or by drinking milk helps the condition.

Orgasm is the most pleasant way to alleviate the symptoms of premenstrual tension and to realize the origin of the problem.

Many women are riddled with feelings of anxiety, fear, and pain, which are triggered by their menstrual periods. In order to alleviate these symptoms, you should be as open as possible about them. Discuss your feelings with friends and close relatives. Exercise, eat a well-balanced diet, and relax, and keep your body in a healthy state. Most women have learned to live satisfactorily by following the above suggestions. Along with understanding the difficulties, women who know they might not feel well a few days prior to menstruation will not plan important meetings or special events on those days.

Dysmenorrhea—Painful Menstrual Cramps

Dysmenorrhea is the medical term for the painful cramps that accompany the menstrual period. A great number of men probably think that it is merely a woman's monthly excuse for acting bad-tempered and pampering herself, but any woman who has experienced dysmenorrhea knows it is a very real and debilitating condition. The cramps accompanying menstruation, particularly during its onset, can be so severe that a woman must be bedridden with her heating pad, feeling sweaty and at times almost in shock. There is usually a general feeling of malaise, lack of energy, and weakness in the legs; some women describe it as feeling as if their insides are falling out. Although the term "curse" is outmoded and Victorian, dysmenorrhea can be so severe that some women undoubtedly view it as such.

There may be an explanation why cramps can be so severe as to cause this condition. Scientists who have studied uterine physiology have found that the strength of cramps during menstruation is as high, and at times even higher, than contractions during labor. However, it is not the contractions per se that cause the severe pain (although they may cause some malaise); it is the dilation, or opening, of the cervix that results in the pain experienced during menstruation. The cervix is richly enervated and extremely sensitive. Each time the cervix stretches to allow passage of a blood clot, extreme pain results.

Prior to the passage of menstrual clots, an increased amount of cramps causes dizziness and sweating similar to that of a woman in labor.

No one knows why some women suffer so much more than others from menstrual cramps, but it may have something to do with uterine anatomy. Some women have longer cervices than others, with tighter openings. If the cervix is tight, dilation is more difficult, often resulting in more severe pain. The cervices of certain women with dysmenorrhea are so tight they allow only a trickle of blood to pass, and the bulk of menstrual waste is instead pumped into the abdominal cavity, where it could grow and lead to *endometriosis* (see Chapter 12, Infertility and Chapter 13 on Uterine Abnormalities). This is more common if the woman is very tense.

Hormones called *prostaglandins* are another possible factor in dysmenorrhea. These hormones are used to induce labor and abortion. A recent British study showed that women with dysmenorrhea produced and excreted more prostaglandins with the menstrual blood than women with normal cramps. Since these hormones can cause strong cramps, this might be the cause of the dysmenorrhea.

Pain during menstruation is also related to a woman's mental state. A tense person usually complains of more severe menstrual cramps than a relaxed person. It is often noted that highly strung women have a higher degree of dysmenorrhea.

Tolerance to pain varies greatly from one person to another, as it does from one culture to another. Eastern women, such as Chinese and Japanese, are more conditioned to tolerate pain than are Western women. When they are in labor, these women usually require much less pain medication than their Western sisters.

Cultural background and religious upbringing also have some bearing on a person's tolerance for pain. Jewish, Moslem, and Catholic women usually experience a higher degree of menstrual difficulty than Protestants. Several psychologists believe this difference is directly due to religious beliefs. Jewish women are brought up to believe that menstruation is unclean: Orthodox Jewish women must even take a ritual bath *(mikvah)* before resuming sexual relations after menstruation. This same custom applies throughout the Middle East for Arab women. Religious Arab women are not allowed to bathe during their menstrual periods. Catholicism, with its strict emphasis on purity and its rigid rules against premarital sex and birth control, tends to give Catholic women a negative view of menstruation. Protestant women, on the other hand, are raised to suffer less in this aspect, as the Protestant church is more liberal in its view on women's sexuality.

Occasionally there is a clear pathological reason for severe menstrual pain. Women with pelvic infections sometimes develop extreme pain during menstruation, since the pumping movement of the uterus rapidly spreads the infection. There are several other causes for a painful menstrual period, such as fibroid tumors, which are occasionally located in such areas in the uterus that they interfere with the menstrual flow. A woman with a tilted uterus often has painful menstrual cramps, particularly when the cervical canal is bent backward to an extreme degree. If the menstrual period is delayed a week or two, tissue builds up inside the uterus. This subsequently results in a heavier flow and more menstrual pain.

Cramps tend to decrease in severity as a woman gets older. They might even disappear completely. After childbearing, when the cervix has been opened, many women have fewer or no symptoms of pain. However, some still continue to have severe dysmenorrhea even after giving birth.

At times, menstrual cramps can be so severe that some women feel menopause will be a welcome relief.

Treatment of Dysmenorrhea

There is no specific treatment that completely alleviates the misery connected with dysmenorrhea. Each woman with severe cramps usually finds her own special remedy, but her formula might not work for another woman. Menstrual cramps are often relieved to some extent by heat. A hot water bottle or heating pad placed on the abdominal area or on the lower back often lessens the pain. Some women find relief soaking in a hot bath. This relaxes the muscles and the heat also helps open the cervix, which facilitates the blood flow and subsequently alleviates the cramps. A hot bath is not dangerous. You should not use a tampon at this time, allowing the blood to flow normally. In fact, you should never use a tampon if you have severe dysmenorrhea. Many women find that a few drinks lessen menstrual pain. This can be recommended, since alcohol is found actually to decrease uterine contractions.

Exercises are also recommended to alleviate pain. There are several types of abdominal exercises which should be done a week prior to menstruation. These exercises strengthen the abdominal muscles and keep the body in better physical shape. It is well known that dancers and athletic women have fewer menstrual complaints.

Many women find that lying on their backs with their legs elevated on a pillow, or with their knees bent, often alleviates pressure and pain. Other women find relief by pulling their knees up toward their chests. The "fetal position," lying on the side with the knees pulled up tight to the chest and the head bent forward, is also strongly recommended.

As with premenstrual tension, some women have found that orgasm is the most enjoyable way of alleviating severe menstrual cramps. This is actually in accord with medical research, since the severe pelvic congestion which occurs immediately before the onset of menstruation can also be alleviated by an orgasm. The orgasm drains the pelvis and, therefore, causes relaxation and comfort.

Recent research has demonstrated a clear connection between the severity of menstrual cramps and the blood levels of a hormone called *prostaglandin*. Drugs such as aspirin, Motrin and Naproxen are the most effective new treatment for the control of dysmenorrhea. These drugs prevent prostaglandin release from the body tissues and thus prevent propagation of menstrual cramps. It is important to take these agents before the prostaglandin enters the system. A woman might be advised to take two aspirin four times a day twenty-four hours prior to the expected onset of menstruation through the first days. The other antiprostaglandins, Motrin and Naproxen, are even more effective, but can only be obtained by prescription. The compelling evidence on the potency of Motrin and Naproxen in the treatment of dysmenorrhea is very recent and some physicians may not be aware of these new findings.

Another possible treatment of dysmenorrhea is the birth-control pill. Actually, the reason not as many women suffer from dysmenorrhea today as years ago is that millions of women take the pill. The hormones in the birth-control pill replace a woman's own hormones and thus prevent ovulation. The pill, particularly one with a low estrogen content, does not stimulate the endometrium as much as the woman's own hormones; therefore, there will be less menstrual flow and less pain. A woman suffering from severe dysmenorrhea should take the pill if she has no contraindication to it. The minipill and a low-estrogen pill are preferred for this purpose, since menstruation on these pills is limited to very little bleeding or spotting.

As previously stated, having a period is not altogether necessary. A woman can take the birth-control pill continuously; this avoids menstruation. If cramping and bleeding occur, she can even double up on the pills.

Another suggested treatment for dysmenorrhea is injection of long-acting progesterone once every couple of months. This causes a cessation of bleeding and, thus, pain.

The newly released medication for endometriosis—Danazol—can also be used successfully for dysmenorrhea. Danazol also stops bleeding. Thus a woman will not experience premenstrual tension or dysmenorrhea.

The menstrual cycle usually renews spontaneously when a woman stops taking these drugs. Because of this, these drugs will prevent conception only while they are being taken.

If there is a clear medical reason for dysmenorrhea, such as pelvic infection or fibroid tumors, the condition should be treated by antibiotics or surgery. If a tilted uterus causes severe dysmenorrhea, surgery might be indicated to pull the uterus forward. Several physicians perform a D&C (dilation and curettage) which alleviates symptoms due to a very tight cervix. There have even been cases in which all alternative treatments have failed and a hysterectomy has been unavoidable. However, this should be the last resort and done only if a woman does not want any more children.

Sometimes cramps will respond to none of the non-surgical remedies suggested here and women turn to narcotic drugs, such as codeine. If cramps are that severe, and persistent, consult your physician in order to determine the medication best for you, and remember that narcotic drugs are habit-forming and should be used with caution.

Dysmenorrhea is real. It is important that your colleagues, as well as your husband or boyfriend, understand this and are supportive. Do not be embarrassed or feel guilty about this condition. Instead, be more open and free yourself from the social, cultural, and religious factors that might have precipitated your situation. Try to understand the physiological and psychological factors responsible for dysmenorrhea. This enables you to cope better with the situation. And remember: keep yourself in emotional balance, get plenty of exercise, and learn to relax.

ABNORMAL UTERINE BLEEDING

Abnormal uterine bleeding can be any abnormality, from amenorrhea (no bleeding whatsoever) to irregular bleeding occurring either too infrequently (oligomenorrhea) or too often (menorrhagia), and is completely unrelated to ovulation or menstruation.

Most women experience abnormal bleeding sometime in

their lives. This could be due to an abnormality, but often it is just a symptom of a hormonal imbalance or even of a stressful situation.

Amenorrhea

This is a condition in which there is no menstrual bleeding. There are two types of amenorrhea: *primary,* in which a woman has never had a menstrual period although she is past puberty; and *secondary,* in which a woman stops menstruating after regular bleeding.

Primary amenorrhea can be caused either by congenital abnormalities (absence or abnormality of the vagina, the uterus, or the ovaries) or by a malfunction between the pituitary and the ovaries. A young girl with this condition should be taken to a gynecologist by the time she reaches sixteen to determine why she does not menstruate. If there are any congenital abnormalities, these should be corrected surgically. If there are no abnormalities, the physician usually administers hormones to initiate the menstruation.

The most common cause of *secondary amenorrhea* is pregnancy, but it can be due to many other reasons. Menstruation depends on a very delicate hormonal interaction between the ovaries and the brain. If this is upset by weight gain, weight loss, poor nutrition, emotional trauma, birth-control pills, or serious diseases, bleeding may not occur. If secondary amenorrhea persists longer than two or three months, you should see a doctor.

Diagnosis and Treatment of Amenorrhea

If you miss more than one period and have been sexually active, you must have a pregnancy test, since pregnancy is the most common cause of secondary amenorrhea. If the pregnancy test is negative, you should have a hormone analysis (to determine the body's estrogen level) and a biopsy of the endometrium (to determine if you have ovulated). This can be done either in the office or in a hospital under general anesthesia. You should also have an X-ray taken of your brain, since a brain tumor could disturb the interaction between the pituitary and the ovaries. Weight gain or loss can also cause the problem, and you must report to your physician if this is the case. Prolonged use of the birth-control pill can, as mentioned above, cause amenorrhea. Therefore, the pill should be stopped until bleeding occurs. There are also certain cases in which these conditions are due to pituitary damage occurring as a result of severe hemorrhage or infection during previous deliveries. This usually can only be treated by hormone replacement.

Amenorrhea is frequently caused by nervousness and tension. Mental mood can influence brain hormones, also called the *releasing hormones* (R-FSH and R-LH), which regulate ovulation through FSH and LH. Bleeding usually reoccurs as soon as the woman relaxes or moves to a more peaceful environment.

Oligomenorrhea

Oligomenorrhea is a condition in which a woman has only occasional periods, perhaps just one or two a year. This is usually due either to a pituitary malfunction or to polycystic ovaries (Stein-Leventhal syndrome). In this condition, the ovaries are enlarged. This prevents regular ovulation and development of the corpus luteum, inhibiting menstruation.

This condition can be treated with birth-control pills or other hormones. Bleeding is usually initiated after progesterone administration, either in the form of injection or Provera tablets of 10 milligrams, administered twice daily for five days. If the estrogen level is sufficient, the progesterone results in a sloughing off of the endometrial lining a few days after the injection or the last tablet. The condition can also be regulated by Clomid administration or after a surgical procedure called a *wedge resection of the ovary*, in which a part of the ovary is removed so the size of the ovary is reduced to normal and ovulation resumes. If untreated, a woman with oligomenorrhea *can* conceive, but it is more difficult since she does not know when she ovulates. This condition can also occur after discontinuation of the birth-control pill or by irritation from an IUD. It could be a sign of a threatened miscarriage or an ectopic pregnancy.

Menorrhagia—Irregular Periods

Frequent and irregular bleeding can have a variety of causes: hormonal imbalance, abnormal ovulation, stress and nervousness, uterine trauma, polyps, fibroid tumors, or cervicitis. It can also be caused by inadequate hormone dosage in the birth-control pill or by irritation from an IUD. It could be a sign of a threatened miscarriage or an ectopic pregnancy. Abnormal bleeding should, however, always be evaluated since it can be a sign of cancer.

Bleeding Abnormalities in the Young Woman

The onset of menstruation (menarche) varies markedly from woman to woman. In the last decade, the onset seems to be arriving earlier. It is not abnormal to see a girl start menstruating at twelve years of age. It is not known if this is due to better nutrition or if it is entirely due to a woman's weight. During the first few years, menstrual periods may be rather irregular, light periods may be followed by very heavy ones, and menstrual periods may be absent entirely for a few months. This is due to inadequate ovulation and abnormal hormone levels. A young girl does not ovulate regularly or have regular menstrual periods until she becomes sexually mature. Such menstrual irregularities might continue for three or four years. This often causes uneasiness and nervousness, as well as fear of pregnancy if the young woman becomes sexually active. This nervousness can again influence the brain hormones, thus causing absence of bleeding. If this is the case, menstruation can usually be brought on by progesterone (Provera tablets). When menstruation starts after a prolonged absence, too much tissue has often built up inside the uterus, resulting in heavy menstrual bleeding. This can usually be controlled with progesterone administration, which is often more effective than a D&C.

Dysfunctional Bleeding

Abnormal bleeding is usually not serious, but if it persists, it should be evaluated. It could be a sign of danger and could even result in anemia. If minimal bleeding occurs, you should not do anything about it for a month. If it persists, you must see a gynecologist.

Any malfunction in the delicate hormonal balance can cause abnormal bleeding. Menorrhagia is usually characterized by prolonged menstrual bleeding or spotting.

Many physicians treat this condition with a D&C. Women should be aware that a D&C does not often cure menorrhagia if the problem is a hormonal one. A hormonal cause must often be treated by estrogen and progesterone administered in a cycle regimen, or by progesterone administrated for a few days to bring the body back to its regular cycle. Sometimes birth-control pills will also be effective.

Bleeding Due to Trauma

A young woman often experiences severe bleeding during the first intercourse. This is usually a result of the tearing of the hymen. Some women do not experience this, whereas others bleed during their first *several* times of intercourse, or until the hymen is completely open. Older women, who have more fragile vaginal tissue, often experience tearing of this vaginal tissue, especially if they have not had sex for a long time and have become too tight. This is particularly true if they did not have time to lubricate sufficiently. It is common to experience some bleeding during the first intercourse, after childbearing, or after different types of vaginal surgery. This is usually due to tearing or laceration of the scar tissue. Many women describe bleeding after intercourse, particularly if the man is well endowed. This could be a sign of cancer and should, of course, be evaluated, though it is more likely to be due to an infection of the cervix (cervicitis) or to a cervical polyp that has been irritated during the sexual activity. Women with IUDs might also experience some bleeding, particularly after strenuous intercourse. This is due to strong uterine contractions immediately after intercourse, which can cause part of the endometrium to shed.

If you develop severe bleeding after your first intercourse and it does not stop spontaneously, you should insert a tampon into the vagina and squeeze your legs together. If the bleeding is uncontrollable, you should go immediately to the nearest emergency room, since you may need a few stitches to control the bleeding. Do not be embarrassed about this; it happens quite frequently. The same advice applies if you have any form of bleeding after intercourse, no matter what your age.

Bleeding Associated with Pregnancy

Abnormal uterine bleeding can also be due to an abnormal pregnancy or threatened miscarriage in which the placenta has not implanted firmly in the uterine wall and has started to slough off. This bleeding is usually pinker and brighter than menstrual bleeding, and can often start painlessly. However, if a miscarriage is on the way, severe cramps follow, and a physician should be consulted immediately.

This type of bleeding also occurs as a result of an *ectopic* pregnancy (pregnancy outside the uterus, often in the fallopian tubes). If the egg is growing in a fallopian tube, the hormones which maintain the uterine lining in pregnancy are inadequate and bleeding occurs, though usually without pain at first. As the tubal involvement becomes more extensive, there will be severe lower abdominal pain. If this occurs, particularly in association with bleeding, a woman must see her physician immediately.

Polyps and Cervicitis

A cervical polyp can cause menorrhagia, especially if it is irritated by sexual intercourse. A polyp in the uterus can also cause abnormal bleeding. Either of these conditions can be treated with a D&C, with the polyp being scraped off. However, the removed polyps should always be sent to a pathology laboratory to make sure they are not cancerous.

Cervicitis, an inflammatory condition of the cervix, often causes bleeding or spotting. This is particularly true after a Pap smear or intercourse. This should be treated with either coagulation or freezing of the cervix.

Bleeding Associated with IUDs and Birth-Control Pills

An IUD is a foreign object in the uterus and can irritate the uterine wall and cause bleeding. This is quite common for the first few months, or until the uterus adjusts to the IUD, but if it persists, a gynecologist should be consulted. Bleeding due to an IUD is usually treated with either progesterone or birth-control pills. Progesterone decreases the cramps that contract the uterus against the IUD. Birth-control pills help relax the uterus in the same way. This bleeding is also sometimes due to a low inflammatory reaction, in which case antibiotics should be added to the treatment.

Birth-control pills can also be responsible for abnormal bleeding. Usually, the first few months a woman takes the pill, particularly the minipill, the hormones in the pills are not strong enough to take over the woman's ovarian function and bleeding results. This is called *breakthrough bleeding* and is usually treated by doubling the dosage of the pill temporarily and, sometimes, doubling it again. This may be done for several months before the cycle comes under the pill's control (see Chapter 10 on Contraception).

Bleeding and Fibroid Tumors

If a fibroid tumor breaks through into the uterine cavity, it affects the endometrium (uterine lining) in the same way a polyp would, causing bleeding. This is the only time a fibroid tumor is potentially dangerous, because it can cause severe hemorrhage and necessitate transfusion. In this case, the tumors usually must be surgically removed by a myomectomy. A hysterectomy is not necessarily indicated. (See Chapter 13, Uterine Abnormalities.)

Postmenopausal Bleeding—A Warning

Nowadays, the menopause occurs later than in the past, probably because of better nutrition and living conditions. However, if a woman experiences menstrual bleeding after a cessation of at least six months, she should see a gynecologist immediately to have a D&C or a biopsy of the uterus. This bleeding could be a sign of cancer and early diagnosis leads to more successful treatment. Therefore any bleeding, small or large, after change of life should be evaluated immediately. This is even more important if you are in estrogen-replacement therapy. Then you should have a biopsy from the endometrium every one or two years, and a D&C as soon as bleeding or spotting occurs, to rule out any premalignancies.

Bleeding as a Sign of Cancer

Of course, abnormal bleeding *can* be an indication of uterine or cervical cancer. If this bleeding occurs after menopause, you should see a gynecologist immediately, since older women are especially susceptible to genital cancer. Extra caution is necessary if you are in a high-risk group. Abnormal bleeding is the first sign of such cancers, because the uterus tries to slough off the tumors. Cancer of the cervix causes bleeding in its advanced stage, but if a woman has her Pap smear regularly, cancer is usually detected before the cancer advances to stages in which it causes postcoital bleeding.

MENOPAUSE

Of all the mammals on earth, human females are the only ones to stop menstruating in midlife. The "change" usually occurs around age fifty, but variations are great. Genetic factors are important in determining when a woman will reach menopause; if your mother stopped bleeding in her forties, so, probably, will you.

Women are born with about half a million oocytes, ovarian cells which can theoretically grow into an egg. Every month after puberty, one of these oocytes forms into a Graafian follicle and ovulation occurs. These cells also produce the female hormone, estrogen. As the woman approaches middle age, the oocytes begin to degenerate and their estrogen production decreases. This process varies from woman to woman, and might be responsible for the great difference in menopausal symptoms between women. Many women have minimal symptoms because their *ovarian stroma* (supporting tissue) continue to produce estrogen after ovulation ceases. Testosterone also continues to be produced in the ovaries.

The average lifespan for an American woman is seventy-five years, so during the last third (twenty-five years) of her life, she will not ovulate and probably will not have menstrual bleeding.

WHAT HAPPENS DURING MENOPAUSE

The first sign that menopause is approaching is usually abnormal menstrual bleeding ranging from skipping just one period to intramenstrual spotting, to a sudden cessation of menstruation for several months or permanently. This pattern can persist for several years, depending on the individual's estrogen level. Irregular menstruation can, however, be a sign of several conditions and a woman who experiences those symptoms should see a gynecologist to have the bleeding abnormality evaluated and her estrogen level checked. This is particularly true for a middle-aged woman who experiences a resumption of vaginal bleeding after more than a six month cessation of menstruation. She should be alerted to the fact that this could be an early sign of uterine cancer (see Postmenopausal Bleeding, p. 105).

Other symptoms of menopause include a change in skin tone or texture, an abnormal vaginal discharge or pain due to atrophic vaginitis (see Vaginitis after Menopause, p. 125), a decrease of breast size and firmness, back pain (which should alert women to the possible onset of osteoporosis, a decrease in bone substance and a lowering of the bone calcium content), and arthritic symptoms.

SEVERE MENOPAUSAL SYMPTOMS

Only twenty-five percent of American women suffer any significant menopausal symptoms other than cessation of ovulation and menstruation. The most severe and abrupt changes occur in women who have undergone surgically induced menopause via hysterectomy and oopherectomy (removal of the ovaries).

This 25 percent suffer two distinct types of symptoms. One type is due to vascular instability and is characterized by hot flashes and sweating, especially at night. The other type is primarily psychosomatic, and can manifest itself in a variety of ways. These latter symptoms are generally consistent with what a woman has been brought up to expect during menopause, and can include heart pain, hysteria, constipation, ulcers, and severe depression.

To the extent that they are physical, menopausal symptoms are probably due to low levels of estrogen and high levels of gonadotrophins, FSH and LH. These hormonal changes affect the brain, and it should be understood that although many symptoms may be psychosomatic, they are grounded in physiological imbalance.

Treatment of Menopausal Symptoms

The best treatment is often psychological counseling and understanding. Tranquilizers can help a woman over the tense period of adjustment, which can last from one to ten years.

The most severe symptoms are often seen in women with surgically induced menopause who have hysterectomies with removal of the ovaries. Many gynecologists insist that the ovaries are useless after menopause, but this is not altogether true. Despite the loss of their reproductive value, they probably still function to maintain a hormonal balance, and their absence is felt.

With or without estrogen treatment, women should understand that the change of life takes time—probably a few years—and that they will eventually adapt and have no further symptoms.

Good nutrition is essential to minimizing menopausal symptoms. Dietary supplementation of vitamins B and D, calcium, and iron can help protect against cardiovascular diseases, diabetes, osteoporosis, and obesity. Some physicians report that the use of 400 to 1600 international units of vitamin E daily cures hot flashes. It is important for women to watch their weight after menopause, as the risk of heart disease increases greatly at that age and obesity multiplies the risk geometrically. A proper dietary supplement of vitamins and minerals will keep the bones strong and supply the energy that many women feel they lose at menopause. Protein is also important, though excessive animal fats should be avoided. Large amounts of water will flush the system and keep all the cells in balance.

Does Estrogen Replacement Cause Cancer?

Estrogen is thought to protect against *arteriosclerosis* and *cardiovascular diseases*, as well as arthritis and *osteoporosis* (a condition characterized by a loss of calcium in the bones, making them brittle and weak and easily broken). Despite this, many physicians are against estrogen treatment for menopause because of the risk of cancer. Estrogen is said to keep the skin and breasts looking young and firm and to keep the vagina soft. For these reasons, many women consider it a rejuvenating drug. Research, though, has revealed that the same results can be obtained with calcium pills or placebos!

Still, if a woman wants estrogen treatment, she should be aware of the dangers. Estrogen has been linked to both uterine and breast cancer. It is said to increase the chances of endometrial cancer sevenfold. However, endometrial cancer is relatively simple to treat when caught early, and many physicians feel the risk is worth taking. The first symptom of this type of cancer is bleeding. If a gynecologist is consulted immediately and he diagnoses endometrial cancer, the cure rate is almost 100 percent. It is thought this *cancer* is caused by an abnormal buildup of the uterine lining and *can be prevented by prescribing estrogen in three-week cycles, each cycle followed by a week of progesterone treatment* to prevent the endometrium from thickening very much. This, too, is a controversial treatment. Of course, a woman who has had a hysterectomy needn't worry about cancer of the uterus, but she does have to consider the danger of breast cancer.

Women with higher amounts of estrogen in their bodies have a greater tendency toward breast cancer. However, many physicians feel that women who take estrogen treatment offset the risk of death from breast cancer by visiting their gynecologist more often, thereby catching any tumor early enough to treat it effectively and prevent its spread.

Some scientists believe estrogen might actually have some preventive effect on the development of ovarian cancer. This is the worst type of female cancer, because there are no warning signs and by the time it is diagnosed, it is usually too late to cure. Some gynecologists, therefore, feel that even if estrogen might stimulate the development of uterine or breast cancer, it is worthwhile if it aids in the prevention of ovarian cancer. Probably the most widely prescribed estrogen replacement is Premarin, manufactured from the urine of pregnant mares. It is used by an estimated three million American women, and is the fifth most prescribed medication in America.

Unfortunately, there are no definite answers. Until there are, every woman should be informed of the possible risks and/or benefits of estrogen treatment by her physician in order to make an informed and appropriate decision.

Other Hormonal Treatments

Some women take progesterone to alleviate the symptoms of menopause. It has apparantly been effective, but the side effects have not yet been fully explored.

Male hormones have been used therapeutically on menopausal women for many years. Certain women gain energy and maintain a positive calcium balance, making their bones stronger, when treated with testosterone. This hormone also has an aphrodisiac effect on many women. However, testosterone treatment may initiate hair growth on the arms, legs, and face. Again, the pros and cons must be weighed in each case.

Should a Woman Take Estrogen, the "Antiaging" Pill?

The change-of-life symptoms can be so horrendous that many women become extremely depressed. These women cannot control their own minds, and life becomes a misery for both the woman and her family. The change-of-life symptoms can range from mild headaches to symptoms of heart attacks, asthma attacks, and severe abdominal pain. A woman with severe symptoms often visits many physicians, who perform a series of unnecessary tests and X-rays without any further solution or treatment. Many of these women can benefit from love, care, and understanding, but some women do not feel better until they start estrogen treatment. After initiation of hormone replacement, one can often see a complete transformation of these women; from being tired, depressed, and miserable, they become happy, energetic, and in good spirits. For women who respond well to estrogen replacement, the treatment can only be strongly recommended. If a woman does not take estrogen, her skin will get thinner and start to sag. Her vagina will get dry, she will lose her hair, and her bones will be affected with osteoporosis, a condition causing pain and, occasionally, a collapse of the vertebrae. A woman will then start to shrink in stature and experience increasing pain. Therefore, if a woman either has symptoms that warrant estrogen treatment or if she is well-motivated and does not want aging to accelerate when she is at her best age, she could take the estrogen-replacement treatment. If the estrogen is taken in a three-week cycle, followed by one week of progesterone treatment, the chances of developing uterine cancer should be very slim. During hormone administration, it is now recommended to have a Pap smear and a biopsy from the uterus once a year to detect any early cancer sign. A woman should examine her breasts thoroughly every month and perhaps have a mammogram once every one or two years.

If a woman knows about the natural changes that take place in her body during menopause and the therapies available to modify or nullify the less acceptable of these changes, then "change of life" can be, in many ways, a change for the better, a time when she is free from the problems of contraception and wise in the ways of life.

chapter 6

VAGINITIS — THE MOST COMMON COMPLAINT

One out of every two women visiting a gynecologist's office is suffering from vaginitis. In the broadest sense, vaginitis is any type of vaginal infection. It is usually characterized by an abnormal vaginal discharge and symptoms such as vaginal pain, itching, irritation, painful intercourse, and painful urination.

Women always have some type of normal vaginal secretion. This secretion depends on a number of factors: age, time of the menstrual cycle, sexual stimulation, type of contraception, and mental state.

NORMAL VAGINAL SECRETION

A delicate balance of microorganisms, bacteria, and yeast coexist in the vagina. The *Döderlein* bacillus, one of the most important components of the vaginal flora, is responsible for the maintenance of the proper vaginal pH, which should be between 4.5 and 5.0. The normal vaginal milieu, which is slightly acidic, is produced via the fermentation of lactic acid from glycogen (sugar) by the *Döderlein* bacillus. When a woman receives antibiotic therapy for infection, the *Döderlein* bacillus can be killed. If this happens, the acidity of the vagina diminishes, providing an ideal environment for the growth of yeast. The yeast can multiply, creating a yeast infection.

The quantity and quality of normal vaginal secretions change throughout the menstrual cycle. Secretion is thick and sticky just after the end of menstrual bleeding and immediately prior to the next menstrual flow. Secretions are influenced by estrogen; when the estrogen level rises prior to ovulation, the vaginal secretion becomes clear, watery, and slippery. These are sometimes called the wet days.

After menopause, as a woman's estrogen level decreases, vaginal cells usually atrophy and the amount of normal vaginal secretion decreases. The vagina becomes dry and the protective vaginal flora disappear, leaving postmenopausal women more susceptible to vaginal infection. The same situation occurs in prepubescent girls, who also have no estrogen production and are susceptible to infection.

Sexual intercourse allows transmission of the microorganisms which cause vaginitis. As the use of the condom has decreased and the number of a woman's sexual partners has risen, the occurrence of vaginitis has sharply increased. During sexual intercourse, the friction produced by the penis on the walls of the vagina can cause the sloughing off of the cells of the vaginal surface, and thus permits microorganisms to be pushed into the vaginal mucosa and become a source of vaginal infection. The more frequent the intercourse and the more numerous the partners, the higher are the chances of vaginal infections.

An IUD sometimes causes uterine irritation and the formation of a clear, watery discharge secreted through the vagina. This is a normal side effect and should not be a source of concern. Birth-control pills, particularly those with low estrogen content, can decrease the amount of acidity, predisposing the user to monilia vaginitis. Pregnancy also alters vaginal secretion, making a woman more susceptible to vaginitis.

Tension, anxiety, and insufficient rest can cause a decrease in normal secretion, upsetting the balance and rendering the vagina more susceptible to infection. Extreme tension can tighten perineal muscles (the muscles around the vagina) to such an extent that normal vaginal secretions cannot drain. These secretions can become a source of irritation and even infection.

You can examine normal vaginal secretions by placing a finger within the vagina to obtain a small amount of secretion. You can then look at this secretion on a glass plate. If you know what normal secretion looks like, it will help you to spot abnormal secretions. You should examine your vulva with a mirror if you suspect vaginal secretions are abnormal in any way.

LEUKORRHEA

If vaginal secretion increases to an abnormal amount, loosely defined as any secretion truly bothersome, the condition is called *leukorrhea*. Leukorrhea is a white vaginal discharge containing white blood cells and excreted dead, or damaged vaginal cells. Leukorrhea can be caused by a vaginal infection or irritation by a foreign body, such as an IUD, a forgotten tampon, or even a vaginal tumor. When leukorrhea becomes a source of vaginal pain or irritation, a woman should see her gynecologist.

HOW TO PREVENT VAGINITIS

The vagina is the perfect environment for the growth of microorganisms. It is warm, dark, wet, and provides sufficient nourishment and oxygen. The normal vaginal flora offer some protection against vaginitis, and a woman should do everything she can to maintain the balance. She should stay in good physical condition, getting proper nourishment and sufficient rest. She should avoid stress and deal appropriately with tension.

A woman should learn voluntary control of her perineal muscles so that she can relax these muscles to permit the passage of vaginal secretions. Some women can gain voluntary control of the perineal muscle by simply being told they are there, but most women need further help. One method is to start and stop the flow of urine (see Kegel's exercise, Chapter 21). Another is to place a clean finger within the vagina, tensing and relaxing the muscles around it. Once a woman learns the feeling of tension and relaxation of the perineal muscles, she can relax these muscles two or three times a day. Some find it a pleasant feeling—a warmth in the perineal area when the muscles are relaxed.

While on antibiotic therapy, a woman should also receive antiyeast pills or suppositories to prevent disturbance of the vaginal milieu.

A woman should keep herself clean, washing the area of the vulva at least once a day. After urination or bowel movement, a woman should wipe from front to back—*never* from back to front—to prevent the passage of bacteria from the anus to the vulva.

She should make sure that her sexual partner is clean. A man should wash his penis once a day. Women could learn a useful trick from the professionals by carefully inspecting and milking the penis prior to intercourse. This is particularly appropriate with a new sexual partner. The use of a condom may not be a bad idea for the primary sexual encounter. If a couple engages in anal sex, the penis must be cleansed prior to vaginal intercourse.

Diabetes and obesity predispose a woman to vaginitis by causing changes in the vaginal milieu. Diabetics should avoid excessive sugar intake and obese women should lose weight.

A foreign body in the vagina can cause irritation. Therefore, a diaphragm should not be worn for longer than the required time. A forgotten tampon can also be a frequent source of vaginal infection.

Excessive douching can disturb the protective balance of the vagina and predispose a woman to vaginitis. If a woman wishes, she can douche safely approximately once a week with an appropriate solution (see Douching at the end of this chapter).

Panty Hose and Vaginitis

The constant wearing of panty hose can increase a woman's chances of getting vaginitis. When panty hose are worn, the

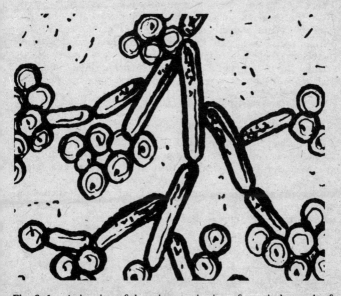

Fig. 6–1: A drawing of the microscopic view of a typical growth of monilia *(Candida albicans)*. The yeast microorganisms multiply by forming new "branches," and can thus spread very rapidly. *Candida albicans* grow better in a moist, warm environment with only a mild degree of acidity.

temperature and moisture of the vagina are increased. The vagina becomes more susceptible to infection. This is a particular problem in the summer. Panty hose also stimulate the growth of bacteria by preventing the circulation of air in the vulvar area. If a woman has vaginitis or has had recurrent episodes of vaginitis, it is recommended that she refrain from wearing panty hose, or wear panty hose with a cotton crotch.

MONILIA OR YEAST INFECTION

Monilia (or *Candida albicans*), a fungus of the yeast family, is a normal resident of the oral cavity, the vagina, and the rectum. When the normal balance among the vaginal flora is disturbed, particularly when the vaginal acidity decreases, monilia starts an uncontrolled growth. The result is a monilia infection.

About half of all vaginitis is due to monilia or yeast infection. There has been an increase of monilia in recent years, thought to be the result of increased use of antibiotics and oral contraceptives and a decrease in the use of condoms and diaphragms. Antibiotics kill the *Döderlein* bacteria and the pH of the vagina becomes more conducive to yeast growth. Low-estrogen birth-control pills also alter vaginal acidity. Pregnancy, diabetes, and obesity all produce a hospitable vaginal environment for yeast.

Transmission of Yeast Infection

A monilia infection need not be transmitted. It can flare up spontaneously whenever the vaginal milieu is disturbed. However, a yeast infection can be transmitted through sexual intercourse. Yeast is viable for some time outside the body if moisture is available. A common site is moist towels. Infection often spreads this way in such places as college dormitories, where women sometimes share the same towels.

Symptoms of Monilia Infection

The symptoms of monilia vaginitis are discharge, itching, burning, and painful intercourse. The discharge is white and curdy, looking something like cottage cheese, and is easily discovered by self-examination. It has a yeasty odor. The vagina, which is usually pale pink, turns bright red. This redness often spreads to the vulva, which you can see with a mirror. The discoloration can reach all the way to the anus. It can cause

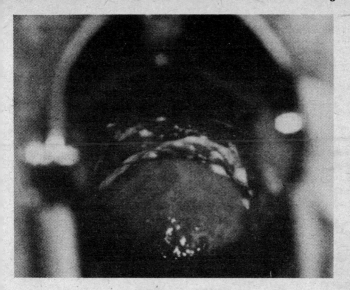

Fig. 6–2: A physician's view of the cervix through a speculum. The cream cheeselike discharge on the cervix and on the top of the vagina is characteristic of a monilia vaginal infection. (Reproduced by permission of the Emko Company, St. Louis, Missouri.)

swelling and become very painful. Sometimes the irritation becomes so severe that walking is difficult. Often there are whitish or grayish areas or spots either in the vagina or on the vulva.

It is possible to have monilia in the mouth. This is usually caused by antibiotic therapy, although sometimes also by oral sex. It looks like curdy white patches in the mouth, which bleed if scraped. Oral pain and fever can occur.

Diagnosis of Monilia

The diagnosis of monilia vaginitis can be made by the characteristic appearance and odor of the discharge, the presence of white or gray patches in the vagina, and the inflammation of the vulvar area. To substantiate this clinical diagnosis, the physician microscopically examines a wet smear of the vaginal discharge for the typical yeastlike organisms. A swab of the vaginal discharge can also be placed on a special culture medium, such as Nickerson's medium. The culture will grow within a few days, even at room temperature, if it contains *Candida albicans.*

Treatment of Monilia Vaginitis

Antiyeast suppositories and creams are the most common treatments for monilia infection. Nystatin suppositories (mycostatin) are the most commonly prescribed and are very effective. The usual dosage is two suppositories a day for fourteen days. The suppository melts, coating the vagina with medication which may leak from the vagina and stain underwear. Follow insertion of the suppository with a vaginal tampon, cut in half and placed in the lower part of the vagina, or use a minipad to protect your clothing.

Mycostatin can be taken orally, but high doses are needed for effective treatment of monilia infection. Oral mycostatin can be used to treat men who have monilia infections.

There are a number of other very effective antiyeast suppositories available. There is a new vaginal cream, Monistat, which appears effective and needs only a single application daily.

If the monilia infection causes swelling of the vulvar tissue and irritation, symptomatic relief may be provided by local application of a soothing medicated cream such as Mycolog. This cream may also be applied to the penis of a man who has a yeast infection.

These antiyeast suppositories and creams should be stored in the refrigerator, and it might be wise for a woman who is subject to recurrent monilia infections to keep medication on hand. When she identifies the initial symptoms of the monilia infection, she can then immediately initiate treatment before she becomes too uncomfortable.

If a monilia infection resists treatment with any of the antiyeast suppositories or creams, successful treatment may be achieved by the use of gentian violet, probably the most common treatment for monilia before the development of the antiyeast drugs. Gentian violet is a deep purple dye that can either be painted on the cervix, vagina, and vulva by the physician twice weekly for three weeks or can be applied by the woman in the form of a suppository with one application daily for three weeks. Although effective, this treatment is extremely messy.

In recurrent cases of monilia infection, it is important to restore the proper acidity of the vagina to inhibit the uncontrolled growth of yeast. This can be accomplished by vaginal administration of acetic and boric acid gel (Aci-jel), or by douching with a vinegar-and-water solution. Some physicians recommend douching with a one-percent potassium sorbate solution to inhibit yeast growth (this chemical is used to inhibit yeast growth in wine making). Still others suggest douching with an iodine solution like Betadine, an agent used for preoperative cleansing.

It would be a good idea for women to eat yogurt while taking antibiotics. In fact, yogurt is a useful addition to the diet of any woman who has or is predisposed to yeast infections. She must, of course, eat yogurt that contains *live* cultures; this counterbalances the yeast in the vagina. It has been suggested that plain yogurt (again, only yogurt with live cultures) could be applied like a vaginal cream for the treatment of a monilia infection. The effectiveness of this yogurt treatment has not been tested.

Oral monilia infection can be treated with an antifungal mouthwash. Mycostatin comes in the form of a mouthwash, and although its taste is anything but appealing, gargling two or three times a day until symptoms disappear cures an oral monilia infection.

TRICHOMONIASIS VAGINITIS

Trichomoniasis vaginitis is caused by a single-cell parasite called *Trichomonas vaginalis*. This organism lives only in the female vagina and the male urethra. The organism is usually transmitted by sexual intercourse. The *Trichomonas* organism can dwell within the reproductive tract without causing any symptoms. It is estimated that approximately 15 percent of men have trichomoniasis within the urethra. The organism can be detected by Pap smear in asymptomatic women.

Transmission of *Trichomonas*

Trichomoniasis is usually spread by sexual intercourse directly from an infected person to her or his partner. After transmission, the organisms can remain dormant in the body for extended periods of time. Alterations in the vaginal milieu can trigger the reproduction of this organism, with subsequent appearance of symptoms. Nonvenereal transmission of trichomoniasis is possible from contaminated toilets, towels, and instruments.

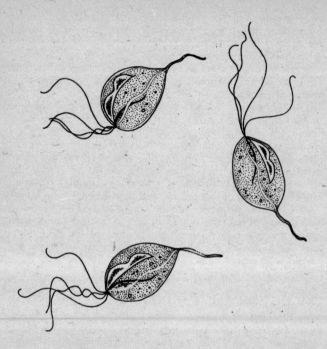

Fig. 6–3:   The form and the shape of *Trichomonas* organisms as they appear under the microscope. The trichomonads are identified by their characteristic form, also by their active twisting movement, caused by swinging movements of the four threadlike tails.

Symptoms

The vaginal discharge that accompanies a trichomoniasis infection is frothy and greenish yellow. The *Trichomonas* organism ferments the carbohydrates in the vagina, producing a gas which is the source of both the froth and the foul smell of the discharge. Trichomoniasis causes an irritation of the membranes of the vagina, producing severe itching. Since the membranes are irritated and sensitive, intercourse is painful, and so, sometimes, is urination. The inflammation can spread to the uterus, causing pelvic pain and a general feeling of malaise.

Diagnosis

The presence of the characteristic greenish, foul-smelling discharge leads a physician to suspect a trichomoniasis infection. A pelvic examination should confirm the diagnosis. If *Trichomonas* is present, the vagina is usually inflamed with a typical strawberry-red color, and there are often numerous small, deep red spots throughout the vagina. The inflammation can even spread to the vulva. The conclusive step in the diagnosis is to take a small amount of the discharge, place it in a drop of saline on a slide, and immediately examine it under a microscope. This should reveal the presence of the *Trichomonas,* a motile, unicellular, pear-shaped organism with a number of flagella (tails). Since it is possible to have trichomoniasis without symptoms, a Pap smear can also reveal the presence of the organism.

Treatment

The most effective treatment for trichomoniasis in women is 250-milligram tablets of metronidazole or Flagyl, taken orally three times a day for ten days. The dose for an infected man is two of the 250-milligram tablets taken daily for ten days. This drug results in a 90 percent cure of patients when the full ten-day course is undertaken. Intercourse should be avoided during the treatment period to prevent contamination or reinfection. A person on Flagyl should not drink alcohol during the treatment period. Alcohol does not inhibit the effectiveness of the drug, but the combination of alcohol and Flagyl can cause changes in body metabolism resulting in nausea and vomiting. Metronidazole can be administered via vaginal suppositories, which, although they have a somewhat less systemic effect, are less effective and recommended only for the most minimal trichomoniasis infection.

It has been reported that fetal abnormalities have occurred in the offspring of pregnant laboratory animals given Flagyl. Therefore Flagyl is not recommended for women during the first three months of pregnancy, and if possible, should be avoided throughout pregnancy. A pregnant woman with a trichomoniasis infection is best treated with a nonmetronidazole suppository.

There have been reports that cancer developed when high doses of metronidazole were given to laboratory rodents over a period of time. There has been no evidence that metronidazole is carcinogenic in humans. Still, it is prudent to avoid overexposure to this potent drug. A woman should be sure to take the full course of metronidazole treatment to control the trichomonal infection completely and, most importantly, to avoid reinfection. She should also be sure that her sexual partner or partners are simultaneously treated. In this way, overexposure to metronidazole is avoided.

Warning!

Symptoms of vaginitis often elicit a diagnosis of trichomoniasis without proper identification of the infecting organism. Many women who have monilia infections are incorrectly treated for trichomoniasis and are given Flagyl, which can actually exacerbate the symptoms of monilia. If trichomoniasis cannot be clearly demonstrated, therapy for trichomoniasis should not be initiated.

HEMOPHILUS VAGINALIS VAGINITIS

Hemophilus vaginalis is a bacterial infection of the vagina now believed to be the third most common cause of vaginitis.

Transmission of Hemophilus Vaginalis

Hemophilus vaginalis is a Gram-negative bacteria that may be part of the normal vaginal flora. The uncontrolled reproduction of this bacteria, triggered perhaps by a change in the vaginal acidity, produces the infection. On the other hand, since the *Hemophilus* can occur in both women and men, the infection may be transmitted by sexual intercourse with an infected partner.

Symptoms of Hemophilus Vaginalis Vaginitis

In the earliest stage of the infection, a woman notices a scant vaginal discharge associated with mild burning and itching. As the infection spreads, the discharge becomes more profuse, either white or gray, and carries a foul smell. Vaginal itching and irritation increase, intercourse may become painful, and there may be a sensation of burning during urination.

Diagnosis of Hemophilus Vaginalis Vaginitis

A pelvic examination by a trained physician is required to diagnose hemophilus correctly. The symptoms of this infection are similar to the clinical symptoms of a trichomoniasis infection, often resulting in a misdiagnosis. The examination should reveal inflammation of the membranes of the vagina. Occasionally there will be small spots of hemorrhage. A sample of the discharge is examined under a microscope, where the absence of either *Candida albicans* or *Trichomonas* rules out these two organisms as being implicated in the infection. Hemophilus vaginalis is difficult to identify, but the presence of granular epithelial cells, called clue cells, and numerous white blood cells helps establish the diagnosis.

Treatment of Hemophilus Vaginalis Vaginitis

A mild hemophilus vaginalis infection can be successfully treated by intravaginal administration of triple-sulfa cream twice a day for two weeks. In more advanced cases, oral antibiotics are indicated. Ampicillin in doses of 500 milligrams, four times a day for five days, or tetracycline in doses of 250 milligrams four times a day for seven days, or other broad-spectrum antibiotics, is usually effective. When oral antibiotics are administered for treatment of a bacterial vaginitis, antiyeast suppositories should be given to prevent the overgrowth of yeast and a flare-up of monilia vaginitis. Intercourse should be avoided during the treatment period, and a woman's sexual partner or partners must be treated simultaneously to prevent reinfection.

NONSPECIFIC VAGINITIS

If the cause of vaginitis is not identifiable as trichomoniasis or monilia, it is often designated as nonspecific. This is usually a nonvenereal bacterial vaginitis with a gray, homogenous, foul-smelling discharge. It can be caused by poor hygiene in the vulvar area, which allows the growth of bacteria, which are then pushed by penile penetration into the vagina. Poor hygiene in the man has had the same effect.

Hemophilus vaginalis is still classified by many physicians as a nonspecific vaginitis, but the frequency of this rather specific infection merits its consideration as a separate entity.

E. coli bacteria are also found in some vaginitis discharge smears. These come from the rectum; they are normally in the intestines and are involved in the digestion process. *E. coli* can reach the vagina because of poor hygiene or mixing anal and vaginal intercourse. Women should be careful after defecation to clean themselves from front to back, not from back to front, to ensure that *E. coli* do not get into the vagina.

Mycoplasma is a microorganism associated with vaginitis; alone it causes no symptoms, but it has usually been found with bacteria. It can cause infertility.

When these bacteria infect a man, they grow inside the urethra and occasionally spread to the prostate. If either sex partner is diagnosed as having nonspecific infections, both should be treated.

A great number of bacteria can cause nonspecific vaginitis—too many to be listed here. The treatment for nonspecific vaginitis is the same as for hemophilus vaginalis vaginitis.

MIXED VAGINITIS

Vaginitis can have more than a single cause, and a woman may be infected with *Monilia, Trichomonas,* and *Hemophilus* bacteria all at the same time. Vaginitis must be carefully diagnosed, and a woman must be treated for *each* of the infecting organisms in order to achieve an effective cure.

CERVICITIS

Cervicitis is an inflammation of the tissues of the cervix, caused by a variety of infecting microorganisms. Cervicitis is classified as either acute or chronic.

In *acute cervicitis,* the inflammatory reaction is fresh and the symptoms are a purulent discharge and pelvic pain. Gonorrheal infection is one of the main causes of acute cervicitis, but it can be caused by any number of bacteria.

Chronic cervicitis is extremely common and may be present to some degree in ninety of every hundred women after childbirth. Chronic cervicitis can be very mild and the symptoms so minimal that a woman does not suspect anything. On the other hand, a woman may experience discharge, backache, and urinary problems. Chronic cervicitis is often associated with pregnancy or the use of birth-control pills with high estrogen levels. This is probably due to an increased blood supply to the cervix secondary to the increased hormone levels.

The cervix is extremely vulnerable to infection, since it is traumatized during childbirth and can even be mildly affected during sexual intercourse. Any infection within the vagina is easily passed to the cervix, where the infecting organism can be harbored. The tissue of the cervix can be so inflamed by the infection that *cervical erosion,* an open sore on the cervix, is formed. With cervical erosion, the outer, protective layer of cervical tissue has been destroyed and the cervix becomes even more vulnerable to infection. One of the symptoms of cervical erosion is a puslike vaginal discharge which, when cultured, often yields *E. coli* bacteria or any of the bacteria found in mixed vaginitis.

Chronic cervicitis can lead to cervical erosion. There may be a minimal, yellow discharge with early chronic cervicitis, but the amount of discharge increases appreciably when cervical erosion develops. As tissue destruction becomes more severe, cervical erosion may develop into a *cervical ulceration,* which can be a source of intermenstrual bleeding and spotting and bleeding after intercourse.

Diagnosis

The diagnosis of acute cervicitis is made after obtaining a smear of the cervical discharge during pelvic examination. The smear is cultured and the infecting organism identified. The cervix is red and swollen with a purulent discharge. In the diagnosis of chronic cervicitis, it is most important to differentiate this condition from cervical cancer, since some of the symptoms of cervical erosion are identical to the symptoms of a cervical malignancy. A Pap smear must be obtained; and any suspicious area should be biopsied during the pelvic examination. The biopsy can be obtained during a culposcopic examination or after the cervix has been stained with an iodine solution. A culture of the cervical discharge should be obtained to identify the infecting bacteria.

Treatment

Acute cervicitis is treated by administration of the appropriate antibiotics to eliminate the infecting organism.

Mild *chronic cervicitis* often spontaneously subsides, even without treatment, once the proper vaginal milieu is reestablished. This can be achieved postdelivery or when a woman stops use of birth-control pills. As with acute cervicitis, the infecting organism associated with chronic cervicitis must be eliminated by the administration of the proper antibiotic. If cervical erosion is present in a mild state, the physician may apply silver nitrate, which destroys the damaged cells and permits the growth of new, healthy cervical cells. When the cervical erosion is more advanced, electrocauterization or cryosurgery is performed to eliminate the damaged cells, making way for new, healthy tissue growth (see Chapter 16 on Operations).

Chronic inflammation of the cervix might predispose a woman to cervical cancer. Therefore, if symptoms of cervicitis appear, a woman should consult her physician.

CERVICAL POLYPS

Cervical polyps are small, fragile protrusions of tissue that grow from the inside of the cervix, sometimes protruding from the cervical opening into the vagina. Polyps usually grow when there has been a persistent cervicitis or other minor cervical abnormalities. The symptoms of cervical polyps are bleeding or spotting following intercourse or bowel movements, and some vaginal discharge. Since any abnormal vaginal bleeding is considered a potential sign of cervical cancer, a Pap smear must be obtained when the presence of polyps is suspected. Some cervical polyps can be removed by forceps in the physician's office. However, since the polyps usually have their origin within the cervix, they are more often removed during a D and C. A physician can then easily scrape the bases of the polyps to ensure that they do not grow back. Polyps are sent for pathological examination to rule out any malignancy.

VAGINAL DISCHARGE IN CHILDREN

A vaginal mucous discharge is not uncommon in girls around the time of menarche, the beginning of menstruation. This discharge signals the onset of estrogen production by the ovaries during the maturation process. Both trichomonas and monilia infections are seen in children. Mothers and elder sisters can spread these infections through towels and contaminated clothing, as can girls in boarding schools. Early sexual experimentation must also be considered, and any persistent vaginal discharge should be examined for gonorrhea. Cancer can also cause vaginal discharge. Although vaginal cancer is very rare in children, there have been cases of clear-cell carcinoma reported in the young daughters of women who received the antimiscarriage drug known as DES during pregnancy.

The combination of discharge, odor, and scant bleeding often means a foreign object in the child's vagina. Children have a tendency to satisfy their natural curiosity by exploring their bodies. Little girls may actually stick some small object into the vagina, which may catch inside the hymen, causing irritation, discharge, and odor. Physicians have extracted a wide variety of objects from girls' vaginas, such as hairpins, pencils, apple cores, and small toys.

When diagnosing a vaginal discharge in a child, the physician should probably perform a rectal examination rather than chance breaking the hymen with a vaginal examination. However, the findings may indicate the need for a vaginal examination, either to confirm the diagnosis of an infection or to remove a foreign body. The treatment of vaginitis in a child must be determined by the child's physician on an individual basis.

Intestinal parasites such as pinworms can also cause vaginal discharge in children, and there are oral medications for the adequate treatment of these conditions.

VAGINITIS AFTER MENOPAUSE

The vaginal milieu is enormously dependent upon hormonal influences. As the level of estrogen in the blood drops drastically during and following menopause, the cells of the vagina change. The vaginal tissue becomes atrophic, the mucosa loses its normal pink color and becomes gray, and the vagina is more easily traumatized, with slower healing due to decreased blood supply. These atrophic changes in the vagina later spread to the tissue of the vulva, and the skin becomes thin and loose. These changes can be accompanied by symptoms such as itching and burning. These symptoms vary enormously from one woman to another.

The atrophic changes which occur following menopause significantly alter the normal vaginal milieu and render the vagina very susceptible to infecting organisms such as yeast, *Trichomonas,* and even gonorrhea.

Treatment

The best treatment for simple *atrophic vaginitis* is local application of estrogen cream. This results in a thickening of the vaginal mucosa, an increase in blood supply to the vaginal tissue, and may help in the restoration of the vaginal milieu. The usual course of therapy involves daily applications of the vaginal cream until the symptoms have subsided. It is then advised that estrogen cream be applied at least once or twice weekly to prevent recurrence of symptoms. There is some systemic absorption of the vaginally applied estrogen; therefore, this treatment cannot be used by women for whom estrogen is contraindicated. If a woman is receiving estrogen-replacement treatment for menopausal symptoms, there is very little chance she will develop atrophic vaginitis.

If a woman contracts a secondary infection such as yeast, trichomoniasis, or gonorrhea with atrophic vaginitis, it should be treated by the usually prescribed medications.

VAGINAL DISCHARGE DUE TO FOREIGN BODIES

One of the most foul-smelling discharges results from a retained tampon. Quite often a woman uses two tampons during heavy bleeding, then removes only one of them. After a while, she notices an odor, and has a discharge that no amount of douching stops. When she finally goes to a gynecologist, the tampon is simply removed, and the symptoms immediately abate.

This same type of discharge can be caused by anything that becomes lodged in the vagina. It is surprising how many things gynecologists find in the vagina. Masturbatory objects are extremely common, and quite embarrassing to the patient. Small vibrators and bottles are frequently found.

Women with prolapsed uteri are often given pessaries, which act like crutches to hold the uterus in place. These, too, are foreign bodies, and can cause irritation and discharge. Retained and forgotten diaphragms do the same thing.

Some women use their vaginas as secure hiding places for money and gems, then either forget their valuables or can't get them out. This used to be a more common practice than it is today, but gynecologists in high-crime areas still extract a sizable booty from vaginal banks.

PSYCHOSOMATIC VAGINITIS

As with many other illnesses or disorders, the origin of vaginitis can be psychosomatic. This does not mean the vaginitis should be ignored or that it is not real; psychologically caused vaginitis is physically identical to any other type of vaginitis.

This type of vaginitis often has a sexual basis. Itching of the vulva or vagina may occur in women who are lonely, sexually frustrated, guilty about certain sexual practices, or overly fearful of venereal disease. Any of these can be especially acute when the woman engages in casual sex with a new partner.

When a woman has intercourse after a long abstinence and then experiences a discharge, it can be very upsetting. She can easily persuade herself that she has VD when her discharge actually stems from emotional stress. Unfortunately, the fear of VD only increases the symptoms.

The same thing can occur when a woman has an abnormal discharge and suspects cancer—the anxiety can easily affect hormonal balance and produce more discharge. On the other hand, some women ignore a discharge, afraid they might have cancer. The reasoning is that what they don't know can't hurt them. Of course, this is dangerous, even if there is no cancer, because any untreated infection can develop into serious physical problems.

Tension is a common cause of vaginitis. Stress causes more steroids to be produced by the adrenal glands, which decrease the body's formation of antibodies (immunoglobins). Thus, stress can make the body especially susceptible to infection by weakening its natural defense system.

The only way to treat tension-produced vaginitis is to learn to relax. Relaxation is not a luxury for the idle rich alone; it is a vital function of good health. It doesn't matter whether you are involved in organized relaxation—yoga, transcendental meditation, hypnosis, biofeedback, psychoanalysis—or whether you just sit back and enjoy music with a glass of wine. Relaxation is good for you and should be done regularly, every day.

One recommended method of relaxation is sex. Orgasm is a normal release of built-up tension, and it can relieve the entire body of anxiety. A healthy life most definitely includes a healthy sex life.

URINARY INFECTIONS

Because a woman's urethra is so much shorter than a man's, she is much more susceptible to urinary infections. These can be caused during intercourse by the penis pushing dirt and bacteria from the vagina into the urethra, or they can occur when a woman cleans herself after bowel movement from back to front rather than front to back, spreading rectal bacteria into the urethra.

Urinary infection is usually an infection in the bladder or kidneys. If it is left untreated, permanent damage may occur. Usually, symptoms are burning during urination, pressure on the bladder, fever, and backache.

If a severe urinary infection is suspected, tests should be performed to determine the source. Urine should be obtained for culture. Kidney X-ray and cystoscopy (examination of the bladder by introducing a scope through the urethra) may be performed. A thorough examination is especially important in children with recurrent infections.

When the clinical symptoms present the characteristic portrait of a urinary tract infection (UTI) with burning during urination, bladder pressure and pain, and low back pain, treatment is usually initiated immediately with one of the sulfa drugs such as Gantrisin. However, once the urine culture returns, treatment may be altered. If the infecting organism is more susceptible to a different antibiotic, it will be prescribed. While on antibiotic therapy for UTI, a woman must drink at least six to eight ounces of fluid every hour during her waking hours. She might also drink orange juice and take vitamin C to render the urine more acidic and less hospitable to the growth of bacteria.

If a woman suffers from recurrent urinary tract infections, she should have a careful evaluation by a qualified urologist to determine if these recurrent infections are the result of any urinary tract abnormality or kidney damage.

HONEYMOON CYSTITIS

A common bladder condition is called *honeymoon cystitis;* it is usually the result of very frequent intercourse, hence the name. The symptoms of this condition are bladder cramps, burning during urination, and blood in the urine. Honeymoon cystitis need not be the result of a bladder infection; it may be caused by an inflammation of the wall of the bladder. Excessive stimulation of the cervix during sexual intercourse can lead to a low-grade cervicitis, and the inflammation can spread via the lymphatic pathways to part of the bladder wall, resulting in honeymoon cystitis. Honeymoon cystitis may also be caused by an infection, with bacteria pushed up the urethra into the bladder during sexual intercourse. Adequate personal hygiene on the part of a woman and her partner may help prevent bacterial honeymoon cystitis.

Treatment of Honeymoon Cystitis

If it is suspected that honeymoon cystitis is not of bacterial origin, the first step in the treatment is to abstain from sexual intercourse. A woman should drink large amounts of water and increase her intake of orange juice and vitamin C. If the bladder pain is severe, pain killers such as Darvon and aspirin may be prescribed. If a urine culture reveals that the cystitis is of bacterial origin, appropriate antibiotic therapy is initiated.

BARTHOLIN'S GLAND INFECTION

There are two small glands inside the opening of the vagina, midway between the anus and the lower edge of the opening of the vulva. These are the Bartholin's glands, and their principal role is to secrete mucus to lubricate the vagina and facilitate penetration of the penis.

An infection or inflammation in the vulval area can cause swelling and irritation of any of the genital glands. The little ducts of the Bartholin's glands can become so inflamed that they will swell shut, trapping the mucous secretions. The trapped secretions cause the glands to swell into lumps the size of small eggs (Bartholin's gland cysts). This swelling is usually not painful, but often frightens a woman. If the Bartholin's gland becomes infected with a virulent organism, it leads to an abscess (Bartholin's gland abscess). This condition can be so painful that the woman is unable to walk. Abscess of the Bartholin's gland is most often caused by gonorrheal infection, but any kind of bacteria can be responsible.

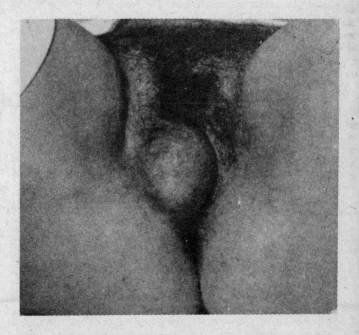

Fig. 6–4:   A view of the vulva area. The woman's legs are resting in the stirrups. The large egg-shaped mass seen in the lower aspect of the right *labia majora* is an abscess of the Bartholin gland. (Reproduced by permission of Edmund R. Novak, M.D., from *Textbook of Gynecology*, 9th edition, The Williams and Wilkins Company, Baltimore, Maryland.)

Treatment

Bartholin's gland cysts and inflammation of the duct can heal spontaneously and, as the swelling of the duct subsides, the trapped secretions drain and the gland usually returns to normal size. This initial inflammation of the duct may be treated with oral antibiotics in combination with local application of an antibiotic-antiyeast cream. Sitz baths may also be advised. In some women, the gland may remain somewhat enlarged over a period of years, but this enlargement is not painful and requires no medical treatment. If reinflammation of the duct occurs, drainage of the cyst is impaired and the cyst will swell. If this reenlargement is asymptomatic, sitz baths may be the only treatment required, but if there are symptoms of pain, antibiotics should be taken. Women with Bartholin's gland cysts should be particularly attentive to their personal hygiene to avoid infection.

When the Bartholin's gland becomes abscessed, the pain usually becomes so severe that hospitalization is necessary. Cultures are obtained to determine the infecting organism and intravenous therapy with the appropriate antibiotic is initiated. Sitz baths are given to help reduce and ease the pain and swelling and aid the drainage of the gland.

In cases of very severe infection, a surgical procedure is required to drain the gland; this procedure is called *marsupialization*. A ortion of the cyst wall is removed, the purulent material is drained, and the incision is sutured in such a fashion that the gland drains directly into the vagina, bypassing the ducts. Antibiotic treatment and sitz baths are continued postoperatively until complete healing has occurred. This procedure should have no sequel.

DOUCHING

Women have probably been douching, or instilling various fluids in the vagina, as long as they have been cleansing other parts of their bodies. In the past, douching was thought to have therapeutic effects, from the control of pelvic infections to the prevention of conception. The types of douches are widely varied and women have to the present day used everything from wine and garlic (as reported in the Ebers Papyrus of 1450 B.C.) to the perfumed and even flavored solutions available in today's pharmacies. In the past, one of the most common reasons for douching was contraception; recipes for the prevention of pregnancy were handed down from mother to daughter rather like a prized recipe for apple pie. Today, douching is used almost solely for cleanliness.

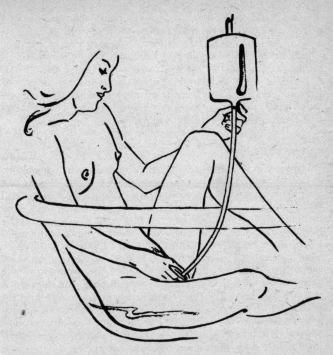

Fig. 6–5: Douching should be done in the bathtub. The douche tip is within the vagina and the labia are held by one hand to keep the fluid in the vagina. In this drawing, the douche apparatus is slightly higher than it should be, no more than 2 feet above the hips.

About fifty percent of American women douche at least occasionally. Most of them douche when they notice excessive or bad-smelling discharge. If this discharge is the result of an infection, douching will probably not help. On the other hand, it will probably do no harm, and although it does not treat the infection, it can clean out excess vaginal secretions.

Is Douching Recommended?

Douching is not necessary to cleanse the vagina, since the normal, healthy vagina cleans itself. If a vaginal discharge is present, douching usually increases, rather than decreases, the amount of vaginal secretions. Too-frequent douching can alter the vaginal milieu and render the vagina more susceptible to infections. Douching tips and the douching solutions are seldom sterile and can even be a source of infection.

However, in general, douching is a benign procedure. If a woman feels it is personally necessary, she may douche perhaps once a week with little problem. On the other hand, the *perineal area* should be carefully washed every day as an essential part of personal hygiene. The Europeans have a good system in the bidet, which washes the external perineal area to prevent infection from spreading into the vagina.

How to Douche

If a woman wishes to douche, she should douche lying down in the bath tub rather than sitting on the toilet. The douche bag should be filled with one to two quarts of douching solution and placed no more than two feet above the level of the hips. The tip is inserted gently into the vagina as far as it will go, and the labia are pressed against the tip with one hand to keep the tip in place and to keep the douching solution from leaking out. The woman uses her free hand to release some of the solution from the douche bag and allows it to flow into the vagina until she feels a sense of fullness in the lower abdomen. She then stops the flow and holds the labia shut for fifteen to twenty seconds, during which time she tries contracting the muscles of the vagina to circulate the solution. The labia are then opened and the solution drains from the vagina. This procedure is repeated until all the douche solution has been used.

Douche Apparatus

There are three important don'ts when it comes to douching apparatus:

1. Don't use anyone else's douche apparatus—it is the perfect way to spread infection from one woman to another.
2. Don't douche with an apparatus that has been used at any time for an enema—bacteria from the rectum can live inside the tubing and easily be spread to the vagina.
3. Don't use a positive-pressure, bulb-type apparatus—if the pressure is too high, the douching solution, and possibly infection, can be forced into the uterus and even into the abdominal cavity.

A douche apparatus should be carefully cleaned and dried following each use, and should be placed where it will be as free from contamination as possible. A disposable douche bag is highly recommended, since their tips are sterile.

Douching Solutions

An enormous variety of commercially produced douching solutions is available, but probably one of the best, most benign solutions is one quart of ordinary tap water containing one tablespoon of plain white vinegar. If a woman wishes to use a commercially available preparation, she should carefully follow the instructions concerning the preparation of the solution to avoid damage to the vaginal tissue resulting from too strong a solution. An iodine solution, such as diluted Betadine, can be used as an effective cleansing douche and may alleviate the symptoms of herpes Type II infection. The FDA is expected to propose that commercially produced solutions carry an insert stating that their only proven therapeutic effect is that of cleansing.

Douching and Pregnancy

Douching is not recommended during pregnancy, since it is feared that if the douching solution enters the uterus it can harm the fetus and perhaps cause miscarriage. There is the possibility that some of the chemicals in the douching solution might enter the general circulation, pass the placenta, and even cause fetal abnormalities. Some douching solutions contain phenylmercuric acetate (PMA), and it has been shown that mercury can be damaging to a developing fetus.

chapter 7

VENEREAL DISEASE

WHAT IS VD?

Basically, venereal disease (VD) is an infection contracted and transmitted primarily through sexual intercourse. The organisms which produce the various types of VD are extraordinarily fragile and cannot survive for any length of time outside the body. Air, light, lack of moisture, and even minor variations in temperature will destroy *most* VD organisms.

VD cannot be contracted from inanimate objects such as toilet seats, bed linen, or clothes, despite the stories you may have heard. It is transmitted directly from one partner to another in the act of sexual intercourse. These organisms invade the body where tissues provide a favorable environment (dark, moist, and warm), and are susceptible to the organism. These tissues are the mucous membranes of female and male genitalia, the mouth, the eyes, and the anus. VD in a pregnant woman can infect her unborn child.

Most VD is either a *bacterial* or a *viral* infection. Syphilis is caused by a microscopic, unicellular, spiral bacteria called *Treponema pallidum*. Gonorrhea is a bacterial infection caused by the bacteria *Neisseria gonorrhoea*. Other venereal diseases are discussed later in this chapter: *chancroid, lymphogranuloma venereum, granuloma inguinale,* and *herpes simplex* virus. All but the last are relatively rare, but herpes is a major problem as it becomes widespread because there is no known cure.

Venereal disease may be detected by the appearance of certain symptoms after intercourse with an infected individual. The symptoms vary, and the interval, or incubation period, between the time of exposure and the onset of the active disease may extend from two days to as long as six months, depending on the type of infection. The early signs of venereal infection are usually obvious in the male, although they may be ignored, tolerated, rationalized, or perhaps even unrecognized due to ignorance of the disease. In the woman, however, manifestations of venereal infection in the genital tract are often neither felt nor seen and cause no distress. Unknowingly, she becomes a *carrier of the disease,* completely unaware of the infection spreading inside her that she, in turn, may transmit to others.

You Can Have VD Without Knowing It

In women, both syphilis and gonorrhea can be asymptomatic (without symptoms). Gonorrhea can be asymptomatic eighty percent of the time, but a syphilis sore can also go unnoticed, since these sores are not painful and often disappear spontaneously. For this reason, women should be checked frequently for VD if they engage in sexual activity with many partners. If you do not know where to obtain information regarding VD symptoms and treatment, call the National VD Hot Line (Operation Venus) at the following toll-free numbers, 9:00 A.M. to 9:00 P.M. 7 days a week:

(800) 523-1885 (National)
(800) 462-4966 (For Pennsylvania)

VD on the Rise

With the discovery of penicillin, it appeared that venereal disease had finally been conquered. The past decade, however, has seen a dramatic resurgence in venereal disease. Today, the number of cases reported far surpasses the number reported before the advent of antibiotic treatment. Venereal disease is now considered an epidemic and reportedly strikes one person every two minutes in this country.

The term venereal disease (VD) refers to both syphilis and gonorrhea. These two diseases are, however, different; syphilis can, in its final stage, cause death, whereas gonorrhea is rarely fatal but can cause permanent sterility in both women and men. The required premarital blood test, VDRL (Venereal Disease Research Laboratory), detects only syphilis. Gonorrhea can be detected only by a culture obtained from the infected area.

Both syphilis and gonorrhea (GC) are on the rise, but there are about twenty-five cases of GC reported for each case of syphilis. The reported incidence of VD is higher in men than in women, particularly among male homosexuals.

HISTORY OF VD

At the end of the fifteenth century, the first documented epidemic of syphilis ravaged Western Europe, spreading rapidly from the southern countries to their northern neighbors. The Europeans had not acquired immunity and the initial stages of the disease were far more severe and deadly than what is seen today. People fearfully recalled the Black Death, which had decimated the population of Europe 150 years earlier.

When syphilis was first reported, it was not known by that name but labeled differently in each country, usually by a form of political epithet. In France it was *le mal de Naples* or the Neapolitan disease; the Italians reciprocated by calling it the French pox. Depending on an Englishman's political preference, he suffered from either the French or Spanish disease. The Turks indicted all of western Europe by calling it the disease of the Christians.

By 1530, it appeared that the epidemic was over, and an Italian physician and philosopher, Hieronymus Fracastorius, left descriptions about the disease in the form of a poem, "Syphilis, Sive Morbi Gallici." In this poem the author invented the myth of Syphilis, a shepherd in the land of Opyhre who cursed Apollo, the Sun, and led his people from the worship of Apollo to that of their king, Alcithous. Reacting to this blasphemy, Apollo

> was vexed in spirit, and shot forth harsh rays of angry light . . . Forthwith a pestilence unknown before sprung up on the unhallowed earth.

The shepherd was the first victim of the new disease; his name was Syphilis.

The poem achieved such widespread popularity that the name of the unfortunate mythical shepherd, Syphilis, later on became the name of the disease.

There are two theories on the origin of syphilis: *the Columbian* and *the pre-Columbian. The Columbian theory* holds that syphilis is the gift of the New World to the Old. While there is no evidence that syphilis existed in Europe prior to the voyage of Columbus, ancient skeletons bearing the marks of syphilis infection have been discovered in the Americas. In 1492, Columbus explored the island of Hispaniola. Syphilis was present among the native population; the crew of Columbus acquired the infection through intercourse with native women and carried it back to

Europe. A physician, Ruy Diaz de Isla, wrote in later years that he had treated Columbus's men for syphilis when they landed in Barcelona in 1493. More members of the crew were infected after the second voyage in 1494, and the contagion spread rapidly to groups of Spanish mercenaries.

These soldiers were sent to help King Alphonso II, a Spaniard who held the throne of Naples and was being threatened by King Charles VIII of France. As King Charles besieged Naples with an army of fifty-thousand men gathered from all the countries of Europe, the city was being infected with syphilis from the troops of Alphonso. Naples surrendered to King Charles on February 22, 1495, and it is generally accepted that the fall of Naples marks the beginning of the first epidemic of syphilis in Europe.

King Charles was eventually defeated and his army was disbanded in November, 1495. The troops returned to their respective countries carrying with them the contagion. Cases of syphilis were reported in France, Germany, Switzerland, Holland, England, and Greece in 1496. The pestilence reached Scotland by 1497 and Hungary and Russia by 1499.

The *pre-Columbian theory* recognizes the role played by the siege of Naples and the armies of Charles in the spread of syphilis but holds that the disease was present in Europe prior to the voyage of Columbus, though it went unrecognized or was confused with other diseases such as leprosy. It was the great flux of armies and people precipitated by Charles's invasion and the subsequent retreat from Naples that probably initiated the epidemic.

Syphilis has not readily yielded the secrets of its nature. In many parts of Europe, it was originally thought that syphilis was spread by any form of contact with an infected individual. Cardinal Wolsey was accused of infecting Henry VIII with syphilis by whispering in his ear. In other areas, the transmission of syphilis through sexual intercourse was acknowledged quite early.

The ultimate recognition of the venereal aspects of syphilis both promoted a clearer understanding of the disease and led to further confusion. In the sixteenth century, the history of syphilis was intertwined with that of a far more ancient condition, gonorrhea. For centuries following the first syphilis epidemic in Europe, GC and syphilis were regarded as variations of the same ailment. This fallacy was perpetuated by the tragic self-experimentation of John Hunter in the eighteenth century. He thought that gonorrhea and syphilis were two different diseases, and he deliberately innoculated himself with pus from a gonorrheal patient. Unfortunately for both Hunter and science, the gonorrheal patient also had syphilis, and the pus with which he infected his own body was contaminated with syphilitic organisms. In his report of the experiment, Hunter objectively described how he developed gonorrhea and then syphilis, erroneously convinced that they were indeed the same disease. Hunter eventually died of syphilis and so great was his reputation that evidence opposing his theories was disregarded for the next half-century. Finally, in 1838, Philippe Ricord, after studying the results of 2,500 human innoculations, published a report which irrefutably established the distinctions between syphilis and gonorrhea and identified them as separate diseases.

SYPHILIS

Transmission of Syphilis

Syphilis is known in the vernacular as lues, pox, syph, or bad blood.

The nature of the infecting organism, the *Treponema pallidum,* dictates the mode of syphilis transmission. *T. pallidum* is an anaerobic microbe; that is, it cannot survive or be transmitted through the air. Syphilis is spread by direct contact; the *T. pallidum* must be transmitted from the infectious syphilitic lesion of a carrier to the susceptible body surface of her or his partner. The most infectious syphilitic lesions, those swarming with *treponomes,* are located in the area of the genitals. The most susceptible body tissues, those which provide the proper environment for treponemal survival, are the membranes which line the reproductive tract. Sexual intercourse provides the opportunity for contact between infectious genital lesions and susceptible genital tissue and is the most efficient means for the transmission of syphilis. Nine out of ten cases of acquired syphilis are contracted through sexual intercourse.

Syphilis can be spread without sexual intercourse. Infectious syphilitic lesions can appear in the throat, and the lining of the oral cavity also offers the proper conditions of susceptibility—warmth and moisture—required for treponemal survival. In these cases, the infection may be passed by kissing. It is doubtful that the *T. pallidum* can pass directly through the skin into the body, but the slightest break in the skin, even a cut or abrasion of microscopic size, permits treponemal invasion. Thus, contact between broken skin surface and an infectious syphilitic lesion allows passage of the infection.

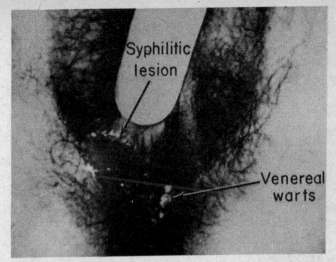

Fig. 7–1: A primary syphilitic lesion on the right labia of a woman, with the characteristic sharp edge of the chancre. This woman also has venereal warts on the perineum, the area between the vagina and anus. The presence of venereal warts should lead a physician to check for venereal diseases such as syphilis or gonorrhea. (Reproduced from *Syphilis: A Synopsis*, by permission of the Dept. of Health, Education & Welfare; Public Health Service; Center for Disease Control; Atlanta, Georgia.)

Finally, a pregnant woman infected with syphilis can transmit the disease to her unborn child. During the first five months after conception, the fetus is protected by the developing placenta, which blocks passage of the treponomes. After the fifth month, this barrier weakens and syphilitic organisms can invade the body of the infant and cause congenital malformations, miscarriage, or infant death.

Primary Syphilis

When syphilis first invades the body, some of the treponomes spread through the lymphatic system. Most of them, however, remain at the point of infection. The organisms alter the tissue surrounding this point, producing a *chancre*—a painless, hard, open sore—which occurs between three to four weeks after exposure. This is the characteristic sign of primary syphilis.

Chancres can appear singly or in groups. They look like small craters, ranging from an eighth of an inch to an inch in diame-

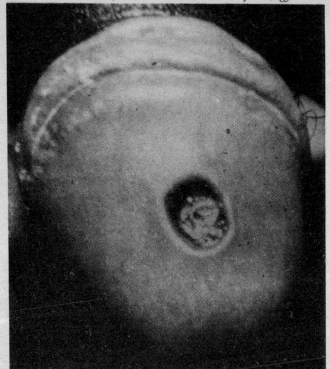

ABOVE
Fig. 7–2:   A primary syphilitic lesion on the glans of the penis, with the characteristic smooth and sharp edge of the chancre. This type of sore heals very slowly but is not painful. (Reproduced from *Syphilis: A Synopsis*, by permission of the Dept. of Health, Education & Welfare; Public Health Service; Center for Disease Control; Atlanta, Georgia.)

RIGHT, TOP
Fig. 7–3:   A primary syphilitic lesion on the shaft of the penis. This type of sore can be mistaken for venereal herpes lesion. Any abnormal sore in the genital area that does not heal easily should be immediately evaluated. Herpes lesions are, however, painful. (Reproduced by permission of Robert Boyers, M.D., from *Hospital Medicine*, July, 1972.)

RIGHT, BOTTOM
Fig. 7–4:   A primary syphilitic lesion on the upper lip. This is a characteristic chancre with sharp edges. Oral syphilitic chancres are frequently painful. (Reproduced by permission of Robert Boyers, M.D., from *Hospital Medicine*, July, 1972.)

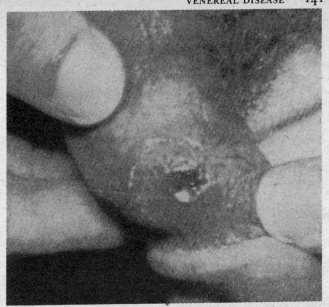

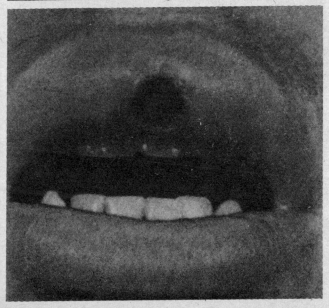

ter. The raised edges are firm, but the surface is shiny red, raw, and sometimes crusted. When chancres occur in the genital area, they are usually painless. They generally develop in men on the shaft of the penis, but sometimes they develop invisibly beneath the foreskin or within the urethra. In women, genital chancres are often hidden within the vulva, on the walls of the vagina, or on the neck of the cervix. Chancres of the anus are becoming increasingly common as a result of homosexual intercourse. Extragenital chancres—on the lips, tongue, tonsils, or lining of the mouth—are frequently painful. These can also develop elsewhere on the body where syphilis has invaded a break in the skin, occurring most frequently on the nipples and fingers. Lymph glands near chancres often become infected and swell, aiding in diagnosis.

The chancre, or *primary syphilitic lesion,* appears to heal spontaneously one to five weeks after its appearance. This does not mean the syphilis has gone away. Instead, it signals a passage from primary to secondary syphilis.

Secondary Syphilis

In this stage of the disease, the effects of the spread of the infection throughout the body are first seen. Although transmitted locally, usually through the mucosa of the genitalia, syphilis is a *systemic* disease. In the secondary stage, its effect on the organs of the body becomes more evident. This stage usually occurs about two and a half months after initial exposure to the disease. In approximately one fourth of the cases, the signs of secondary syphilis appear before the chancre has healed, while in some cases these symptoms may be delayed for up to six months. The symptoms include fever, general malaise, and loss of appetite. Some may experience headaches, pain in the joints and long bones (which seems to worsen at night), sore throat, and swollen lymph glands.

There is also a skin eruption in the secondary stage. First, a rash called *macular syphilide* appears in small, round, rosy spots on the upper torso and arms. This rash may be so light that the discoloration of the skin cannot be seen under artificial light. It may disappear after a few days, or it might develop into a more common and prominent rash called *papular syphilide.* This rash is characterized by dull red, slightly raised spots from an eighth of an inch to half an inch in diameter, appearing all over the body, on the arms, legs, palms, soles, and face.

The treponomes may attack the hair follicles (*follicular syphilides*), causing the hair to fall out in patches, looking moth-eaten. Hair loss may also occur at the outer edges of the eyebrows.

Papular, or raised, lesions, may occur where skin surfaces meet in warm, moist areas—between the buttocks, or the inner surfaces of the upper thighs. These can become large, fleshy masses with broad bases and flat tops *(condylomata lata).* Initially dull red, they become grayish white. As the dead surface skin is shed, the lesion may ooze fluid swarming with infectious treponomes. A very rare form of secondary syphilis, malignant syphilis, a condition reminiscent of the first syphilis epidemic of the fifteenth century, is characterized by deep, ulcerating lesions which, if left untreated, can lead to death.

Mucous patches, or lesions of the mucous membranes, are also common in secondary syphilis, occurring in the throat and mouth or on the tonsils. These are round, grayish white lesions with dull red areolas. They can cause sore throat and, sometimes, deepening of the voice. Mucous patches resembling chancres can also appear on the genitals. Whether in the oral cavity or on the genitals, these lesions are extremely infectious.

Even if untreated, the symptoms of secondary syphilis disappear after two to six weeks, although the skin rashes may reappear. Syphilis then enters the latent stage.

Latent Syphilis

This stage is basically a symptomless period in which the only indication of the disease is a positive serological test (VDRL). During this phase, the disease cannot be transmitted except by a pregnant woman to her fetus. In one third of the cases, the disease disappears entirely. There is a spontaneous cure. In another third of the cases, the syphilis will never progress past the latent stage and no further manifestations of the disease occur, even though the blood tests remain positive. In the final third of the cases, the latent syphilis takes its time invading the various organs of the body. This can take up to forty years, or it may take only a year. Then the late, or *tertiary,* stage begins.

Late or Tertiary Syphilis

Twenty-five percent of all victims of *tertiary syphilis* die of the disease. One of the symptoms is *gummas,* relatively benign skin lesions appearing anywhere on the body. Gummas on the skin are disfiguring, but not deadly. If they occur on the spinal cord or in the brain, gummas can cause blindness, insanity, paralysis, or death. The *T. pallidum* shows a preference for cardiac tissue, and eight of every ten syphilis deaths result from cardiac problems. Syphilis can weaken the aorta, causing a huge *aneurysm* (a ballooning in the wall of the artery) which may burst and cause death. Likewise, the aortic valve may be attacked, causing the blood to back up into the heart instead of being pumped into the body, resulting in cardiac insufficiency. By this stage, damage is irreversible, and treatment can only slow down deterioration or perhaps stem it.

Congenital Syphilis

Congenital syphilis is a misnomer, since it is not an inherited genetic defect but rather an infection that is transmitted from mother to fetus. Since the placental barrier prevents the transmission of syphilis to the baby during the first five months after conception, congenital syphilis is a preventable disease. Early detection and treatment of syphilis in the mother completely protects the fetus, while an undetected syphilitic infection in a mother can result in death or permanent damage to the infant. The more recent the syphilitic infection in the mother, the greater the chance that she will miscarry or deliver a stillborn infant. If the mother has had the disease for an extended period of time, there is less chance that she will pass it to her child, but if passage of the infection does occur, it is more difficult to detect without the proper serological tests.

The manifestations of congenital syphilis are varied, since syphilis is a systemic disease and can attack any organ system. The effects of syphilitic infection on the developing organs of the fetus can be particularly devastating, and death *in utero* is commonly seen in cases of congenital syphilis. During the seventeenth century, congenital syphilis was probably the major cause of fetal mortality. If a child with congenital syphilis survives, it may suffer anything from skin lesions to blindness and deafness. Congenital syphilis detected before the age of two years is often characterized by a bloody nasal discharge called the snuffles. In some children, the signs of syphilis do not appear until after the age of two, but the destructive disease processes have been occurring since birth and these children often bear "stigmata" of congenital syphilis. These are often bone malformations, such as notched teeth, perforated palate, and disfigurement of the nasal bone called saddle nose. Congenital neurosyphilis is one of the most serious forms and may lead to paralysis and mental retardation.

Diagnosis of Syphilis

The symptoms of syphilis vary, and the incubation period (the length of time between the infecting intercourse and the onset of symptoms) may extend from ten days to as long as three months. The early signs of syphilis are usually obvious in men, although they may be ignored or tolerated. Conversely, a woman can be a carrier of syphilis but not be able to see or feel anything abnormal.

Serological blood tests are the most valuable tools in the diagnosis of syphilis. During certain stages of syphilis, for example, they are the only way to detect the presence of the disease. These blood tests fall into two categories: *specific* and *nonspecific*. The nonspecific tests (the famous Wasserman test, now largely replaced by the more accurate VDRL, or Venereal Disease Research Lab), are useful for general screening and searching for antibodies produced by the body to fight this invading organism. Such tests are required in most states before issuance of a marriage license.

Specific tests are required when the nonspecific test results are positive but no further clinical evidence is available to pinpoint the disease. This frequently occurs with syphilis, in which certain stages exhibit no symptoms. Tests like the TPI *(Treponema pallidum* immobilization) and the FTA—ABS (Fluorescent Treponemal Antibody—Absorbed) can detect the specific antibodies the body develops to fight syphilis.

The serological tests not only indicate the presence of syphilis, but also serve as guides to treatment. When serology reverses from positive to negative, VD has been cured.

When there is a fresh lesion, syphilis can also be diagnosed by scraping the surface of the lesion and examining this material with a specific microscope (dark field microscope). Only venereal-disease specialists have access to this diagnostic technique.

Treatment of Syphilis

Fifteenth-century physicians discovered ancient Arabic writings that prescribed an ointment containing mercury to cure scabies. Since syphilis produced similar skin ulcerations, this treatment was applied to VD for the next four hundred years. Patients were anointed, swathed in heavy clothing, and confined in hot, vapor-filled rooms for up to thirty days to sweat out the disease. Many were given overdoses of poisonous mercury by unknowing physicians. The patients salivated continuously, their lips and mouths became covered with sores, their gums swelled, and their teeth fell out. Many chose to die of syphilis rather than undergo this rigorous treatment.

Today, penicillin is the most effective antibiotic in the treatment of syphilis. The *T. pallidum* is particularly sensitive to this drug. The amount of penicillin depends on the stage of syphilis, but the usual dosage in primary and secondary syphilis is 2.4 million units of benzathine penicillin G given intramuscularly at one time and repeated seven days later. Early, active syphilis responds very rapidly to this therapy, but the more advanced stages of syphilis require higher doses. The treatment, however, varies individually and should only be administered by specialists in venereal disease who check the response to treatment. If the response is not satisfactory, a higher dose of penicillin will be administered. If the treatment is initiated prior to a positive serology in primary syphilis, the serology remains negative, since the infecting organism is destroyed before it can effect major tissue changes. If the serology is already positive, the effectiveness of the treatment can be judged by a serology reversal and by the disappearance of symptoms. It is prudent to advise patients to refrain from further intercourse for one week after the relief of the clinical symptoms and reversal in serology. In patients sensitive to penicillin, other antibiotics are employed, such as erythromycin and tetracycline. In late syphilis and congenital syphilis, the effectiveness of antibiotic treatment is not as great; the syphilis may be cured but the destructive effects of the disease cannot be reversed. Syphilis is such a dangerous disease that it should only be treated by specialists familiar with the latest developments in diagnosis and treatment of this condition.

GONORRHEA

History of Gonorrhea

Gonorrhea, the most common form of venereal disease, is perhaps also the most ancient. It is referred to several times in the Bible and is described in the writings of most ancient civilizations. Gonorrhea is recognized as a purulent, or pus-filled, discharge arising from the reproductive organs.

The name *gonorrhea* is derived from the Greek, meaning a "flow of seed," and was first applied by Galen in 300 A.D. The venereal origin of gonorrhea was recognized during the Middle Ages by Guillaume de Salicet, a physician who believed that the

vidual over a period of several weeks. They should be brought in for specific testing for the organism. If there is some doubt about the contact, treatment with injectible penicillin should be instituted within a ten-day period. The only way to control the gonorrhea epidemic is by being honest about the disease and making sure all contacts are treated before they contaminate others.

The Incidence of Gonorrhea

The reported incidence of GC has increased by 15 percent per year in the past decade. The incidence of the infection in men is three times greater than in women. Gonorrhea in the male is usually a symptomatic disease, with clear symptoms of the infection. Since 80 percent of the women with gonorrhea are asymptomatic, a great number of women are, therefore, unknowing carriers of gonorrhea.

A great number of venereal diseases are not reported to the authorities, but it is estimated that there are approximately two to three million new cases of gonorrhea in the United States every year, and more than one hundred million new cases worldwide.

The chance of being infected is high, particularly if a person has many sex partners. Any suspicious discharge should be immediately evaluated by a physician to rule out VD.

Diagnosis of Gonorrhea

Gonorrhea can be diagnosed either by microscopic examination of the discharge or by culturing of the organism.

For many years, the most frequently used diagnostic technique was the microscopic detection of the *gonococci* bacteria. The obtained smear was treated with a series of complex chemical dyes (Gram stain) to reveal the presence of the bacteria. This rather involved procedure was lengthy and did not offer great accuracy in diagnosis. This technique was only correct in 30 to 40 percent of the cases and, therefore, is rarely used today.

Gonorrhea is almost entirely diagnosed through the culture technique. The gonorrhea bacteria is extremely fragile and can only survive in an atmosphere that contains very little oxygen. Immediately after being obtained, gonorrhea cultures are placed in a special transport medium, Trans-grow; the culture is taken as soon as possible to a special laboratory, where it is placed on a selective medium called Thayer-Martin (T-M) medium. The T-M is a growth medium which provides nutrition to the multiplying bacteria. The specimen in the T-M medium is placed in an incubator, where the cells multiply over a period of one to two days. After this time, the characteristic growth pattern of the gonorrhea can be diagnosed by specialists.

Unfortunately there is no quick, foolproof method that can diagnose gonorrhea within a few hours, and there is no simple blood test for the detection of this condition. When gonorrhea cultures are obtained, they must be sent to the specialized laboratories immediately, and if a culture is taken in a private physician's office or in a small clinic, it must be immediately transported for accurate diagnosis.

If a single smear is obtained from the cervix, it will detect gonorrhea in 90 to 93 percent of infected women. To improve the chances of detecting the condition, three cultures are obtained, one each from the cervix, from the urethra and from the anal canal.

Research is being performed to provide simple and inexpensive methods of gonorrhea screening. In one such program now in operation throughout the country, women come to a special clinic during the second or third day of their menstrual cycles. They are asked to use a vaginal tampon for at least fifteen minutes, and then the tampon is employed as the source of a smear for a gonorrhea culture. This simple technique eliminates the need for a pelvic examination by a trained physician, but is still only being carried out on a limited basis in a few institutions.

Treatment of Gonorrhea

For centuries, the most common treatment for gonorrhea was weekly injections of sandalwood oil, forced up the penis or into the upper vagina and female urethra.

Today, if caught in the primary stages, most VD is easily cured with antibiotics. Since this treatment was begun in the 1940s, however, the dosage has increased tremendously as various strains of VD have built up immunity to penicillin and other drugs. In the late 1950s and early 1960s, penicillin dosage was gradually increased from 600,000 units to 4,800,000 units. However, no one strain has developed immunity to *all* antibiotics, so gonorrhea can be treated.

The suggested treatment today is a one-time injection of penicillin. The recommended dose for women is 4.8 million units of procaine penicillin G divided into two doses and injected intramuscularly into each buttock. The dose for men is 2.4 million units of procaine penicillin G. If a person is allergic to penicillin, other antibiotics are effective. Procaine penicillin is more potent than regular penicillin because it is more self-sustaining. Oral tetracycline treatment has been widely used and provides an acceptable alternative. The recommended dose is an initial intake of 1.5 grams of tetracycline followed by 500 milligrams orally four times daily for four days. Vibramycin in the dose of 100 milligrams twice daily for five days is also recommended. Kanamycin and erythromycin, as well as other antibiotics, have also proven effective. The most important factor for a successful cure, however, is early treatment.

GENITAL HERPES INFECTION

Infection with genital herpes virus or the herpes simplex virus Type 2, HSV-2, is considered a venereal disease since, in the majority of cases, it is transmitted by sexual intercourse. The infection is characterized by the appearance of painful blisters or sores in the area of the body below the waist, usually confined to the genitalia. The herpes 2 virus is closely related to the herpes simplex virus Type 1, which causes cold sores or fever blisters, usually in the area of the mouth, but they can occur in any area above the waist. Although the two viruses, Type 1 and Type 2, are closely related, they are strictly confined to their respective areas of the body; thus, a cold sore on the mouth cannot be the source of infection during oral sex from a genital blister, and vice versa.

There is an increased interest in genital herpes, both in the lay press and in the medical community. There are a number of reasons for this attention, such as the reported association of herpes Type 2 virus with cervical cancer, reports in medical literature that genital herpes can be transmitted from an infected mother to the child at birth, and reports of the almost epidemic spread of this condition.

In the United States alone, it is estimated that 300,000 people are infected with this disease every year. The estimated number of people exposed to herpes Type 2 virus, determined by a specific blood test, is much higher. This blood test determines the presence of antibodies to the herpes Type 2 virus. Many more people have positive results than ever complain of the symptoms of a genital herpes infection. It is known that if a person experiences recurrent fever blisters around the mouth, her or his body produces antibodies to the herpes Type 1 virus, which appear effective in combating the herpes Type 2 virus, also. Thus, a person can be infected with the herpes Type 2 virus, but experience only minimal and transient symptoms that will not require medical attention. On the other hand, if a person has never had cold sores and is infected with herpes Type 2 virus, the infection is usually quite severe and there is a high incidence of recurrence of the symptoms until this individual has built up his or her own antibodies to the virus.

How Genital Herpes Is Transmitted

Genital herpes can be transmitted during sexual intercourse with a partner in the active phase of the disease, usually immediately after the genital blister has broken and the virus lies free on the surface of the mucosa. The virus can also be spread when there are open herpes sores.

The symptoms of infection can occur as soon as four days after exposure, or the virus can invade the cells of the genital mucosa and lie dormant for varying periods of time. What stimulates the virus from a dormant to an active phase is not clear, but it is known that a variety of stressful situations triggers the growth of the virus. In women, the cause of the stress situation can be the onset of the menstrual period, or perhaps being run down from too much work and too little sleep. Periods of emotional stress also appear to trigger viral growth. Stressful situations inhibit the immune response of the body and its natural ability to hold the growth of the virus in check, and thus the virus moves from a dormant to an active form.

Symptoms of Genital Herpes Infection

The virus in the active stages starts to multiply unchecked, inside the cells in which they have remained during the dormant state, causing the inflamed enlargement of one cell and then a number of cells. This causes the appearance of a blister or series of blisters. The first symptom may be itching and minor irritation in the genital area. The blisters may not appear on the vulva, in the vagina, or on the cervix until the infection has spread extensively in women. In men, the sores or blisters usually appear on the shaft of the penis, under the foreskin, on the glans or within the urethra. The blisters begin to enlarge, irritating nerve endings and causing pain. These soon rupture, becoming shallow, very painful ulcers, which interconnect and become extremely painful sores. These sores develop a secondary infection and then take up to six weeks to heal. During this period, the sores or lesions are extremely painful and are often mistaken by the sufferer for the primary chancre of syphilis. One point can be borne in mind to make the distinction between these two conditions—the chancre of syphilis in the genital area is usually not painful.

The first time a person has a genital herpes infection, the symptoms can be rather severe. High fever, general malaise, enlarged lymph glands, painful or difficult urination, and severe pelvic pain usually occur. These symptoms are often mistaken in women for pelvic inflammatory disease. They can, in various degrees of severity, last from a few days to a few weeks.

After the primary infection, the virus returns to its dormant state; it has not been destroyed, it is merely dormant. If a person has not had a previous herpes infection, this dormant state is usually transient and the symptoms of herpes genital infection may recur at any time from a few days to a year later. In some individuals, there may be up to ten recurrences of the symptoms. It should be emphasized that these recurrences are not caused by reinfection but by the transition of the virus from the dormant to the active state. Fortunately, the recurrent episodes of the disease are usually less severe than the primary infection, since antibodies are developed naturally. In the recurrent episodes, the lesions again appear, the lymph glands swell up, and urination becomes painful. Urinary-tract infections occur when the virus spreads to the urethra. When the body develops sufficient antibodies, the recurrent episodes of genital herpes cease.

Incidence of Genital Herpes Infection

Herpes virus Type 2 infection is very rarely reported in persons before they become sexually active. HSV-2 appears to be prevalent among teenagers and young adults. The mean age for people with a primary infection is about eighteen years and the mean age for recurrence is twenty-five years. There have been extensive studies to screen HSV-2 antibodies in the blood, and it has been found that the incidence of this virus is three to four times higher among lower socioeconomic groups, where it has been found in up to 30 percent of sexually active individuals. In some segments of the lower socioeconomic population, amongst those who have a high rate of sexual activity, the incidences of herpes Type 2 antibodies have even approached 60 percent.

Genital Herpes Infection and Pregnancy

Herpes 2 erupts more frequently in pregnant women, possibly because the body's immune system is weakened during pregnancy. This has caused considerable concern, since the virus can be passed on to the infant during delivery through the vagina or even directly through the bloodstream, causing possible brain damage, meningitis, or death. Many physicians advocate Caesarean section delivery for women who have an acute HSV-2 infection within a few weeks of delivery to minimize the threat to the child.

Genital Herpes Infection and Cervical Cancer

Women with cervical cancer have been found to have HSV-2 antibodies in the blood more often than women without cervical cancer. This may be coincidental, since both cervical cancer and genital herpes infection are associated with an early and active sex life. There is no evidence that the herpes virus causes cancer, but studies indicate that women with HSV-2 antibodies have two to four times the chance of developing cervical cancer than women without these antibodies. There is no proof that if a woman has a genital herpes infection, she is necessarily a candidate for cervical cancer. She should, however, follow the prudent course by having a Pap smear performed every six months. Symptoms of the cancer would be detected while it is in a treatable stage.

How Can Genital Herpes Infection Be Prevented?

As with any venereally transmitted disease, the best prevention is avoidance of sexual intercourse with anyone in the active phase of a genital herpes infection. If there is any suspicion that a person's sexual partner has a genital herpes infection, the use of a condom may prevent the spread of the infection. Spermicides, such as contraceptive jellies and foam, in conjunction with a diaphragm may offer some protection, but the infection could still be transmitted. Any indication of a blister or sore in the genital area must raise the suspicion of genital herpes infection, and intercourse should be avoided.

Treatment of Genital Herpes Virus

At the present time, there is no cure for a genital herpes infection, but it can be treated symptomatically by a trained physician and complications avoided. A physician can prescribe antibiotics to prevent secondary infection, pain relievers, or a combination cream, such as Mycolog (cortisone and antiyeast) to reduce swelling and pain. An increased intake of vitamin A may be helpful, since this vitamin has been proven to stimulate the body's immune system. A person should also try to relax, giving the body a better chance to fight the infection.

There are several experimental treatments being used around the country today, and though none of them has been proven successful, the signs are encouraging. Studies have shown that 90 percent of patients treated with daily douches of a Providone-iodine solution (Betadine) showed symptoms of relief within one to three hours, with relief lasting up to three days. Interest has also been centered on photodynamic therapy, where proflavine, or "neutral red dye," has been painted on the external lesions, then exposed to fluorescent or ultraviolet light. This seems to dry up the lesion and speed healing, giving symptomatic relief and curing the lesions within seven days. The recurrence rate also seems to decrease, although studies show that the virus itself survives the exposure to the light and dye. Vaccination of BCG, a drug used to fight tuberculosis (made of tuberculosis bacteria), also seems to reduce recurrence, since it stimulates a person's immune mechanism.

RARE TYPES OF VD

Chancroid

Chancroid is a rare form of VD that derives its name from the resemblance between its symptoms and those of syphilis. However, the two diseases are distinct. Chancroid is caused by the *Ducrey* bacillus and is easily treated with sulfa drugs over a period of one to two weeks. If untreated, the lymph glands in the groin become infected and enlarged, sometimes requiring incision and drainage.

Granuloma Inguinale

Another rare disease, *granuloma inguinale,* is characterized by large areas of swollen, red, meaty skin around the genitals. The disease is diagnosed by the discovery of an organism, called Donovan bodies, in tissue scrapings from the infected area. This disease is much more common in tropical areas than it is in the United States. The treatment is tetracycline, given four times a day for ten to fifteen days.

Lymphogranuloma Venereum

This is another tropical disease, characterized by small, transient skin ulcers occurring seven to twelve days after sexual intercourse. After the primary lesion, there is a tremendous enlargement of the lymph nodes in the groin, which blocks lymphatic drainage. In women, there is swelling of the labia, and in men, swelling of the scrotum and penis. Sulfa drugs or a broad spectrum of antibiotics are effective in treating *lymphogranuloma venereum*. If it goes untreated, sores of the rectum occur, followed after several months by a narrowing of the rectum, which requires corrective surgery.

PELVIC INFLAMMATORY DISEASE (PID)

Pelvic inflammatory disease (PID) is the term given for any extensive infection in the organs of the pelvic area. Vaginal or uterine infections can spread up into the fallopian tubes, causing an infection in the tubes, or *salpingitis*. The infection occasionally spreads into the abdomen and to the ovaries, causing a pelvic inflammatory disease. PID can lead to an abscess in the fallopian tubes or ovaries, or can spread to the peritoneum, causing peritonitis. This is an extremely serious condition that can lead to death if left untreated.

PID is often caused by a gonorrheal infection. The symptoms of gonorrhea often go untreated in a woman, who sometimes mistakes the gonorrheal discharge for minor vaginitis. Studies have shown that some 5 percent of women have undiagnosed gonorrhea that has spread dangerously far into the fallopian tubes, threatening sterility. It is essential for a woman, for this very reason, to consult a gynecologist whenever she notices an abnormal discharge.

PID can also be of nonvenereal origin due to other bacteria, including streptococcus, staphylococcus, or coli (from the rectum). Many of the anaerobic bacteria, which grow without oxygen, have also been found to cause PID. This type of nonvenereal infection is often found after childbearing or abortion, when bacteria have spread into the uterine cavity and continue into the fallopian tubes. If it is treated correctly with hospitalization and antibiotics, this infection rarely causes sterility. X-ray examination could, however, be conducted several weeks after treatment to ensure that the tubes are open.

With gonorrheal infection, the disease often spreads all the way through the tubes without causing any significant symptoms. The ends of the tubes swell shut, stopping the infection from spreading any further; the tubes then close their

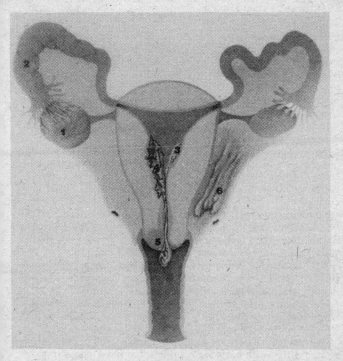

Fig. 7–5: Areas subject to pelvic infection:

(1) Infection in the ovary is called *oophoritis;*

(2) infection in the fallopian tube is called *salpingitis,* and can distend the fallopian tubes, causing adhesions between the fimbriated end of the tube and ovary;

(3) infection of the endometrium within the uterine cavity, called *endometritis;*

(4) infection of placental tissue which has been retained in the uterus after delivery or after miscarriage;

(5) infection of the cervix is called *cervicitis* and could result in a sore or ulceration of the cervix. Cervicitis is usually accompanied by a discharge from the cervical os; and

(6) infection can spread outside the uterus, resulting in advanced pelvic inflammatory disease.

(Courtesy of Eli Lilly and Company, Indianapolis, Indiana.)

ends. This closure is often permanent and causes sterility, since the egg and the sperm cannot meet. Even though it is possible to open the tubes through plastic surgery, the chance of subsequent pregnancy is slim.

An unclean abortion, or intercourse a few days after abortion (allowing the penis to push bacteria into the uterus), can also cause PID. Sterility rarely results if prompt and proper treatment is carried out.

If the fallopian tube or the ovary becomes heavily infected, an abscess can form. The tube may be distended and damaged through the formation of extensive pelvic adhesions, so that the woman becomes sterile. A severe infection of this type is most properly treated with hospitalization, rigorous antibiotic therapy, and, on occasion, surgery (to drain the deeply infected abscess). In rare cases, a hysterectomy is indicated, but this procedure should be performed only as a last resort. It is a sad comment that many unnecessary hysterectomies are performed. A woman who refuses a hysterectomy, is adequately treated with antibiotics, and undergoes plastic surgery to reopen the fallopian tubes has at least a chance of conceiving. If a hysterectomy is suggested because of this condition, another physician should be consulted for a second opinion.

PID leading to tubal or ovarian abscesses occurs in women of any age. Often, when abscesses occur in postmenopausal women, the diagnosis is missed since the symptoms are ascribed to postmenopausal irregularities. Any irregularity at this age should be investigated with blood tests and cultures for VD. Women of any age can contract VD.

Women with IUDs are more susceptible to PID, particularly women fitted with early IUD models that have tails with many *filiforms*, several fibers acting as wicks for bacteria. It is now known that bacteria can climb up these tails into the fallopian tubes causing salpingitis. This often occurs on one side only, so if a woman has an IUD and pain on one side, it may be salpingitis, and she should be treated immediately with high doses of antibiotics. The later-model IUDs do not permit the entrance of bacteria, but tubal infection can still occur.

Peritonitis

The most advanced stage of PID is peritonitis, in which the fallopian tubes, both ovaries and the surrounding tissue, and the peritoneum (the thin, watery membrane covering the abdominal lining and the organs) are totally infected. This is probably the most painful condition a woman can have, and if untreated, it leads to death. The cure involves hospitalization, intravenous treatment with high doses of antibiotics, and several days of fasting to keep normal bowel functions from spreading the infection to other organs.

Pelvic Tuberculosis

Pelvic tuberculosis is very rare, but it can also cause PID. There are two types of tuberculosis: primary and secondary. Primary tuberculosis is probably transmitted through sexual contact. If a man has tuberculosis in his urinary tract, he can spread it to a woman's vagina. From there, it develops through the cervix, the uterus, the fallopian tubes, and often reaches into the abdominal cavity to cause peritonitis. This is rare, but it is probably the only way tuberculosis spreads as a primary infection of the fallopian tube. Years ago, when tuberculosis was spread by unpasteurized milk, it often reached the peritoneum through the intestines. This, of course, is no longer a problem, except in the most isolated instances.

A secondary tuberculosis infection in the pelvic area is spread through the bloodstream from a primary infection in the lungs.

The diagnosis of this disease is usually made after the physician has detected an infection and takes cultures. It is sometimes noticed during surgery, when masses are found and sent for pathological examination. This type of tuberculosis is usually successfully treated with antituberculosis medicines, but should be treated by a specialist in this type of disease. Tuberculosis in the fallopian tubes usually causes sterility.

OTHER SEXUALLY TRANSMITTED CONDITIONS

There are several sexually transmitted conditions that are not considered real venereal diseases. They are, however, spread during sex acts and infect both women and men. These diseases do not have the same damaging consequences as VD.

Venereal Warts

Venereal warts (*Condylomata acuminata*) are caused by sexually transmitted viruses. Some women are not susceptible to venereal warts, while others catch them from only brief exposure. Women with monilia seem to have a higher incidence of contracting them, probably because the pH changes make the vagina more receptive.

Once a woman has venereal warts, it is common for the virus to drain out of the vagina down toward the anus. This causes

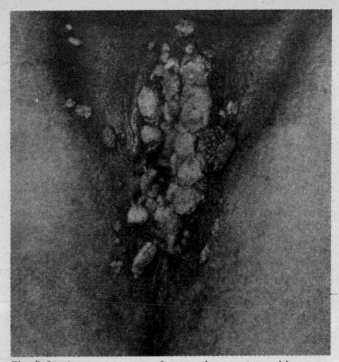

Fig. 7–6: An extreme case of venereal warts, or *condylomata accumulata.* The warts have grown on the vulva all the way down to the anus. These warts can occasionally become so large that they obstruct the entire vagina. (Reproduced with permission by Edmund R. Novak, M.D.; *Textbook of Gynecology,* 9th edition. The Williams and Wilkins Company, Baltimore, Maryland.)

spread of the warts, which look like small lumps, located anywhere from the vagina to the opening of the anus. If you find such lumps, contact your gynecologist immediately. Venereal warts are easy to treat in early stages, but if left untreated, they can overgrow the vagina to the point of closing it up, becoming football-sized lumps in severe cases. During pregnancy, this could necessitate a Caesarean section.

Though they are usually sexually transmitted, there are cases of apparent spontaneous eruption of venereal warts. The exact transmission in these cases is unknown. Normal warts on hands, feet, and so forth usually indicate a susceptibility to venereal warts. Warts on hands and fingers are not, however, caused by the same virus and cannot, therefore, spread to the female or male genitals by touching. Venereal warts on a man are usually located on the mucosa underneath the foreskin or on the glands. A woman who discovers venereal warts should immediately examine her sex partner. He might have only a tiny wart, but it is enough to transfer the virus. He should also be treated when you are undergoing treatment. If he is not treated, the warts will be transferred back, and you will be reinfected time after time.

Treatment of Venereal Warts

When external warts are seen, a speculum examination of the vagina and cervix is required to determine the extent of wart growth. Most venereal warts are treated with a medication called podophyllin, which burns the warts away. This is used for both women and men. This should be administered, only by a physician, directly to the head of the warts. It should never be applied to the skin because it causes painful burning and irritation. After application, the patient must remain on the examining table for a few minutes until the podophyllin dries. Then, after four hours, she should wash the area to remove the remaining podophyllin. To achieve a permanent cure, the milieu of the vagina should also be changed. Venereal warts are often associated with yeast infections. Treatment should, therefore, include antiyeast suppositories or cream.

If the podophyllin is unsuccessful in completely removing the warts even after several applications, your physician may have to coagulate or burn the warts. This is painful, and local anesthesia is used. If the warts are too extensive, this should be done under general anesthesia. If the warts are extremely developed, surgery may be required to cut them out. A vaccine can be developed from excised warts, but this is rarely done. Venereal warts during pregnancy usually disappear after delivery.

Sexually Transmitted Hepatitis B

Recent British studies have shown that 50 to 60 percent of hepatitis B cases not attributed to needles occur in homosexual men. American studies have found ten times as much hepatitis B antigen (a substance which induces the formation of antibodies) in the blood of homosexual men as in heterosexual men. The virus is also known to be present in saliva and semen and can be transmitted even by kissing and oral sex. Because of these findings, hepatitis B is thought to be, at least sometimes, sexually transmitted both in homosexuals and heterosexuals. Vaccines are presently being developed to prevent this disease.

Nongonorrheal or Nonspecific Urethritis

Discharge due to a nongonorrheal or nonspecific urethritis (infection in the urethra) is often identical to gonorrhea symptoms and is often misdiagnosed in both sexes. On closer examination, this infection can be identified as *Chlamydia trachomatis*. If a person has a discharge resembling gonorrhea and a test for that disease is negative, it could signal one of the lesser-known venereal diseases. Many laboratories do not have sufficiently sophisticated equipment to diagnose a *Chlamydia trachomatis* infection, yet an accurate diagnosis is important to ensure proper treatment—the discharge could also be due to trichomonas or other nongonorrheal infections. *Chlamydia trachomatis*, however, is the most common cause of nonspecific urethritis in both women and men. If you have no access to an adequately equipped lab, but gonorrhea has been definitely ruled out, treatment can be initiated against the Chlamydia infection with a fairly high rate of success.

The treatment is consistent with that of many other causes of nonspecific urethritis. A broad-spectrum antibiotic, like te-tracycline, should be administered in a dose of 500 milligrams given four times daily to both sexual partners for seven to ten days.

Chlamydia infection is also common in pregnant women, and should be checked for since it can be transmitted to a child during delivery. It is now considered the most common cause of eye infection in newborn infants.

Crab Lice

Crab lice are tiny creatures which can be transmitted through sexual intercourse. They cause intense itching and, on close examination, can be seen at the base of hair shafts. Scratching often leads to secondary infection, with pus-filled areas in the genital region.

Crab lice survive only in pubic hair, in eyebrows, or in armpit hair. The crabs do not survive on the skin unless there is an extremely thick mat of body hair; they never survive on the scalp or on hairless skin. Though intercourse is generally the

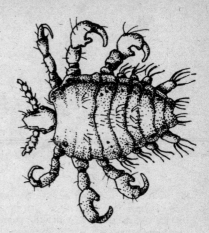

Fig. 7–7: A crab louse *(Phthirus pubis)*. (Reproduced with permission of Beck J. Walter, M.D., and Barrett Connor, M.D.; from *Medical Parasitology*, St. Louis, 1971, The C.V. Mosby Company.)

common method of transferral, crabs can be caught from infested bed linen.

If you begin itching in the pubic region, examine yourself under strong light. If you have crabs, you should be able to see them. There may also be eggs, like little lumps, at the base of hairs. These are black and visible, and can be removed with your fingernails. But be thorough; it takes only one egg to begin a new infestation. The first sign might often be small black spots or bloodstains on the underwear.

You can buy over-the-counter insecticide washes to treat crabs, but they may not be sufficient. The best medication is Kwell lotion or shampoo, available by doctor's prescription only. Use it liberally throughout the infected area, then wash carefully the following morning. Scrape up all the eggs with your nails and send all clothing and bed linen for cleaning. You may have to repeat the Kwell treatment several times until the crabs finally disappear. Your sexual partner should immediately be informed and treated.

There is no need to shave if you are infected with crabs. This will not help get rid of the lice or eggs.

Scabies

Scabies is a microscopic insect, *Sarcoptes scabiei,* that burrows into the skin, causing severe itching. The insects are seldom seen because they lie under the skin, but they spread rapidly

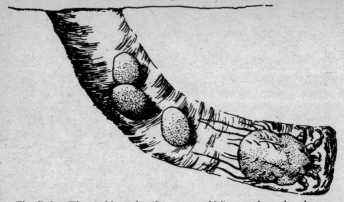

Fig. 7–8: The scabies mite *(Sarcoptes scabiei)* tunnels under the surface of the skin and deposits its eggs. The upper line is the skin surface and the depth to which this parasite can infect the skin can be seen. The scabies are very small and the mite itself is usually not seen, but the infestation is detected by symptoms of itching and, occasionally, minute breaks in the skin. The openings of the mites' tunnels can be seen on very close inspection, particularly between the fingers and the toes. (Reproduced with permission of Beck J. Walter, M.D., and Barrett Connor, M.D., from *Medical Parasitology*, St. Louis, 1971, The C.V. Mosby Company.)

from person to person, even without sexual contact. If one person in a house has scabies, everyone must be treated for it, including children.

The itch gets worse at night, usually attacking the palms, between the fingers, beside the scrotum, the breasts, the genitals, the beltline, and the armpits. Scabies can be found anywhere except the face. The tunnels, though theoretically visible to the eye, are usually obscured by marks, irritation, and infection from scratching. If you have full-body itching, see your doctor. Kwell lotion will effectively treat the condition, working on the scabies overnight. All linen and clothing must be carefully washed the next day.

CONDITIONS OFTEN MISTAKEN FOR VD

Several conditions are often mistakenly thought to be cases of venereal disease, not so much by physicians as by patients who feel they are wise enough to diagnose their own ailments and prescribe their own cures. They may indeed have seen identical sores before and experienced identical symptoms, but that does not mean the cause of the symptoms is the same. This is especially common with skin diseases.

Contact Dermatitis

Contact dermatitis, or *skin eczema*, is an allergic reaction caused by any number of irritants—hair tints, skin creams, detergents, plants, chemicals. The body reacts by releasing its own chemicals and increasing blood flow, producing the characteristic redness of an allergic rash. This condition is often the result of something you have used for a long time. Many people assume that it must be a reaction to something new, since they have had no problems before. But the body may have been developing antibodies that are finally released after months or even years of exposure to a product. If the contact continues, the rash will worsen. Bacteria can infect the area, causing a secondary reaction. An antihistamine administered by your physician may help if you are unable to pinpoint the source of the allergy, and external cortisone cream can be applied for local relief. Most important, however, is to find the source of the allergic reaction.

Heat Rash

In hot, moist weather, the sweat ducts can become plugged, balloon up, and form red blisters. This heat rash usually occurs in folds of skin or in areas covered by tight clothing. It often occurs beneath breasts in women or under the scrotum in men. Women who wear pantyhose often develop it in the pubic area. The primary treatment is to discard restricting clothing in order to let the skin breathe. Keep the skin as dry as possible; powder and heat lamps can help. Cortisone cream helps clear up the rash at first; then proper skin care is required.

Nonvenereal Warts

Nonvenereal warts are caused by susceptibility to wart virus, possibly a hereditary trait. The warts on people's hands and feet are contagious only if a person is susceptible to warts. They are not the same as venereal warts and *cannot* spread to the genitals. Treatment is either special salve or cauterization.

Acne

Acne is a common skin disorder, most often seen during adolescence, on the face and shoulders. It is brought on by a hormonal imbalance. As oil is secreted from the skin and combines with the normal dirt and bacteria lying on the surface, the glands that cover the surface of the body become infected, causing pimples. Good skin care and cleanliness help to an extent, but often it is a matter of waiting for the body to grow into a normal hormone balance. Junk foods should be avoided, especially oily snacks like french fries, potato chips, or chocolate. For sugar, eat fruit instead of candy, and get plenty of vitamin B complex, even if it means taking daily vitamins. Drinking, smoking, and exhaustion all contribute to this skin problem. The skin is a mirror of your body's internal condition, the abuse of your body often manifests itself by breaking out on the skin. Lack of estrogen can cause acne, and women who develop this condition while taking low-estrogen birth-control pills might need a vitamin supplement strong in B complex to prevent breakout. If this does not help, they should change to a pill with higher estrogen content.

More severe cases are treated with tetracycline to prevent secondary infections. Drying therapy with alcohol or other astringent medications, or even heat treatments, is often prescribed. Exposure to the sun also helps. X-ray or radiation therapy used to be prescribed, but this is now considered dangerous because of the threat of cancer.

Boils

Boils are red, hot, swollen areas similar to large pimples. When a hair follicle is plugged and doesn't drain, it becomes a perfect medium for bacterial growth. White blood cells rush to the area to fight the infection and create pus. The blood brings nutrients to the trouble spot, causing redness. The skin stretches from the influx of all these fluids and the nerves stretch, causing pain. Scratching spreads the infection, creating multiple boils.

To treat boils, remove any tight clothing. This stops dirt from being rubbed into the infected area. Then soak a washcloth in hot water and place it directly on the boil to increase pressure and bring the pus out. A heating pad can also be used for this. Antibiotics help prevent further spread of the infection. The boil should drain after application of moist heat, and antibiotics for a few days should keep it from returning.

Ringworm

Ringworm is a fungus, often carried by cats and other animals, that causes itching and small, scaly, gray patches on the skin, sometimes forming a gray ring. It is easily treated with medication, prescribed by a dermatologist, which is applied directly to the irritated areas. If there is a cat in the household, it should be taken to a veterinarian to be treated or the infection will spread all over again.

Fever Blisters—Herpes Simplex Virus Type 1 Infection

Herpes simplex Type 1 causes fever blisters or cold sores, usually in the mouth and nasal cavity, but sometimes elsewhere above the waist. This is a nonvenereal virus, but is spread through direct contact—kissing, touching, and so forth. When the blister breaks, it is highly infectious. Like herpes simplex Type 2, Type 1 can hibernate in the cells, then erupt unexpectedly through the thinner skin surfaces—the gums, the lips, the tongue, the roof of the mouth. When the cold sore finally bursts, it takes a long time to heal and is quite painful. A secondary infection can develop if the area is not kept clean. The body usually heals the sore within seven to ten days and the virus goes back into the cells until it is ready to erupt again.

The virus usually comes to life when a person is in a weakened state—tired, run down, ill, under stress, or about to menstruate. This virus does not grow in the genital area. If you have a herpes lesion on your lips, you *cannot* transmit it to the genitals through oral contact. Although there is no known cure, researchers are looking into promising areas.

PREVENTION OF VD

The best prevention of VD, short of abstinence, is a condom (a rubber sheath over the penis). This protects both the male and the female, providing, incidentally, good and safe birth control if used correctly. Cleaning the genitals with soap and an antiseptic solution following intercourse offers theoretical, but not confirmed, protection. The prophylactic use of penicillin or other antibiotics is not recommended, since the body builds up a sensitivity to the drug necessitating increasingly larger doses until the antibiotic eventually becomes ineffective or subsequently results in an allergic reaction.

Once VD has been identified, it is essential to control its spread by informing everyone with whom the individual has had sexual relations during the previous weeks (this period depends on the type and stage of the disease). Each of these people should be examined and, if necessary, treated. All of these individuals should then contact all of *their* sexual partners, *ad infinitum,* until all possible spread has been checked.

chapter 8

A BRIEF HISTORY OF CONTRACEPTION

Before examining the techniques of modern birth control, it is important to stress that birth control is *not* a twentieth-century discovery. Contraception has been a continuing concern of humanity since the most primitive times. Techniques for birth control were described in the earliest forms of writing, and while most of them were ineffectual, some did provide protection from pregnancy.

Most modern birth-control methods have historical roots, and a review of society's struggle with this age-old dilemma can help us to understand the problems inherent to contraception.

Some of the history is both amusing and horrifying. Above all, it offers insight into society's concept of the position of women and the role of sex.

PESSARIES

A pessary is an object or substance placed in the vagina for contraceptive purposes. Pessaries were used by the ancient Egyptians, and the formula for a pessary described in the Petri Papyrus, dated 1850 B.C., called for a mixture of crocodile dung and honey to be placed in the vagina before intercourse. Interestingly, this mixture not only acted as a barrier to the sperm, but had some broad spermicidal effects. If a convenient crocodile wasn't available, elephant dung could be used.

Elephant dung and honey was used as a contraceptive pessary throughout India and Africa. In fact, this honey and dung compound appeared up to the eleventh century, when it was specifically mentioned by Constantinus Africanus in his Islamic book of surgery.

By the sixth century A.D., pessaries were a widely used contraceptive method; almost every ancient medical book prescribed their use and suggested varying formulas.

In Persia during the tenth century, a pessary was invented which not only acted as a barrier, but acted as a chemical spermicide as well. This pessary mixed rock salt and an oily material. Today, ordinary table salt is still recognized as an effective spermicide.

In his memoirs, Casanova describes the use of a gold ball—18 millimeters in diameter—which was inserted into his partner's vagina prior to intercourse. Unfortunately he did not comment on the actual effectiveness or reasoning of this elegant technique.

The onset of the industrial age in the nineteenth century saw the practice of family planning become an increasingly important social and political issue. Walter Rendell, a London chemist operating his own pharmacy in the 1880s, felt the rising concern. As he listened to his customers' stories of poverty and deprivation, it became apparent to him that an effective birth-control method was urgently needed. After much work and experimentation, he developed a pessary containing quinine, which he distributed freely to his customers with instructions on its proper use.

The results of this new pessary exceeded his expectations. Requests were logged so rapidly that the pessary was marketed commercially in 1886. By the turn of the century, the product was a best seller throughout the world. In fact, until the twentieth century, quinine was the only recognized spermicide which could be used with complete safety.

Today, quinine has been replaced by nonirritating substances in stronger spermicides like foam or antispermicide jelly, which are sold separately or in conjunction with diaphragms. Still, Rendell's discovery was a landmark in the history of birth control—it was the crowning peak of pessaries even as it ushered in a new age of birth-control products.

SPONGES, DIAPHRAGMS, AND CERVICAL CAPS

Diaphragms and pessaries originated from the same idea—to create a barrier to keep semen from entering the uterus. While pessaries were used to block the semen, other early methods were used to absorb it. The earliest reference to such absorption devices was made in the Ebers Papyrus, around 1500 B.C. The papyrus described a tampon made of lint and soaked with acacia and honey to be placed in the vagina before intercourse.

Ancient Talmudists considered the sponge an effective contraceptive device—a method which has persisted almost unchanged for a thousand years. Even as recently as ten years ago, one could still buy sponges for contraceptive purposes in Paris.

Early physicians suggested a round or cuplike device placed in the vagina to block the sperm. In the first century, Discorides prescribed vaginal insertion of a swordlike leaf filled with honey. By the sixth century, Aetius of Amida created a barrier in a natural shape. He suggested cutting a pomegranate, removing the seeds and pulp, and inserting the hollow end into the vagina before intercourse. This was probably the first real diaphragm.

In 1883, Dr. Frederick Wilde, a German physician, described a rubber cap as a blocking contraceptive, but it was Dr. Mensinga of Germany who popularized the method. The function of this cap was to block, or close, the cervical canal to semen. This method spread from Germany to Holland, then to England, where it became known as the Dutch cap.

Once the popularity of the cap-type contraceptive was established, doctors realized that it was necessary to completely seal any gap in its fit against the cervix to prevent sperm from entering.

DOUCHING AND FUMIGATING

Douching and fumigating (in this context, sending fumes or gases into the vagina) were long believed to be effective contraceptive methods. Douching appeared very early in Egyptian literature. Inscriptions have been found giving details of the solutions. Drawings and instructions for douching, plus an actual douching instrument, have also been uncovered.

After coitus, the woman was advised to douche with such ingredients as wine and garlic with fennel. These solutions were administered through instruments made from horns of animals or bills of birds. The most common was the bill of the ibis, which was used as a conductive tube to pour liquid into the vagina.

In the early 1880s, Charles Knowlton, in his book *The Fruit of Philosophy*, offered various recipes for contraceptive douching solutions, such as mixing alum with the juice extracted from hemlock plants or green tea.

Today there are various spermicides available, but these are inserted into the vagina immediately prior to intercourse, not after. Douching is advocated simply as a hygienic, not a contraceptive, method.

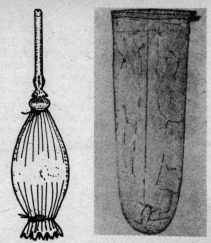

LEFT

Fig. 8-1: A douche bag from the thirteenth century. The bag was constructed of sow bladder and the nozzle of wood. (Reproduced by permission from: *Contraception through the Ages* by B. Finch and H. Greene, published by Peter Owen, London.)

RIGHT

Fig. 8-2: A condom from the eighteenth century. This condom was made from the cecum of sheep. (Reproduced by permission from: *Contraception through the Ages* by B. Finch and H. Greene, published by Peter Owen, London.)

THE CONDOM

The condom, or sheath, was not developed to prevent conception, but to prevent the spread of venereal disease. Even before the connection between intercourse and conception was recognized, people were concerned with disease passed between women and men during coitus.

The earliest known condom was depicted in paintings on cave walls of Cambarelles dating from prehistoric times. One of the drawings showed a man and a woman engaged in the sexual act, the man seeming to have his penis covered with some sort of coat.

In ancient and imperial Rome, the guts and bladders of animals were used to cover the penis. The animal cebum had a fineness, an elastic quality, and a tensile strength which made it an excellent sheath.

Dr. Falloppio, an Italian authority on syphilis, described in his book, *De Morbo Gallico,* first published in 1564, a linen sheath to fit on the glans to help prevent infection. His definitive instructions on the use of this sheath apply even today.

When the connection between intercourse and pregnancy was established, the dual-purpose sheath came into focus, and what is known as the condom was gradually perfected.

Curiously, one of the first manufacturers of condoms was a woman, Mrs. Phillips, who operated a small warehouse in London in the latter part of the eighteenth century. She advertised her wares, made from dried gut of sheep, by circulars and handbills. Gradually the condom was refined and redesigned using rubber and, finally, synthetic rubber.

COITUS INTERRUPTUS

Once it was established that male semen was, indeed, a fertilizing agent, society dealt with means of preventing the semen from reaching the egg. The simplest and least expensive method was simply to withdraw the penis before ejaculation. This was the most widely adopted method in early history and, known as the practice of *coitus interruptus.* It has retained its popularity for over two thousand years, and it is only with the dissemination of more effective methods that coitus interruptus has become one of the lesser-used methods of birth control.

STERILIZATION AS A MEANS OF CONTRACEPTION

One of the more efficient ways to prevent conception has been sterilization of men and/or women.

Men

It was probably in China that the practice of castration had its earliest history. The Chinese studied animals to discover the role of testicles and ovaries in conception. They castrated dogs, cocks, and bulls with remarkable success. They also castrated men. In early Chinese medical history, castration was originally adopted as a means of punishment for certain grave offenders. About 1200 B.C., it was used on servants or attendants of the emperor and his family in the Chou Dynasty.

Other civilizations, including the Assyrians and Babylonians, castrated slaves and made them guardians of the home. These slaves became known as eunuchs, men rendered incapable of the act of sexual intercourse.

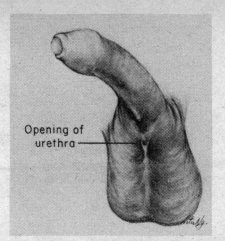

Opening of
urethra

ABOVE

Fig. 8–3: Subincision, or *koopli*. This was a form of male surgical contraception used by Australian tribes. A man in a tribe who had this operation could be easily recognized, since he would have to stand with his legs far apart to urinate.

BELOW

Fig. 8–4: Male *infundibulation* consists of attaching a ring or clasp to the penis. This procedure was performed by the Romans, but only on uncircumcised males, since the ring was placed through the foreskin. The purpose of the ring was to prevent the insertion of the penis into the vagina. The ring was usually larger than the one shown in this drawing and could be considered a type of chastity belt for men, since it prevented intercourse.

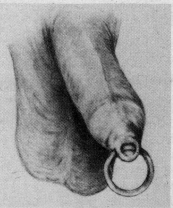

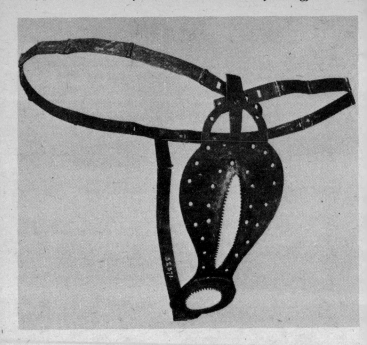

Fig. 8–5: The chastity belt was a frequently used apparatus, apparently introduced in France at the time of the Crusades, circa 1180. The belt consisted of two main parts—a band of flexible metal and a perforated plate (or a pair of hinged plates). The band was worn around the hips. The underportion passed just above the buttocks, with the second part of the apparatus attached by a joint to a band in the front. The second piece (constructed of metal, bone, or ivory) was convex so it could press firmly against the mons Veneris. It extended downward, completely enclosing the vulva. A dentured or plain perforation permitted the natural functions but was too small to admit even the tip of the penis. (Reproduced by permission of Nordiske museet, Stockholm, Sweden.)

Another surgical sterilization means used by aboriginal tribes in Australia was called *Koolpi*, or subincision. Basically, it was a ritual operation in which a slit was cut along the urethra close to the testicles. At the time of ejaculation, the semen would not go into the vagina, but would, rather, spill through the slit.

The Romans are credited with a semisurgical procedure which was a highly effective contraceptive. Called *infundibulation*, it consisted of attaching a ring, or clasp, to the penis. During this procedure, the foreskin was pulled forward over the glans of the penis until it formed a complete cover. Two threads were then drawn through the edge of the foreskin. Each day the threads were moved backward and foreward until two clear holes were formed. A ring was then placed through these holes, making it impossible to have intercourse. Infundibulation was one of the only reversible surgical methods of early times.

In the twentieth century, the X-ray was discovered as a means of sterilization for both men and women, but the harmful effects of radiation and the possibility of it causing cancer in later life ended most research in this area.

Vasectomy (the surgical removal of the *vas deferens*), has become the most popular method of sterilization. Developed in the early 1900s, the procedure has been refined over the years and is now considered a very viable birth-control alternative.

Women

The problem of fertility in women has been researched during all of human history.

Hippocrates, in the fourth century B.C., was one of the first to notice that fat women appeared to bear fewer children than lean women. It followed that fatness was encouraged in women wishing to remain sterile. Curiously, modern medicine has reached the same conclusion. If a woman is too fat, she does not experience normal ovulation and is, therefore, less fertile.

The most drastic measure to insure female sterilization was removal of the ovaries, known as female castration. In ancient Egypt, kings castrated the young women of their harems. It was thought that if women were castrated at a young age, female sex characteristics would not develop and their youth would be preserved.

There were, of course, many other ideas and concoctions and devices, some far-fetched and some fairly sound, used through history to prevent conception. When these failed, more extreme measures, like abortion and infanticide (the slaughter of babies), were instigated. These, of course, were not contraceptive techniques; rather, they were early exercises in population control.

Most of the old methods, though, never really freed women from the worry and concern of unwanted pregnancies. It has only been in the twentieth century that women have been able to approach contraception with any sense of self-dignity, safety, and reliability.

chapter 9

MODERN METHODS OF CONTRACEPTION

Birth control has become increasingly important in an era of dramatically increasing population and changing personal life-styles. Attitudes of greater sexual freedom have been accompanied by growing knowledge of contraceptive methods. Nearly everyone has the ability, and certainly the right, to use their own bodies as they desire. To exercise that right, you must understand how your body functions. Full control of your sexual life means being able to take advantage of the various methods of birth control. The more you know, the greater your personal choices.

In this chapter, the current methods, trends, and notions about birth control are discussed. Some of these methods are effective, advanced, and changing every day, while others are misunderstood, outdated, or just plain ineffective. Several methods are especially well suited to couples planning families and can help in the spacing of children. Couples who have completed their families may find other, more acceptable methods for preventing further pregnancies. People who have infrequent or unexpected sexual relations might find some of the more traditional methods better suited to their needs. Virtually everyone should be able to find contraceptive techniques compatible with his or her thoughts on family planning, not to mention particular sexual desires. This chapter will give you a thorough understanding of the various forms of contraception, as well as of their safety and effectiveness.

Many people have been justifiably concerned with the reported side effects of various contraceptives. Oral contraceptives and intrauterine devices (IUDs) have been criticized for producing harmful side effects, or even fatalities. Many contend that not enough is known about the full effects of such powerful or potentially dangerous methods. Medicine should never be taken for granted; an educated concern about what we do to our bodies is beneficial. The side effects and the changes that contraceptives produce in the body, as well as the risks involved in their use, are discussed here to give you a basis for making your own informed decision.

Control of your body and sexual freedom without the worry of unwanted pregnancy are advances made in the last twenty years. To take full advantage of these, you must know your choices, and what you do not know *can* hurt you!

VAGINAL SPERMICIDES: FOAM, CREAM, AND JELLY

Vaginal spermicides, called a *barrier method* of contraception, have been around a long time. The ancient Egyptians were said to place mixtures of honey, vegetable gum, sodium carbonate, and crocodile dung into the vagina to prevent pregnancy. Aristotle reported using a combination of frankincense, oil of cedar, and olive oil for the same purpose. In the Middle Ages, people were fond of rock salt and alum. Walter Rendell, the founding father of modern spermicides, introduced a suppository of cocoa butter and quinine sulfate to England in 1885. Rendell's, probably the first commercial spermicide, is still available today.

Modern spermicides are made of two basic components: a spermicidal (sperm killing) chemical and a harmless, bulky base. This base is heavy enough to block the cervix, so that even if some sperm are not killed by the chemical, they cannot enter the cervical canal.

Spermicides are available in a number of different forms. There are spermicidal foams, creams, jellies, foaming tablets, and suppositories. Foaming tablets and suppositories are not widely available since they do not work as well as the other methods. Foams are the *most* effective spermicide—they spread quickly and evenly coat the cervix. Creams and jellies are more likely to fail because they do not spread as easily, nor as evenly, throughout the cervix. Emko and Delfen are two of the most popular spermicidal foams, and their names have nearly become synonymous with contraception. Many foams are now available in factory-filled, premeasured doses for easy use.

The Pros and Cons of Spermicides

Spermicides offer several advantages. They are relatively benign to the body and can be purchased in almost any drugstore or pharmacy without a prescription. Almost everyone finds a spermicide quite simple to use, and it can easily be combined with other birth-control methods for added protection. There is no device involved, which may prevent the artificial or physically unsatisfactory feeling that condoms sometimes cause.

On the other hand, a spermicide must be used *immediately* before intercourse, which some people feel interrupts the spontaneity of lovemaking. It also must be inserted before *each and every* intercourse. Some women do not like having to touch their genitals in order to insert the spermicide high up in the vagina. Other users report a mild burning or similar vaginal irritation after application, but this may be relieved by changing to another, perhaps less irritating, brand. Then, of course, there is the complaint of messiness due to the dripping or leaking of the spermicide from the vagina, which is simply unaesthetic. Some men object strongly to the taste of the foam or spermicide.

How to Use Foam, Cream, and Jelly

The first step in the use of a spermicide is to fill the applicator with the preparation. A prefilled applicator, such as Emko's brand Because, can also be used. Creams and jellies usually have applicators that screw onto the top of the tube for easier handling. Next, the woman lies down and gently inserts the applicator as far up into the vagina as it will go. The applicator is then pulled back about a half an inch, the plunger depressed or the tube squeezed to deposit the spermicide near the cervix, allowing the preparation to coat it evenly. Creams and jellies do not spread as easily as foam, so the careful positioning of the applicator is more important with these preparations.

Spermicides should be applied no more than a half-hour before intercourse. If more than an hour passes, there must be a second application. There should be an interval between application of the spermicide and intercourse. Two to three minutes should pass to allow creams and jelly preparations to coat the cervix. Waiting is not necessary if foam is used. After the vaginal spermicide has been applied, a woman must remain on her back to prevent leakage prior to intercourse. After intercourse, she should wait at least six hours before douching. Douching too early dilutes the spermicide, weakening its ability to kill any sperm still left in the vaginal tract.

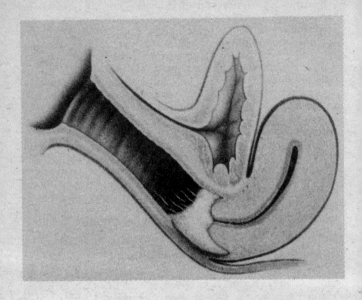

Fig. 9–1: Once a spermicidal foam has been injected, it coats the upper part of the vagina, covering the cervix and preventing the entrance of sperm, which can be seen immediately underneath the foam. (Courtesy of the Ortho Pharmaceutical Corporation, Raritan, New Jersey.)

The spermicide kills sperm by coating the surface and preventing the passage of oxygen into the cell. There is evidence that spermicides may inhibit the growth of VD and herpes organisms spread during intercourse, but they are by no means totally effective as protection against VD. Women who use spermicides, however, have a lower incidence of VD than women who use nonbarrier forms of contraception or no contraception.

ENCARE OVALS AND OTHER FOAMING TABLETS

Foaming tablets and suppositories contain a spermicide that melts and spreads through the vaginal vault at body temperature. Most American pharmaceutical manufacturers have been reluctant to introduce this type of contraceptive to the United States since they felt its effectiveness was significantly below that of contraceptive foam or jelly. The foam and jelly immediately coat the upper vaginal region, forming an effective barrier of spermicide. The tablets, however, must be given time to dissolve and there is no optimal spermicidal effect until at least ten minutes after insertion. This delay in effectiveness from the time of administration until the tablet has time to coat the vagina may be one of the reasons for the number of reported pregnancies by users of foaming tablets. Encare Oval, which has been recently introduced into the American market, is characteristic of the foaming tablets. It appears that more pregnancies occurred than were initially anticipated from the European experience when this suppository was introduced in the United States. This higher rate may be due to the improper use of the suppository. A clinical study sponsored by the manufacturers of Encare Oval demonstrated that the optimal spermicidal activity was from ten minutes to one hour following administration. Many physicians believe that the contraceptive effectiveness of Encare Ovals remains to be demonstrated by closely controlled U.S. studies and, until such data are available, the foams and creams are to be the preferred spermicides. These tablets, however, offer the advantage of being available "over-the-counter" and easy to use. The disadvantages include delay between insertion and effectiveness. Also, the inserter used with vaginal creams and foams permits application of these agents high in the vaginal vault. When a woman uses the suppository she must make a conscious effort to place the tablet high in the vagina. A number of women fail to do this, reducing the effectiveness of the spermicide. Finally, there have been reports of an unpleasant burning sensation experienced by either or both sexual partners accompanying the use of the Encare Oval.

When Should Spermicides Be Used?

Spermicides are more effective when used in combination with condoms, and are acceptable for women who experience infrequent or unexpected sexual relations. They provide some contraceptive protection, as well as convenient lubrication, during coitus. They may be used when nursing children, during the first month on the minipill until the pill becomes effective, or during the time shortly after an IUD insertion for added protection. A spermicide can also be beneficial if more than one pill of an oral contraceptive series is forgotten. Some of the prefilled foams such as Because are ideal in these instances. They are prepacked in a relatively small applicator not much larger than a tampon and are, therefore, very portable.

How Effective Are Spermicides?

They can be very effective, but they often are not. Actually, the pregnancy rate for the foam spermicide is about thirty per one hundred women years. In other words, for every hundred women using spermicide for one year, thirty will get pregnant. The high failure rate results largely from not using the preparation with every intercourse or from not inserting an additional application before a second intercourse. The effectiveness is also higher for women who use the missionary position, since spermicides tend to leak in any other position, thus not covering the cervix completely. It is the user of the method, rather than the method itself, that causes failure. Proper use of a good-quality foam has produced reported pregnancy rates of five pregnancies per hundred women yearly. Because of their high failure rate, however, spermicidal preparations should not be relied on by women who must not get pregnant. These women should choose another more effective means of birth control. Creams and jellies are even less effective than foams.

The use of spermicidal preparations has declined in recent years with the advent of the pill and IUDs. It is estimated that between two to four million women use these products in the United States.

Side Effects

The worst side effect of spermicides is probably a mild vaginal irritation, which can vary from one woman to another. If this happens, change brands. The preparations do not cause cancer, and if you should become pregnant, the baby is not affected in any way.

COLLAGEN SPONGE—A FUTURE BARRIER CONTRACEPTIVE?

Dr. Milos Chvapil of the University of Arizona Medical Center has developed an intravaginal collagen sponge made of bovine skin which is being tested as a new barrier contraceptive. The sponge is placed in the vagina and absorbs the sperm. The natural acidity of the sponge will actively kill sperm for up to one month. It was originally thought that since the sponge was an active spermicide for one month it could be left undisturbed in the vagina for that period of time. However, as sperm were deposited on the sponge during period of sexual activity the problem of malodor arose, and it was determined that the sponge should be removed and rinsed with a vinegar solution periodically. This is only during periods of sexual activity; if a woman is not sexually active the sponge may be left in place. At the present time only patient acceptability of the sponge has been tested on women with tubal ligation or intrauterine contraceptive devices. The contraceptive effectiveness is now being evaluated in a group of women using no other form of birth control. The availability of this sponge is presently limited to the research group at the university where it has been developed.

THE DIAPHRAGM

A diaphragm is a soft, latex rubber dome stretched around a steel spring. Although it acts as a mechanical barrier, preventing sperm from entering the cervical canal, its major contraceptive function is as a container holding a spermicidal jelly against the opening of the cervix. The dome of the diaphragm covers the cervix; in the front it fits snugly behind the pubis bone, and in the back into the posterior fornix, a small pocket behind the cervix. A spermicidal cream or jelly *must* be used with a diaphragm to kill sperm which pass the rim of the diaphragm. The diaphragm acts *primarily* as a container for the spermicide and *secondarily* as a physical barrier to sperm.

How to Be Fitted for a Diaphragm

Each woman must be individually fitted for a diaphragm, either by a doctor or by trained paramedical personnel. With diaphragms, there is no such thing as one size fits all. The doctor first performs a pelvic examination to determine the distance between the pubic bone and the back of the vagina. The doctor then inserts, in sequence, a series of diaphragm rings; these are diaphragm springs covered with latex, with the

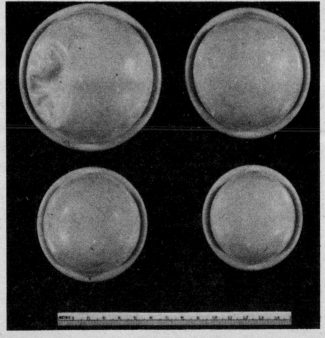

Fig. 9–2: Four different sizes of the Ortho-All-Flex diaphragms, clockwise from upper left: 90, 80, 65 and 70. The number of a diaphragm indicates its diameter in mm.

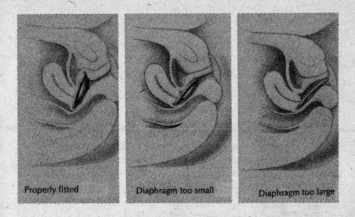

Properly fitted   Diaphragm too small   Diaphragm too large

Fig. 9-3: The diaphragm on the extreme left is properly fitted; the one in the center is too small; the diaphragm on the right is too large. When a diaphragm is not properly fitted, it will not provide proper contraceptive protection and can even interfere with intercourse. (Courtesy of Ortho Pharmaceutical Corporation, Raritan, New Jersey.)

center domes missing. The doctor determines which size diaphragm most correctly suits each woman. Diaphragms range in diameter from 55 to 95 millimeters (approximately 2⅛ to 3¾ inches). The majority of women are fitted with a diaphragm of 70 to 80 millimeters in diameter (2¾ to 3⅓ inches). The type of diaphragm employed depends on the contour and size of the vagina as well as on the position of the uterus and adjacent organs. Some women with anatomical disorders (such as poor vaginal muscle tone, lacerations of the vaginal wall from birth trauma, or a complete uterine prolapse) are not able to use a diaphragm.

To function effectively, a diaphragm must fit properly. If it is too small, it can slip out during coitus; too large a diaphragm may buckle and will be both uncomfortable and ineffective. As a general rule, it is best to use the largest diaphragm that fits properly without the user being aware of its presence.

A diaphragm must be refitted after childbirth, miscarriage, any surgical operation, or a weight change in excess of ten pounds, and routinely every two or three years. The fit of a diaphragm can be affected by the emotions—if a woman is nervous at the time of the examination, her vaginal muscles can tense, making proper fitting difficult. A virgin, with hymen intact, can be fitted for a diaphragm. She should be refitted shortly after she becomes sexually active, since vaginal muscles stretch with intercourse. If you choose to be fitted for a diaphragm, the doctor will ask you to examine yourself so that you recognize the position of the diaphragm in relation to the cervix and pubic bone. You should be able to feel that the cervix is completely covered by the dome of the diaphragm. If it is properly positioned, you can press one side of the diaphragm without tilting the device. It is most important that you know how to insert the diaphragm properly and are able to check its position for a correct fit. Do not leave the doctor's office until you understand this and have tried to insert and remove the diaphragm a few times with a nurse's supervision.

Insertion and Removal of the Diaphragm

Before inserting the device, smear about a teaspoon of spermicidal cream or jelly on each side of the diaphragm dome (the instructions suggest placement of jelly only on the inside of the dome, but since you often do not know how the diaphragm lies inside the vagina, it is safer to apply the jelly on both sides of the dome). Also, smear the cream with your fingertip around the rim of the device to kill any sperm that may slip past. To prevent the introduction of bacteria, you should wash your hands prior to insertion. Read the personal instruction booklet enclosed with the new diaphragm carefully.

The device is most easily inserted if you are crouching, squatting, lying down, or standing with one foot raised on a chair or toilet seat. Insert the diaphragm by squeezing it into a long, narrow shape with one hand, while the other hand holds the vaginal lips open. You slide the device up the vagina until the far rim passes the cervix. Then gently push the front rim up under the pubic bone, checking to see that the cervix is covered. If a woman has short fingers or dislikes handling herself, a plastic or metal inserter may be used. The diaphragm should now be far back in the vagina so neither partner is aware of it during coitus. A diaphragm is held in place by the spring tension of the rim, by vaginal muscle tone, and by the pubic bone. You remove it by hooking your index finger behind the forward rim and gently pulling downward. Be careful not to puncture it with your finger or nail.

A diaphragm should not be inserted more than *two* hours before intercourse. If coitus is delayed for more than two

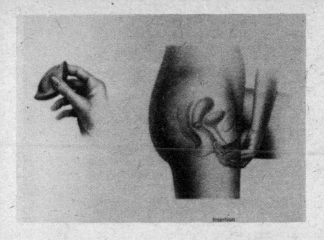

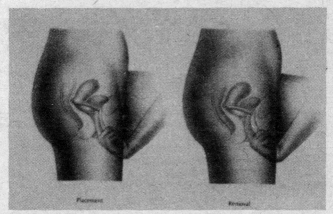

Fig. 9–4: The sequence of insertion and removal of the diaphragm. The diaphragm *must* fit snugly behind the pubis bone in front. (Courtesy of Ortho Pharmaceutical Corporation, Raritan, New Jersey.)

hours, you need to recover the diaphragm with spermicide or to apply a spermicidal foam. Likewise, reapply the cream or jelly before each successive intercourse. *Do not* remove the diaphragm to reapply the spermicide; simply insert some cream or jelly into the vagina. The diaphragm can be left in place overnight, but insert additional jelly before morning intercourse. You may bathe, walk around, or urinate with a diaphragm in place, but check its position after each bowel movement. Leave the diaphragm in place for at least *six hours* after the last intercourse to make certain the sperm in the vaginal tract have been killed. Douching is not necessary, but for that, too, you must wait at least six hours after intercourse or you will rinse away all the spermicide.

Care of the Diaphragm

To clean the diaphragm after removal, wash it with a mild soap and water, dry it, and then put it in its container. Unscented soaps and powders are best, for they will not corrode the rubber. Never use Vaseline or any petroleum products on your diaphragm. Regularly check the diaphragm for holes, cracks, or leaks, especially near the rim. Hold it up to the light, or fill it with water to see if there is any leakage.

Types of Diaphragms

There are four basic types of diaphragms. The most popular, the Ortho-All-Flex, has a spring ring that is flexible and easily adjusts to the vaginal contour. The Koromex has a stronger spring that does not bend much, which gives a better fit with weaker vaginal muscles. Other varieties curve or bend to provide a better fit for women with poor muscle tone or other individual disorders.

The Diaphragm in Historical Perspective

Women have used many things to block the cervical entrance during coitus. Casanova recommended squeezing the juice from half a lemon and placing the lemon shell in the vagina. The lemon shell acted as a barrier, while the citric acid was a spermicide. Dr. C. Hasse, using the name Mensinga, popularized the first modern diaphragm in Germany and Holland in the 1880s. It spread to England, where it was called a Dutch cap, and helped move Victorian women to responsibility for their own contraception. The material and construction of modern diaphragms has improved, but the basic concept goes directly back to Mensinga.

The Pros and Cons of Diaphragm Use

The diaphragm is an attractive form of contraception primarily because it affords protection from unwanted pregnancy without causing physiological or systemic changes in the body, and secondarily because, if used properly, it is a very effective form of birth control. The use of the diaphragm is under the control of the woman and has to be used only when needed. This technique appeals to women who have infrequent intercourse and also to women who have established relationships with intercourse on a routine basis. It is a very acceptable method for spacing children, since the spermicide jelly will not harm the fetus if pregnancy should occur. Since the use of a diaphragm causes no physiological changes in the body, it is also safe to use during breast feeding. Some women find that the cream or jelly used in conjunction with the diaphragm is helpful in providing extra lubrication during intercourse. It is interesting that a number of women employing other methods of birth control such as oral contraceptives or IUDs use a diaphragm when having intercourse during menstruation to contain the menstrual flow.

The major problem with a diaphragm is that it requires a high degree of motivation to make it work. It must be used with a spermicide for each and every intercourse, and this can deprive a relationship of a certain amount of spontaneity. In short, if your diaphragm is at home and you're not, you had better not. The use of a diaphragm requires that a woman handle her genitals; some women find this a problem. Other women have difficulty learning the proper method of insertion, which is all-important to the effectiveness of the diaphragm. Another objection is that the spermicide can be messy and expensive and some sex partners find the taste sour.

Use and Effectiveness

Before the pill and IUDs became popular, the diaphragm was used by about 30 percent of American couples practicing birth control. Today its popularity has fallen behind the pill and IUDs, probably because of the ease and effectiveness of the newer methods. Recently, however, there have been a great number of women who have resumed the use of diaphragms, mainly because of the adverse publicity the pill and IUDs have

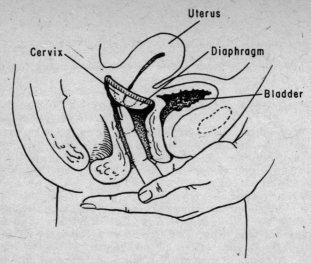

Fig. 9–5: How a woman should check for proper placement of a diaphragm. The cervix must be completely covered with the diaphragm dome, as shown in this illustration.

received. It is, therefore, difficult to estimate the exact number of women who are using diaphragms today. Many women are pleased with the switch from the oral contraceptive and IUDs to the diaphragm, but others have found the diaphragm too inconvenient and have subsequently gone back to newer and more acceptable types of pills and IUDs.

Successful use depends largely on a woman's motivation. There are failure rates of anywhere from six to twenty-nine pregnancies per year per hundred women using the device. If the instructions are carefully followed, however, rates as low as four pregnancies per hundred women a year have been reported, certainly well within the limits of acceptability. Younger women have higher failure rates, perhaps due to their inexperience in using the device. The method may fail for several reasons: improper use, improper fit, slippage during coitus, or a leak in the diaphragm. Diaphragms slip more frequently in woman-dominant positions, as the female organs hang slightly downward. They can also be dislodged by repeated penal thrusts. The vaginal walls expand during sexual orgasm, and the diaphragm can slip out of position. Such failure is the exception rather than the rule, but you should be aware of it. Although the pill and the IUD are highly effective, the diaphragm which causes no side effects, can be equally safe if properly fitted and intelligently used.

THE CERVICAL CAP

The cervical cap is a small, clear, rigid device of thimble-shaped lucite. Unlike the diaphragm, which blocks the entire upper portion of the vaginal canal, the cervical cap blocks only the cervix. Compared to a diaphragm, it is smaller in diameter, deeper, and more rigid. Most importantly, it is held in place by suction rather than by spring tension.

The cap, like a diaphragm, must be fitted by a doctor. To use it, fill the cap about a third full of jelly spermicide. Squatting or reclining, grasp the cap, dome down, separate the vaginal lips, and push it up the vagina as far as it goes. Then press the rim around the cervix until the dome covers the cervical opening and the cervix can be felt under the dome. The cap is then on tightly. You remove it by breaking the suction. It can be used without spermicide, but this decreases the cap's effectiveness. In these cases, the cap can be applied only once a month, after menstruation, and remains on the cervix for the entire cycle. It need only be removed at the next menstruation.

Though not widely popular today, the cervical cap has been around a long time. It was used in England even before the diaphragm, and does have several good things to be said for it. Because it is held on with suction, it is unlikely to slip during intercourse and can seldom be felt by the man. It can also be used by women with abnormalities or poor muscle tone who cannot use a diaphragm. And, because the cap covers only the cervix, you will not need constant refitting as your vaginal muscles change. It is not widely used, however, because it is difficult to insert. As it must be placed deeply within the vaginal canal, many women cannot learn the technique of proper insertion.

There are several varieties of cervical caps to fit women with differing anatomical features or problems. There have been no studies in recent years, but the cap is thought to be about as effective a contraceptive as the diaphragm.

THE CONDOM

The condom, also called a rubber, a prophylactic, and a safe, is a sheath the man wears on his penis during intercourse. This much-celebrated device is still widely used, and when handled properly, is an effective mechanical barrier for contraception.

Most condoms today are made of a strong, thin, latex rubber. Condoms made of animal membrane, usually sheep intestines, are also available. Looking much like a skinny balloon, the condom is slightly thicker near the open end and has a ring around the opening to keep it on the penis. It is possible to get condoms

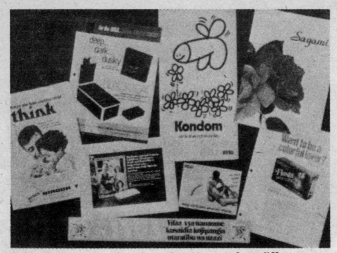

Fig. 9–6: Examples of condom advertisements from different parts of the world. These promotion techniques are used by various family-planning agencies as well as by the condom manufacturers to encourage the use of condoms. (Courtesy of I. Dalsimer, P. Piotrow, and J. Dumm; *Condoms: An Old Method Meets a New Social Need. Population Reports,* Series H, #1. Washington, D.C., George Washington University Medical Center, Population Information Program—1973.)

with reservoir ends to contain the sperm, lubricated to facilitate intercourse, transparent for the latest in the see-through look, or in different colors to match whatever turns you on.

Most condoms come dry and powdered, but, as stated above, lubricated condoms are readily available. The sheep membrane condoms, while considerably more expensive, are said to conduct heat better and to provide more sensation than the latex variety. With proper care, membrane condoms can be reused several times. Condoms may be obtained in virtually any drugstore or pharmacy. The cheaper brands sold in washrooms or gas stations are generally of inferior quality and should be avoided. Tip condoms, or condom caps, which cover only the tip, or glans, of the penis can easily slip off and should *not* be used.

The History of the Condom

The condom has a long history. The name itself may come from the Latin *condus,* meaning a receptacle, or may even date back to the Persian word *kendu* or *kondu,* which refers to long vessels made from animal intestines and used to store grain. Possibly it refers to the unfortunately named Dr. Condom, who supplied England's Charles II with methods to prevent illegitimate children.

In its early days, the condom was probably used primarily to prevent venereal disease, and only secondarily for contraception. Since the days of Casanova, however, it has been associated with secret rendezvous and illicit sex. Its reputation has been tarnished further by being standard equipment issued by many armies, and by American labeling requirements stating it is "for the prevention of disease." For years, the condom has remained one of the most popular methods of birth control in England, Sweden, and Japan. Its unsavory reputation is not worldwide.

How to Use the Condom

Some couples actually incorporate unrolling the condom into their regular foreplay. Whatever your routine, unroll the condom a half-inch and place it on the man's penis, squeezing this half-inch reservoir to keep out the air. This allows the sperm to collect after ejaculation without leaking from the top of the condom. If the man is not circumcised, he should have his foreskin rolled down before using the condom. Roll the condom down the length of the penis, being careful not to tear it with rings or fingernails. It should cover the penis, with a half-inch hanging limply at the end. When inserting the penis, be careful not to catch the reservoir on the outside of the vagina, or to insert it too quickly—you may tear it.

Trying to force the condom into a dry vagina is very uncomfortable. Unless you have a lubricated condom, you will probably want some artificial lubrication, like a sterile jelly, a spermicidal foam or cream, or even saliva. Never use Vaseline or any petroleum jelly or oil, as this quickly *destroys the latex rubber.* For complete protection from unexpected or premature ejaculation, the condom should be worn throughout intercourse.

After ejaculation and loss of erection, the man should hold the condom tight against the base of his penis to avoid leakage. When he wishes to withdraw from the vagina, the condom is held on the penis at the base. If it slips off during coitus, remove it from the vagina immediately, holding the open end closed. To remove it from the penis after withdrawal, stretch the open end and pull down. Quickly inspect it for holes or leakage. If there is a leak, the woman should immediately use spermicidal foam. There is also a high-estrogen "morning after" pill to prevent pregnancy, which is taken for five days following intercourse (see information on "morning after" pill). While this can be used in cases of certain condom failure, this pill has very unpleasant side effects.

A good-quality condom can be used several times. After removal from the penis, drop it in a glass of water. As soon as is convenient, wash it in warm, soapy water, dry it, and powder it with cornstarch to preserve the latex. Skin condoms can be cleaned in a solution of mild household boric acid and water. Inspect all condoms for leaks before reusing them. Condoms should not be kept in a wallet or pocket for any length of time, as heat causes the latex to deteriorate.

The Pros and Cons of Condoms

There are a number of advantages to using condoms; they are inexpensive, completely harmless, compact and disposable, readily available, easy to use, fairly effective, and may inhibit the transmission of venereal disease in people who are very active sexually (there are no studies to support this assumption at the present time). If the man is willing, it is an excellent method for infrequent or unexpected sex. Couples involved in a continuous relationship will probably find that other methods (such as the pill, an IUD, or a diaphragm) are more suitable and more effective as a long-term contraceptive.

The condom is, of course, used by the man alone, although it can be combined with spermicidal foam. Many women, however, are reluctant to trust their protection solely to the man, wondering if he is reliable in the heat of passion. Many men say they dislike a condom because it is a mechanical device which disrupts spontaneity and dulls pleasure. This latter claim is rather dubious, for modern condoms are extremely thin. Nonetheless, some people dislike their artificiality, which is psychologically understandable.

How Effective Is It?

The condom is recognized as an effective method of contraception, and nearly a billion condoms are sold yearly in the

United States and Canada. It can be used successfully by itself, but is more effective when used with a spermicidal foam or cream. Studies have shown this method is about as effective as the diaphragm and jelly technique of contraception. The failure rate has been measured at anywhere from five to twenty-five pregnancies per hundred women per year.

This method depends largely on motivation and on how strongly you wish to prevent conception. Failure is due mainly to not using the condom consistently for every intercourse. Not using the condom "just this once" can be a big mistake, as no contraceptive works well when it's still in the drawer.

Automated machinery produces high-quality condoms which are electronically tested at the factory, so the old "pinhole" problems of the 1940s have been virtually eliminated. Thus, condom failures can be attributed to human mistakes rather than the latex. The shelf life of a condom is about two years, after which time the latex or lubrication has deteriorated, making the condom undependable for use.

THE RHYTHM METHOD

The rhythm method means programed abstinence from sexual intercourse during those days of her cycle that a woman is most likely to become pregnant. It is based on the simple principle that egg and sperm must be in the same place at the same time for conception to occur. The rhythm method is so named because there is a rhythm to the periodic abstinence, and it is still the only method of birth control, short of complete abstinence, officially approved by the Catholic Church. The rhythm method is also referred to as *natural family* planning.

The Theory behind Rhythm

A woman can only become pregnant if she has intercourse during a fertile period of her menstrual cycle. This fertile period consists of those days immediately prior to and immediately following ovulation (the release of the egg from the ovary). Intercourse prior to ovulation must be avoided since the sperm can live in the female reproductive tract for up to seventy-two hours, and intercourse after ovulation must be avoided since the egg can live for up to forty-eight hours. If a live sperm meets a live egg, there is a very good chance for conception.

Since it is almost impossible to determine the *exact* time of ovulation, the principle of rhythm is simple in theory but difficult in practice. In general, a woman ovulates fourteen days

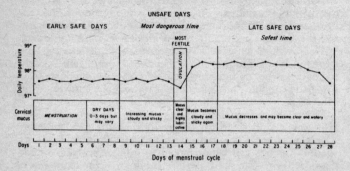

THE RHYTHM METHOD

Fig. 9–7: The Rhythm Method. When using the rhythm method, it is most important to avoid intercourse around the time of ovulation. The chance of conception is much higher with intercourse prior to ovulation than after ovulation, because the sperm can survive for several days prior to ovulation in the female reproductive tract.

before the start of the menstrual period, but not necessarily fourteen days *after* the onset of her menstrual period. Only for the rare woman with a consistent twenty-eight-day cycle is there a good chance that she ovulates exactly mid-cycle at day 14 (counting from the first day of menstrual bleeding). Very few women have twenty-eight-day cycles month after month, and even the most regular women usually have cycles that vary between twenty-seven and thirty-one days. It is with this variation that the problems of rhythm arise. If a woman cannot determine when she ovulates, she cannot determine her fertile period. The estimation of ovulation is all-important to the success of the rhythm method.

Predicting Ovulation—Safe and Unsafe Days

Ovulation occurs in mid-cycle, making this the most likely time of conception. Conversely, the beginning and end of a cycle are the least likely times of conception. A sperm can live within a woman for approximately seventy-two hours, and sometimes longer. An egg can survive up to forty-eight hours after ovulation. This means a couple should not have intercourse for at least three days before the earliest chance of ovulation, to make certain all the sperm are dead by the time the egg is released. Likewise, a couple must abstain for at least two days after the latest possible chance of ovulation, to make certain the egg is no longer viable.

The two most widely used methods for predicting ovulation involve daily charts based either on a calendar or on your body temperature. These methods are complex, involve a large chance for error, and should not be initiated without the supervision of a doctor or a family-planning clinic. There are other methods for ovulation prediction: One involves the estimation of the consistency and amount of cervical mucus, and another is based on the determination of the acidity of the vagina.

The Calendar Method

Often called the Ogino-Knaus method, this method assumes that ovulation occurs at some point during a five-day period approximately twelve to sixteen days before the onset of the next menstruation. Therefore, intercourse must be avoided for three days before this five-day span and for two days following it. For example, if a woman has a completely regular twenty-eight-day menstrual cycle, the length of abstinence during her fertile period will be ten days.

Most women, however, do not have menstrual cycles with textbook regularity. To determine what her individual cycle will be, a woman must keep a calendar record of her cycles for eight months. To determine her cycle variation, she counts the first day of her menstrual flow as day 1. She records on a calendar chart the length of each cycle for eight consecutive months. From the ninth month, she is theoretically able to determine her unsafe period. She subtracts nineteen from the length of her shortest cycle to determine her first unsafe day (ovulation may be a maximum of sixteen days before menstruation plus the three days the sperm can survive). If a woman's shortest cycle was twenty-six days her first unsafe day is seven days after the *onset* of menstrual bleeding ($26-19 = 7$ days). To determine her last unsafe day, a woman subtracts ten from the length of her longest cycle (ovulation can occur a minimum of twelve days before menstruation, minus two days for the life of the ovum). If a woman's longest cycle was thirty-one days, her last unsafe day is twenty-one days after the onset of menstrual bleeding ($31-10 = 21$). There should be no intercourse from the first to the last unsafe day; thus a woman with a cycle varying between twenty-six and thirty-one days must avoid intercourse from day 7 to day 21 of her cycle. For a woman with cycle variation of this degree, the only safe days for intercourse would be the first six days after the onset of menstruation and the last seven days before the beginning of menstruation.

Basal Body Temperature Method

A more accurate procedure for determining the time of ovulation is based on measurement of subtle changes in the normal, or "basal," body temperature. Called the Basal Body Temperature (BBT) method, it resulted from the discovery that immediately prior to ovulation body temperature drops slightly, rising rather sharply directly after ovulation. This change in body temperature (only 0.15°–0.3° Centigrade [or 0.5°–1.00° Fahrenheit]), can give a reasonable estimation of the time of ovulation. The temperature remains elevated for about two weeks if ovulation has occurred. This temperature increase is due to progesterone production by the corpus luteum (these physiological changes are thoroughly described in Chapter 5, The Reproductive Cycle).

If a woman wishes to use the BBT method, she must take and record her temperature every morning as soon as she awakens. This procedure must be performed faithfully before the woman even gets out of bed. The obvious drawback with this technique is that it does not predict when ovulation will occur; it only gives an indication of when ovulation *has* occurred. The safest period for intercourse with the BBT method would be three days, a full seventy-two hours, after the temperature elevation, since by that time ovulation would have occurred and the ovum would have disintegrated. The most unsafe period, as estimated by the BBT method, is the preovulatory time, particularly from five to seven days prior to the expected time of ovulation. Since the BBT method does not attempt to predict ovulation, in order to be completely safe, a woman should avoid intercourse during the entire first half of the menstrual cycle, from the time she bleeds until the seventy-two hours after the rise in Basal Body Temperature.

Because of the prolonged abstinence required in the BBT method and factors such as illness that impair its accuracy, women often combine the BBT with the calendar method to shorten the abstinence period. In this combined approach, the first unsafe day is taken from the shortest cycle on your calendar chart, and the last unsafe day is the third day after the rise in the BBT.

Mucus Method

It has been observed that the time of ovulation can be estimated by changes in the quality and quantity of the cervical mucus. During the period of time immediately following the end of menstrual bleeding, there is very little cervical mucus. These are known as the dry days. As ovulation approaches, there is an increase in the production of mucus, and it becomes cloudy and sticky. At the time of ovulation, the mucus is clear and highly lubricative. During the immediate postovulatory period, it again becomes cloudy and sticky. During the late safe period, more than seventy-two hours postovulation, the amount of mucus decreases, and it may become clear and watery until the time of menstrual flow. With this technique, the post menstruation dry days and the late postovulatory period of decreasing, clear, watery mucus may be considered safe days for intercourse.

The acidity of the vaginal mucus also changes throughout the menstrual cycle. The mucus is slightly acidic throughout the majority of the menstrual cycle, but it changes to a slightly alkaline factor around the time of ovulation. These changes can be determined with the use of litmus (pH) paper to estimate the time of ovulation. With this method, the safe period begins three days after ovulation has occurred.

Effectiveness of the Rhythm Method

The reported effectiveness of the rhythm method varies tremendously from study to study and from country to country. The lowest incidence of unplanned pregnancy, ranging from 0.3 to 6.6 pregnancies per 100 woman years, was observed with the BBT method when intercourse was restricted to the postovulatory period only. When there was intercourse in both the pre- and postovulatory phases of the period, the failure rate was high, ranging from 0.7 in a West German study to 19.5 pregnancies per 100 woman years in a United States study. The failure rate with the calendar method alone was quite high, ranging from 14.4 in the United States to 47 pregnancies per 100 woman years in Colombia. The cervical mucus method also has a high failure rate.

The Pros and Cons of Rhythm

The major and perhaps only advantage of the rhythm method is that there are no devices or medication involved. However, the rhythm method requires an extremely high degree of motivation, since it requires abstinence for a minimum of ten days a month. Furthermore, it has one of the highest failure rates of any of the widely used birth-control methods. This is why this method is facetiously called Vatican Roulette. The rhythm method should not be used by women who must not become pregnant, and cannot be used by women with irregular cycles.

The use of the rhythm method has declined dramatically in the last few years, because of the trouble and effort in predicting ovulation and the development of newer and more effective contraceptive methods. In 1955, approximately 22 percent of American couples practicing birth control used rhythm; the current level is about 6 percent.

Increased psychosexual stress is associated with the rhythm method. Lack of spontaneity and so-called programed sex can put pressure on a relationship. There is also strong evidence that the fertilization of an overaged ovum has been linked to fetal abnormalities. What this means is that the rhythm method fractionally increases the chances for fertilization of aged ova during the late, supposedly safe days. This creates a greater incidence of spontaneous abortion and abnormal children due to chromosomal abnormalities. There is a greater danger of this in older women or those with a history of habitual abortion or miscarriage.

COITUS INTERRUPTUS

Coitus interruptus is a variation on birth control's equivalent of Russian roulette. If you don't get pregnant, you are just plain lucky. This ineffective method allows unprotected intercourse to continue until the male is about to reach orgasm. He withdraws his penis from the vagina as he feels ejaculation coming. In biblical times, Onan threw his semen out to fertilize the land, and forever gave his name to coitus interruptus as the "sin of Onan," or onanism. A male must withdraw completely and ejaculate away from the vagina. Sperm cells move on their own. Sperm deposited anywhere between the labia majora (the external vaginal lips) can move all the way through the vagina to the uterus and fertilize the egg. The hymen need not be broken for conception to occur.

The Pros and Cons of Coitus Interruptus

The primary advantage of coitus interruptus is that it is always available. Since it does not require use of any type of medication or device, it is also physically harmless.

The great disadvantage of coitus interruptus is that it is a most ineffective method of birth control and results in a high pregnancy rate. The exact failure rate of coitus interruptus is not known, since there have been no recent studies of this technique. Some couples use coitus interruptus as a means of sexual foreplay and achieve orgasm either by oral or anal sex or by mutual masturbation.

One of the reasons for the high failure rate is that as orgasm approaches, both men and women find that complete voluntary control of the muscles becomes difficult. A man in the excitory phase just prior to orgasm may forget to withdraw, or he may suddenly decide he does not want to. Also, only about 50 percent of men ejaculate in one single burst; others expel semen sporadically or in a slow stream. Many men do not know exactly when they should withdraw, since there may have been a small ejaculation of semen prior to actual orgasm. Even a small ejaculation can contain millions of sperm, each one capable of fertilizing an ovum.

Some men can maintain an erection for five to twenty minutes, while others ejaculate within two to five minutes of intercourse. Men who ejaculate more quickly have greater difficulty with control and withdrawing. Younger men ejaculate more sperm, and thus have a greater chance of fertilization. They also have less physical control and more difficulty pulling out at just the right moment. All this makes successful coitus interruptus particularly difficult for younger men. If there is a second coitus, sperm left in the urethra (the tube of the penis) from the first intercourse can easily enter the vagina prior to the second orgasm.

Coitus interruptus also presents some psychological problems. Some women find it difficult to trust completely their sexual partners to withdraw in time. The man must be aware of when he will ejaculate, and must then be willing to withdraw. A woman may find that withdrawal interrupts her attempts to reach orgasm and causes her frustration. Both men and women may fear that ejaculation will occur before withdrawal. This subconscious fear of unwanted pregnancy does nothing to help the pleasure of the moment.

THE INTRAUTERINE DEVICE

An intrauterine device, or IUD, is a small object placed in the uterus to prevent conception. Intrauterine types of devices have been used in one form or another for centuries.

There are three basic types, or generations, of modern IUDs: The first generation was a *closed circular ring,* first developed by Gräfenberg in the 1920s and modified by Ota. The second generation is *open devices* of various shapes, such as the popular Lippes Loop or Saf-T-Coil, and devices such as the Dalkon Shield, which is a single, closed plane. It should be noted that because of their serious side effects, the closed ring devices are not recommended for use. The Dalkon Shield is used in special cases, but requires extra supervision. The third generation devices are either devices of improved design, such as the Ypsilon or Antigon-F, medicated IUDs such as the Copper-T or -7, or progesterone-impregnated devices such as the Progestasert.

Most modern devices are made of plastic, a body-friendly substance. All devices made exclusively of stainless steel have been removed from the market. The malleability of plastic is a great advantage, as it can be bent and threaded into a narrow "introducer," which inserts it into the uterus with a minimum of pain. Metallic salts are usually molded inside the plastic so the position of the IUD can be checked with X-ray. Many IUDs also have little tails made of nylon to facilitate their removal. The tail, extending from the cervix (the mouth of the womb), can be felt by the woman or seen by the doctor to be certain the device is still in the proper position.

History of IUDs

IUDs in one form or another have been used for a variety of purposes over the past twenty-five hundred years. Hippocrates reportedly used a hollow tube to insert medication or pessaries into the uterus. Translations vary as to whether this was for contraception or some other purpose. For centuries, nomads placed stones in the uteri of their female camels prior to a long caravan trip across the desert. This prevented these animals from becoming pregnant on the trip. It was many years before the contraceptive potential of a foreign object in the human uterus was widely recognized.

In the late nineteenth and early twentieth centuries, devices made of wood, glass, ivory, silver, gold, pewter, ebony, and other materials were inserted into the cervical canal. Some of these were inserted into the uterus, with the bottom of the devices extending into the cervix. The lower portion acted as a ladder, enabling bacteria and infection to climb from the cervix into the uterus. These devices may have prevented conception, but they generally functioned as uterine supports or were attempts to correct irregular or delayed menses. In 1902, a wishbone-shaped IUD was developed for contraception; it was implanted in the uterus. Some variations of this were supplied with instructions for self-insertion. Many complications resulted from their use, and they were quickly and unanimously condemned by the medical profession.

In the late 1920s, Dr. Ernest Gräfenberg developed a silver ring that was placed entirely within the uterus. In 1934, a ring with a center disc connected by three spokes was developed by Ota in Japan. The medical profession, aware of the problems of previous crude IUDs, did not accept the first generation IUDs of Gräfenberg and Dr. Ota. Gräfenberg subsequently abandoned his ideas, and the Ota Ring was banned by the Japanese government in 1936. Research in the late 1950s and early 1960s by physicians such as Margulies and Lippes finally encouraged reexamination of the theory of IUDs. Variations of the Gräfenberg Ring are still used today, and the Japanese lifted the ban on the Ota Ring in 1974. Today the IUD has an acknowledged place in the modern birth-control program.

How Does the IUD Work?

There is disagreement over exactly how the IUD prevents pregnancy. Some doctors maintain that it disrupts the dynamic muscular balance between the uterus, the cervix, and the fallopian tubes, interfering with the movement of the sperm up into the tubes and with the ovum's transport down toward the uterus. Fertilization would, thus, be prevented. Another theory maintains that the IUD causes cellular changes in the uterine lining, the endometrium. The development of the endometrium is disrupted, so even if the egg is fertilized, implantation is prevented.

Research has also shown high concentrations of *macrophages* in the uteri of women with IUDs. A macrophage is a normal cell which attacks invading cells, such as bacteria, swallowing and destroying them in a process called phagocytosis. What is most interesting is that macrophages do not normally exist in the uterus, and it is thought that they may destroy the fertilized egg in a process similar to phagocytosis.

Of course, uterine contractions increase with an IUD and this may prevent the normal implantation of a fertilized egg into the uterine wall. It has also recently been postulated that an IUD works simply by acting as a partition between the uterine walls. The highest contraceptive effect is obtained when the largest area of the uterine wall is covered. The more closely an IUD molds to the uterus, the more effective it is as a contraceptive.

Whatever the answer, an IUD does not work by causing early abortion or by creating a low-grade infection in the uterus. Both of these occur in a small percentage of women with IUDs, but they are not related to its contraceptive properties.

Types of IUDs

Intrauterine contraceptive devices are divided into two types: *inert* devices, usually most suitable for multiparous women

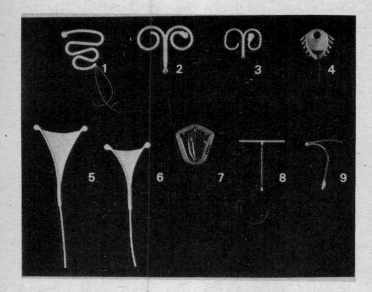

Fig. 9–8:   Different types of IUDs. (1) Lippes Loop-D, the largest of
the four sizes of this device; (2) Saf-T-Coil for a woman who has had
children; (3) Saf-T-Coil for a woman who has never had a child; (4)
Dalkon Shield, nulliparous size; the use of this IUD has been linked to
septic spontaneous abortion; (5) Ypsilon, multiparous size; and (6)
Ypsilon, nulliparous size, still under investigation; (7) Antigon-F,
under investigation, chiefly effective in multiparous women; (8)
Copper-T, still under investigation; (9) Cu-7, found to be very effective particularly in nulliparous women.

(women who have given birth), and *bioactive* devices, which have
a better acceptance rate in nulliparous women (women who
have never given birth).

The inert devices depend largely on configuration and size
for their contraceptive effectiveness. One of the most widely
used devices of this type, the Lippes Loop, is a very effective
contraceptive. The device is made of flexible plastic in a complex S-shape and measures little more than an inch across; it is
available in several sizes to afford the best fit for the individual
woman. The Lippes Loop has low expulsion and pregnancy

rates combined with acceptable side effects. The Saf-T-Coil is constructed of plastic similar to the Lippes Loop, but is molded into a quite different shape. This device has a success rate similar to the Lippes Loop. The Antigon-F, a comparatively new inert device, is still being investigated in a limited number of institutions. Since it is a somewhat larger IUD and covers a greater area of the uterus, it appears to have a lower pregnancy rate than either the Lippes Loop or the Saf-T-Coil. These three devices are particularly well accepted as contraceptives by multiparous women.

There is one inert device which has, in initial testing, been shown effective and acceptable in both multiparous and nulliparous women; this is the Ypsilon. The Ypsilon, a Y-shaped IUD, has an inner core of stainless steel and is completely covered by silicon. The stainless-steel frame makes the device a bit rigid and more difficult to expel. In addition, the Ypsilon has a silicone web between the forks of the Y and, thus, covers a large area of the uterus. The Ypsilon has been tested for several years and has a good performance record, with a high acceptability rate and a low pregnancy rate, particularly in nulliparous women.

The bioactive IUDs are also acceptable by nulliparous women because they are usually smaller than the inert IUDs. Bioactive IUDs depend not so much on configuration for contraceptive effectiveness; instead, they act as delivery systems for certain material with contraceptive properties. The Copper-T and Copper-7 are small IUDs made of plastic with copper wire wound around the outside of their plastic stems. Copper has antifertility effects which are not completely understood, but which render these IUDs effective contraceptives. The devices are smaller than inert devices and therefore provide a better fit for the smaller uterus of the nulliparous woman. Of course, being small and flexible, they tend to be more easily expelled than some other IUDs. The copper is depleted from the device within two or three years after insertion, so the device must be replaced at least every three years.

A new bioactive IUD, Progestasert, contains progesterone, the hormone of pregnancy (see Chapter 5, The Reproductive Cycle). This IUD slowly releases the progesterone over a period of one year; thus, two methods of contraception are combined, the IUD and the minipill. The progesterone probably exerts its contraceptive effects by altering the cervical mucus, which interferes with the passage of sperm. It may also interfere with ovulation, but this has not been shown. Women who have the Progestasert have less cramping and bleeding during the menstrual period. This device has only recently been released, and, as yet, it does not appear to be appreciably more effective than copper-bearing devices. Since the progesterone is depleted one year after insertion, the device must be replaced yearly.

Who Can Have an IUD?

Most women can be fitted with and use an IUD. Multiparous women usually tolerate the IUD better than nulliparous women. After a woman has a child, an abortion, or a miscarriage, the cervix is slightly dilated, making it much easier to insert an IUD. Also, after childbirth, the uterus appears to be less irritated by the presence of an IUD, so multiparous women do not usually experience severe episodes of pain and bleeding with IUDs. Multiparous women can usually employ an IUD with good success and high acceptance rates.

Insertion into nulliparous women is more difficult because the cervical canal is narrower and the uterus is smaller. Postinsertion cramping and pain, are, therefore, more severe. Nulliparous women are more likely to have the device removed because of pain and cramping, and they have a higher rate of spontaneous expulsion than multiparous women. Many nulliparous women accept the IUD very well with a minimum amount of problems, but some are very sensitive and have persistent cramping and bleeding. Women with smaller uteri or women who have had a decrease in uterine size due to longterm use of oral contraceptives often have problems when fitted with a large IUD.

It is really impossible to predict how a woman will respond to the presence of an IUD before it is inserted. There are a few women with congenital uterine malformations who cannot use an IUD. If a woman is fitted with the proper size and type of IUD, as determined by her physician, and has a minimum number of side effects, she has found a very acceptable and convenient form of contraception. If, however, despite proper choice and fit of IUD, there is excessive pain and bleeding, the IUD should be removed and the woman must seek some other form of contraception.

Who Should Insert the IUD—Can the Doctor Make a Difference?

While there is a difference in the effectiveness and tolerability of various devices, a difference in performance can often be traced to the skill of the person inserting the device. To place the IUD properly, the doctor or technician must take into account the great differences in internal anatomy and position the device correctly for the location, size, and shape of a woman's uterus. Clinics or doctors with excellent follow-up programs for postinsertion examination and encouragement have much better success records, regardless of the device they are using. If you are considering an IUD, check into the technical skill, reputation, and rate of success for your clinic or physician. In this case, the doctor makes a big difference.

How Is an IUD Inserted?

The insertion of an IUD is a relatively quick procedure, but requires a skilled physician or paramedic. It usually entails a degree of discomfort. In general, it is wise to have an IUD inserted only by a competent physician familiar with IUDs.

An IUD can be inserted at any time during the cycle, but it is *best* done on the second to fourth day of menstrual flow. In this way, a woman can be certain the device is not interfering with an unsuspected pregnancy, since menstruation is the best evidence that a woman is not pregnant. Also, during the early part of the menstrual flow, the uterus is already contracting, and the cramps associated with the insertion of the device will be less severe. The IUD causes additional bleeding and spotting for several days following insertion, and this is less of a problem during menstruation. Most importantly, the cervical canal is

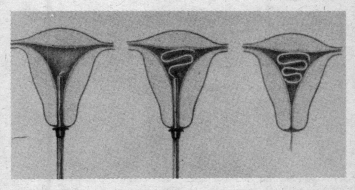

Fig. 9–9: The insertion of a Lippes Loop in three different phases. The loop unfolds inside the uterine cavity as it is inserted with the introducer. The cervix does not have to be dilated during the insertion. (Courtesy of Ortho Pharmaceutical Corporation, Raritan, New Jersey.)

slightly dilated during menstrual bleeding, so insertion is easier and less painful. The advantages of insertion of an IUD during the early part of the menstrual cycle are such that a woman should *only* have an IUD inserted during this period of the cycle, even if this entails an extra office visit.

Since insertion of an IUD is not without a degree of discomfort, it might be advisable for a woman to take a tranquilizer, such as Valium, and perhaps a painkiller, approximately an hour prior to the procedure. It is also advisable for a woman to take two aspirins. There is a theory that prostaglandin causes the cramps associated with IUD insertion; aspirin inhibits the synthesis of prostaglandin and, therefore, reduces the cramps. A woman's physician must be advised of the type, amount, and strength of any medication that is taken prior to the IUD insertion.

The insertion is preceded by a physical examination in which the physician determines the position, size, and shape of the uterus. It is important for a woman to get the IUD best suited to her body. Immediately prior to insertion, the IUD is threaded into a sterile, hollow instrument, an introducer. A vaginal speculum is used and the physician gently inserts the introducer through the cervical canal into the lowest part of the uterus. The physician may steady the uterus with a *tenaculum,* a special forceps, applied to the cervix. The application of the tenaculum may cause a minimum of pain, like a pinprick. The IUD is ejected from the introducer into the uterine cavity, where it regains its original shape. The introducer is withdrawn, leaving the IUD tail (plastic threads hanging from the IUD, which pass through the cervix into the upper part of the vagina). The threads are carefully trimmed so that only an inch or two remains visible.

The Immediate Postinsertion Period

A number of minor problems associated with IUDs occur immediately after insertion. Many women experience nausea and vomiting after insertion. For that reason, it might be advisable for an IUD candidate to avoid a heavy meal prior to the procedure. Women may also feel faint, become pale, sweat profusely, experience cramps, have heart palpitations, or have a drop in blood pressure. These "vaso-vagal" symptoms are well known and are caused by the manipulation of the cervix, but are transient and certainly not as serious as they seem. They can be somewhat alleviated by medication—tranquilizers, aspirin, and painkillers, as previously described. A woman should remain on the examining table for at least five minutes following insertion, and she should not get up until these symptoms have passed, even if she stays there an hour. Once a woman feels well enough to stand, she should sit in the doctor's office for a short time, or until she feels completely confident in venturing out into the street. On the other hand, some women, particularly those who have had children, have no problems with the insertion and find the procedure as simple and benign as a routine pelvic examination.

A woman should not have any sexual intercourse for a few days after insertion. She should let the bleeding subside and allow the mucus of the uterus to form around the device, lowering the chances for infection. A woman should not use a tampon for several days following insertion, but should, rather, rely on a sanitary napkin. Foreign bodies should not be inserted into the vagina soon after the IUD.

During the first few months, a woman may experience some bleeding after intercourse. The penis may touch the uterus, causing contractions and bleeding from the irritated endometrium. In addition, the cycle might be shorter, so a woman might experience her menstrual period more often. Most low-grade infections that do occur can be treated quickly with antibiotics, and progesterone can be given to relieve cramping. A woman should, however, see a doctor about any severe cramping or pain.

The IUD should be checked by a physician after the first menstrual period following insertion, so that it can be ascertained that the device has not been displaced or expelled. The position of the IUD should be evaluated by a physician every six months.

The Pros and Cons of IUDs

The intrauterine device is probably the most effective form of contraception, after the oral contraceptive. The failure rate of the IUD ranges from 1.0 to 5 pregnancies per 100 woman-years of use and is dependent upon the type of device employed and the clinic or doctors who perform the actual insertion. IUDs provide extremely effective contraception without the introduction of drugs into the system (with the exception of the progesterone-bearing IUD). After the initial insertion and an occasional check that the IUD is still in place, a woman with an IUD is freed from continuous conscious concern over contraception; there is no need for daily medication or any type of device such as a diaphragm or a condom, and sexual intercourse can be completely spontaneous.

An IUD is usually an effective contraceptive from the moment of its insertion, but there is a marginal chance of pregnancy during the first month. It is usually advisable to use a spermicidal foam or a condom during the first month after insertion. If a woman is changing from an oral contraceptive to an IUD, it may be best for her to continue taking the birth-control pills for the first month after insertion. The pill prevents any accidental pregnancy and also helps reduce the amount of bleeding that normally accompanies the first month of IUD use. For some former users of oral contraceptives, this will not be possible. Since the birth-control pills have a tendency to diminish the size of the uterus, a woman's physician may suggest she stop taking oral contraceptives one or two months prior to insertion of an IUD to make the insertion somewhat easier.

The pregnancy rate with the IUD is higher in younger women, and declines with increasing age and decreasing fertility. In general, the greatest number of pregnancies occur during the first year after insertion. The pregnancy rate decreases with each succeeding year of use. The contraceptive effect is completely and immediately reversible simply by removing the IUD.

Can a Man Feel the Tail of the IUD?

Men occasionally say that they can feel the tail of an IUD during intercourse. This may be just the power of suggestion or, for the first time, they may notice they are touching the cervix. The cervical tails on the IUD can be cut shorter, and the doctor can check this to make certain the device has not actually slipped out of position. There is a greater chance that a man might feel the tail in the woman-dominant position, as the uterus does hang down slightly.

In general, however, a partner *cannot* feel the tail.

Bleeding and Pain

Many women with IUDs experience an increase in the amount and length of the menstrual flow for the first few periods after insertion. In some women, the menstrual cycle becomes temporarily shorter, so for a few months, a woman who has had a period every twenty-eight days may have her period every twenty-six days. Other IUD users experience bleeding and spotting between the menstrual periods soon after the insertion of the device. Since an increase in bleeding, both menstrual and intermenstrual, is not uncommon with an IUD, a woman must be aware of the possible development of a

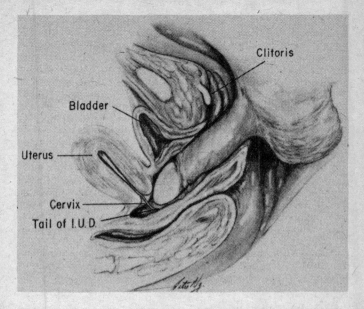

Fig. 9-10: The relationship between the female and male genitalia during intercourse. An IUD is located inside the uterus. The tail of the IUD is located high in the vagina, behind the cervix, and should not be felt by the man during intercourse. The location of the clitoris is compared to the penis; friction between the clitoris and the penis does not occur in the male superior position.

mild anemia. She might, therefore, find it advisable to take an iron supplement.

Increased uterine cramping at the time of the first few post-insertion menstrual periods is not uncommon. This cramping usually subsides as the uterus adjusts to the presence of the device. However, approximately one in ten women has the device removed within the first year of use because of side effects such as bleeding and pain. Other effective forms of contraception are available and no woman should go to heroic extremes to retain an IUD if her body does not tolerate it. In fact, if an IUD is still causing trouble four to six weeks after insertion, you are either one of the ten percent who cannot use IUDs or you are using the wrong type for you. In such a case, demand the removal of the IUD.

Expulsion

The IUD is a foreign body within the uterus, and the increased cramping (increased uterine contractions) is an attempt by the uterus to get rid of this foreign body. At times, it is successful and the device is expelled. About one in ten devices is expelled within a year of insertion. There is no way to predict who will tolerate an IUD and who will expel one. If a woman has expelled her first IUD, there is a very good chance she will expel a second. The majority of expulsions occurs during the first months following insertion—the period of increased bleeding and cramping. The longer the device remains in the uterus, the less is the chance of spontaneous expulsion.

A woman with an IUD should be particularly observant during her menstrual period. She should return to her physician after the first postinsertion menstrual period to have the position of the IUD checked. During the first and all successive menstrual periods, a woman should check tampons or pads after removal to make sure the device has not been expelled with the menstrual flow. If an IUD has threads leading into the vagina, a woman should check these threads after each menstruation. If they cannot be felt, she should see her physician to determine if the device is still in place.

IUDs and Pelvic Infection

There is no evidence of an increase in the incidence of simple vaginal infections, such as monilia, in IUD users. However, there have been reports that there is an increased incidence of the more serious pelvic infections in women with IUDs. Since they are sterilely packaged and inserted, the pelvic infections do not come from the IUDs themselves. The infection usually comes from the vagina. It has been theorized that the presence of the IUD, and particularly the vaginal threads of the IUD, causes the cervical canal to remain slightly more dilated than it normally would. It is this minimal dilation of the cervix that permits passage of bacteria from the vagina, via the IUD threads and the cervical canal, into the uterus.

The most common type of pelvic infection in IUD users remains localized in the uterus. This type of infection, called *endometritis,* results in discharge and severe pain which worsens during intercourse. Fortunately, this condition is usually successfully treated with antibiotics on an ambulatory basis. If it is left untreated, the infection can spread to the fallopian tubes, causing *salpingitis.* There appears to be an increasing number of infections in one fallopian tube, *single-sided salpingitis,* in women with IUDs.

If an IUD user feels a sharp pain on one side, she should immediately have this condition examined to determine if it is single-sided salpingitis, tubal pregnancy, or some other condition, such as appendicitis. If salpingitis is diagnosed, it can often be successfully treated with antibiotics without the removal of the IUD. However, if the physician determines that the response to antibiotics is not satisfactory, he may remove the IUD, which often speeds recovery. If the salpingitis is left untreated, tubal abscesses can develop, and can lead to sterility.

Salpingitis could also spread into the pelvic cavity and lead to pelvic inflammatory disease, PID (See Chapter 7, Venereal Disease). Mild PID can be treated on an outpatient basis with antibiotics. In severe cases, the patients must be hospitalized and treated with intravenous infusions of antibiotics, and the IUDs must be removed. The insertion of an IUD in a woman who has had a previous PID can cause a flare-up of symptoms if the previous infection is not completely under control. Women who have had PID can use an IUD, but their physicians must make certain that the previous infection has been totally eliminated. It is unfortunate, but almost all forms of PID, particularly gonorrhea, are more severe in women with IUDs. A woman with an IUD must be aware of her increased susceptibility and, thus, must be more vigilant concerning any signs of infection.

Perforation by the IUD

In rare instances, an IUD can pass through or perforate the wall of the uterus and travel into the abdomen. The reported incidence of uterine perforation varies from report to report and with the type of IUD used—from 0.5 in 1000 to as high as 5 in 1000 insertions. A major factor in the incidence of perforation appears to be the skill with which the IUD is inserted. Particular care must be taken with postabortion and postdelivery insertions of IUDs. Since the uterine wall is soft and thin, it is very easy for the device to be pushed through the wall at this time. An IUD with a less rounded edge tends to perforate the uterine wall spontaneously, perhaps as it is pushed out of the uterine cavity by contractions. Perforation by an IUD is not usually dangerous. The device is usually caught by the *omentum*, which encapsulates the device and prevents complication. However, if one of the copper-bearing devices perforates, there is a chance it will cause a dense adhesion in the peritoneal cavity; it should, then, be surgically removed. If there is suspicion that an IUD has perforated the uterus, its location should be determined by X-ray. An IUD which has perforated can

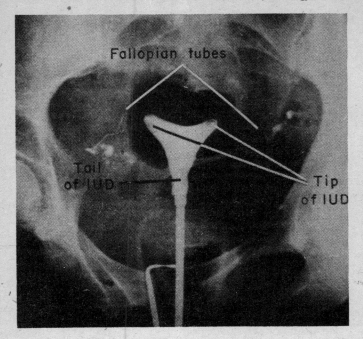

Fig. 9-11: This X-ray of the uterus and fallopian tubes (hysterosal-pingogram) illustrates how the Ypsilon conforms to the uterine cavity. The uterus and the fallopian tubes are completely normal. If a physician cannot see the tail of the IUD, he usually suggests an X-ray of the uterus to determine if the IUD is still in place.

usually be removed with the aid of a laparoscope (see Laparoscopy, in Chapter 10).

Pregnancy and the IUD

If an IUD user becomes pregnant, she has a relatively higher chance for an ectopic (tubal) pregnancy than a woman who becomes pregnant without an IUD. There are two possible explanations for this. In general, the incidence of tubal pregnancy ranges from 1 in 120 to 1 in 200 pregnancies. The presence of an IUD usually prevents implantation of the fertilized egg in the uterus, but may have no effect on implantation in the fallopian tube. Therefore, while preventing most uterine pregnancies, the IUD is not able to prevent extrauterine pregnancy. Secondly, since an IUD renders the wearer more susceptible to tubal infection, the normal passage of the egg down the fallopian tube can be impeded by tubal inflammation. An ectopic pregnancy can result. An IUD user should be aware of these possibilities and alert to any delayed period, particularly when accompanied by one-sided pain. She should seek immediate attention with the onset of any such symptoms.

If uterine pregnancy occurs in a woman using an IUD, there is about a 50 percent chance that she can carry the infant to term and deliver without any ill effects either to herself or the infant. Approximately half of all IUD wearers spontaneously abort uterine pregnancies.

There have been a number of cases of septic abortion among IUD users, some associated with *septicemia* (severe infection in the blood), septic shock, and even death. Septic abortion has been particularly related to the Dalkon Shield, perhaps due to its particular configuration and its braided vaginal strings, which may render it a more efficient vehicle for the transmission of infection. There have been reports of severe infection and even death due to septic abortion with other IUDs, but to a lesser degree. It is estimated that 15 in 1000 pregnancies occurring with the IUD result in death from septic abortion.

It is strongly suggested that an IUD be removed as early as possible in any woman who becomes pregnant with the IUD. The fertilized egg in an IUD pregnancy usually implants higher up in the uterus than the IUD. Because of this, an IUD can usually be removed easily without disturbing the developing pregnancy. This is particularly true if the vaginal strings are visible. If the strings are not visible, the IUD may have to be removed under general anesthesia and, perhaps, in combination with termination of pregnancy.

Cancer and the IUD

There has been some concern that because the IUD is a foreign body within the uterus it might act as a constant irritant to this organ and increase the user's chances of developing cancer. However, there is no difference in the incidence of cervical cancer among women with IUDs, women on oral contraceptives, and women who use no form of birth control. Women who regularly use a diaphragm have a somewhat lower incidence of cervical cancer.

Removal of the IUD

The removal of an IUD is much easier than its insertion, particularly if the string is visible and the IUD is not imbedded in the uterine wall. The Dalkon Shield appears to have a propensity for imbedding and, on occasion, has to be removed under general anesthesia. The majority of other IUDs have a smooth surface and are easy to remove. The removal is usually associated with cramping, which subsides within a few minutes after the procedure. It is probably better for the device to be removed during the menstrual period. If the threads are not visible, removal is somewhat more difficult and is accomplished with a long, narrow metal device, similar to a uterine sound, with a smooth hook at the end.

Summary

An intrauterine contraceptive device is recommended for women who do not want to take oral contraceptives but wish to have a contraceptive technique more effective than barrier methods such as the diaphragm and the condom. The IUD offers the added advantage of contraception without the need of conscious control. Not every woman can tolerate the presence of the IUD in the uterus, and there is no way to predict who can tolerate an IUD and who cannot. IUDs are generally a more successful form of contraception for multiparous women (women who have already given birth). These women seem to have fewer problems with irritation and contractions of the uterus and are less likely to expel an IUD. If a nulliparous woman (one who has not given birth) is fitted correctly with the appropriate IUD and does not expel the device, this can offer an excellent method of contraception. As a general rule, IUD users are somewhat older than users of oral contraceptives.

If you decide to use an intrauterine device, be sure to ask your physician what type of device is to be used. Once your device is inserted, *remember its name*. If it has to be changed periodically, as with the copper and progesterone-bearing devices, if any type of complication should occur, or if you simply wish to have it removed, it is imperative that you know what device you are using.

ORAL CONTRACEPTION

The development of the oral contraceptive is one of the most far-reaching and socially influential discoveries of modern science. Birth-control pills are the most widely prescribed drugs, currently used by more than fifty million women throughout the world. Their popularity is evidence of their general acceptance and enormous social impact.

It is easy to see why oral contraceptives are so popular. Short of sterilization, they are the most effective way to prevent unwanted pregnancy; they are nearly 100 percent effective. In fact, far more pregnancies result from forgetting to take the pill than from an actual drug failure. Although there are still many unanswered questions, oral contraceptives appear relatively safe. The contraceptive effects of the pill are usually reversible, making it useful for family planning. Women do not have to rely on either the promises of their partners or tedious preparations. Although some have called the pill an insult to the physiology of a woman's body and have proved its serious, and sometimes fatal, consequences, the benefits of this form of contraception still seem to outweigh its admitted dangers.

History of Oral Contraceptives

The search for an effective oral contraceptive is centuries old. Hundreds of years ago, women took arsenic and strychnine to prevent pregnancy. More women probably died from ingesting these poisons than would have died from the resulting pregnancies.

The discovery of the modern oral contraceptives is based on a simple but obvious fact of nature: Once a woman is pregnant, she will not become pregnant again during this pregnancy. Hormones produced in the ovaries are responsible for the development of a woman's secondary sexual characteristics. The possible role of these hormones in the maintenance or the prevention of pregnancy was clarified in the 1900s. It was then observed by a German scientist that if the corpus luteum, which secretes progesterone, was removed from the ovary following ovulation, implantation of a fertilized egg would not occur. On the other hand, if the corpus luteum was left intact, the egg would implant, but the development and release of other eggs from the ovary was prevented.

American investigators in the late 1920s identified progesterone as the active ingredient in the corpus luteum that maintained the pregnancy of a released and fertilized egg. In 1929, the hormone estrogen was isolated from the Graafian follicle of the rat ovary. Initially, progesterone was obtained in limited amounts only from animal sources and then purified. This made it a relatively expensive substance which was active only in an injectable form. The discovery, in 1944, that proges-

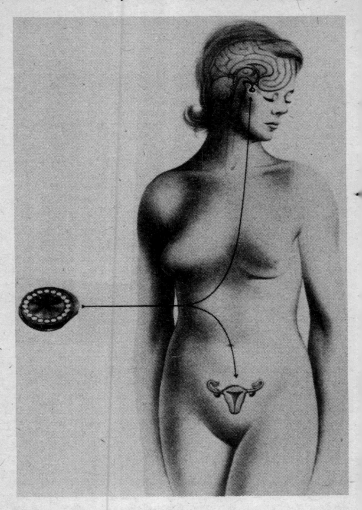

Fig. 9–12: Birth-control pills affect both the brain hormones and the uterus. The hormones in the birth-control pills suppress the body's hormones and, thus, control the menstrual cycle and prevent ovulation. (Courtesy of Ortho Pharmaceutical Corporation, Raritan, New Jersey.)

progesterone could be synthesized from plant steroids found in the root of the wild Mexican yam made an orally active and relatively inexpensive synthetic progesterone available.

Once these hormones were available, their effects on menstrual disorders and the inhibition of ovulation were investigated. In 1953, Dr. Pincus reported that ovulation could be inhibited in animals with a synthetic progestin. These results were confirmed in a group of volunteer women in the Boston area by Dr. Rock. In 1956, the famous Puerto Rican studies were undertaken with Enovid, an oral contraceptive containing both estrogen and progesterone. Their effectiveness as contraceptives was proven and the first birth-control pill, Enovid-10, was released in the United States four years later.

How Does the Pill Work?

Most simply, oral contraceptives produce a state of pseudopregnancy, which prevents the development and release of an ovum. This state of pseudopregnancy is produced by interference with the delicate balance of hormones produced in the brain and in the ovary during the normal menstrual cycle (see Chapter 5, The Reproductive Cycle).

Ingestion of the *combined oral contraceptives,* those containing both estrogen and progesterone, produces a constant level of estrogen and progesterone in the blood, which, in turn, replaces the normal hormonal variation during the menstrual cycle. The combined oral contraceptives exert their contraceptive influence at two different points, making them particularly effective. Primarily, the steady level of estrogen inhibits the release of FSH (follicle stimulating hormone) from the pituitary. FSH stimulates the maturation of eggs in the ovary; by inhibiting FSH, the estrogen inhibits ovulation. The progesterone in the combined pill produces changes in the cervical mucus, which prevent the passage of sperm into the uterus. The progesterone makes the mucus thick and acts almost as a natural diaphragm.

The steady level of estrogen-progesterone produced by the combined birth-control pill causes a change in the lining of the uterus. The endometrium does not build up under the steady level of hormones from the pill, as it does during the normal menstrual cycle. The bleeding experienced by a woman on oral contraceptives is a withdrawal bleeding, resulting from the drop in the estrogen-progesterone blood level when the pills are not taken for seven of the twenty-eight days. It is not a true menstruation, and this withdrawal bleeding is usually less than that experienced with normal, or true, menstruation.

The sequential oral contraceptives reflect an attempt to produce an effective contraceptive that more closely mimics the flow of hormones during the normal menstrual cycle. Estrogen alone is taken for fourteen days; this prevents ovulation. Progesterone is then taken with the estrogen for seven days to cause a build-up in the endometrium similar to the buildup following ovulation. No pills are taken for the next seven days, during which menstruation occurs.

The sequentials, which are no longer available in the United States, were particularly attractive to women with low tolerance for progesterone, but they were less effective than the combined pills, because the secondary contraceptive effect of progesterone on the cervical mucus was absent for the first two weeks of the cycle. Also, if a single pill of the sequential series was forgotten or missed, ovulation could occur.

The minipill contains no estrogen, only progesterone. It exerts contraceptive effectiveness primarily by causing the cervical mucus to thicken and act as a natural diaphragm or barrier to the passage of sperm. The progesterone also interferes with the normal buildup of the uterine lining; thus, if fertilization does take place, the endometrium will not be receptive to implantation. It is believed that the minipill does not interfere with ovulation. For that reason, the pregnancy rate with this oral contraceptive is higher than with the other birth-control pills.

Types of Oral Contraceptives

The first oral contraceptives released in the United States in 1960 contained ten to twenty times more progestin and two to three times more estrogen than needed. The reported severe side effects related to the oral contraceptives were, in most cases, related to the high-dose contraceptive initially released. As the estrogen level in birth-control pills was lowered, there was a decrease in occurrence of severe side effects. A woman should know which birth-control pill she is taking and how much estrogen is in that pill. If her oral contraceptive contains more than 50 micrograms of estrogen, she should request a lower dose from her physician. If a woman is new to the pill, she should start on a low-estrogen dose; if side effects occur, the estrogen can then be altered accordingly. A list of the presently available combined oral contraceptives follows.

Name	Year Released	Estrogen	(in micrograms)	Progestin	(in milligrams)
Enovid-E	1964	Mestranol	100 mcg	Norethynodrel	2.5 mg
Ortho-Novum-2	1963	Mestranol	100 mcg	Norethindrone	2.0 mg
Norinyl	1964	Mestranol	100 mcg	Norethindrone	2.0 mg
Ovulen	1966	Mestranol	100 mcg	Ethynodiol diacetate	1.0 mg
Ortho-Novum 1 + 80	1968	Mestranol	80 mcg	Norethindrone	1.0 mg
Norinyl 1 + 80	1968	Mestranol	80 mcg	Norethindrone	1.0 mg
Enovid-5	1962	Mestranol	75 mcg	Norethynodrel	5.0 mg
Ortho-Novum-10	1963	Mestranol	60 mcg	Norethynodrel	10.0 mg
Norlestrin-2.5	1964	Ethinyl estradiol	50 mcg	Norethindrone acetate	1.0 mg
Demulen	1970	Ethinyl estradiol	50 mcg	Ethynodiol diacetate	1.0 mg
Norlestrin 1 + 50	1967	Ethinyl estradiol	50 mcg	Norethindrone acetate	1.0 mg
Zorane 1 + 50	1974	Ethinyl estradiol	50 mcg	Norethindrone acetate	1.0 mg
Ortho-Novum 1 + 50	1967	Mestranol	50 mcg	Norethindrone	1.0 mg
Norinyl 1 + 50	1967	Mestranol	50 mcg	Norethindrone	1.0 mg
Ovral	1968	Ethinyl estradiol	50 mcg	Norgestrel	0.5 mg
Ovcon-50	1976	Ethinyl estradiol	50 mcg	Norethindrone	1.0 mg
Brevicon	1975	Ethinyl estradiol	35 mcg	Norethindrone	0.5 mg
Modicon	1975	Ethinyl estradiol	35 mcg	Norethindrone	0.5 mg
Ovcon-35	1976	Ethinyl estradiol	35 mcg	Norethindrone	0.4 mg
Loestrin 1.5 + 30	1973	Ethinyl estradiol	30 mcg	Norethindrone acetate	1.5 mg
Zorane 1.5 + 30	1974	Ethinyl estradiol	30 mcg	Norethindrone acetate	1.5 mg
Lo-ovral	1975	Ethinyl estradiol	30 mcg	Norgestrel	0.3 mg
Loestrin 1 + 20	1973	Ethinyl estradiol	20 mcg	Norethindrone acetate	1.0 mg
Zorane 1 + 20	1974	Ethinyl estradiol	20 mcg	Norethindrone acetate	1.0 mg

Oral contraceptives contain one of two types of estrogen, either *ethinyl estradiol* or *mestranol*. Ethinyl estradiol is slightly more potent than mestranol.

There are basically five different types of progestin currently used in the combination oral contraceptives: *norethynodrel, norethindrone, norethindrone acetate, ethynodiol diacetate,* and *norgestrel.* These synthetic progestins, with the exception of norgestrel, have some estrogenic effect. On a weight-for-weight basis, norgestrel is the most potent progestational agent, and, in addition, it has the highest androgenic activity of all the progestins.

It is both the amount of estrogen and the characteristics of the progestin in the oral contraceptive that contribute to the effects of the pill on a woman's system. If the oral contraceptive produces nausea, breast soreness, and water retention—the estrogen-related symptoms—a pill with lower estrogen should be taken. On the other hand, if side effects such as amenorrhea or acne occur, it is advisable to change to a pill with higher estrogen or a progestin with less androgenic activity. The option in relation to what type of oral contraceptive to use when side effects occur will be discussed more fully under the individual side effects.

These sequential birth-control pills were taken by approximately 1 million women in the United States in 1976:

Name	Year Released	Estrogen	(in micrograms)	Progestin	(in milligrams)
Oracon	1965	Ethinyl estradiol	100 mcg	Dimethisterone	25 mg
Ortho-Novum SQ	1966	Mestranol	80 mcg	Norethindrone	2 mg
Norquen	1967	Mestranol	80 mcg	Norethindrone	2 mg

These pills all contain more than the recommended 50 micrograms of estrogen and have a failure rate of 2 pregnancies per 100 woman-years of use. For years, many physicians have not recommended sequentials and, because of their high levels of estrogen and high failure rates, they have been banned from some European countries. Recently, there was evidence of a link between uterine cancer and the sequential oral contraceptives. The FDA subsequently recommended that drug companies withdraw these pills from the market. Any woman still taking sequentials should consult her physician and change to a combined contraceptive.

The *minipills* contain no estrogen and have a high rate of irregular bleeding. The three minipills presently marketed are:

Name	Year Released	Progestin	(in milligrams)
Micronor	1973	Norethindrone	0.35 mg
Nor-Q.D.	1973	Norethindrone	0.35 mg
Ovrette	1973	Norgestrel	0.075 mg

The failure rate on the minipill is higher than with the combined pills, ranging from 1.1 to 3.7 pregnancies per 100 woman-years of use. Women who cannot tolerate estrogen should be the only users of the minipill. It should not be taken by women who experience irregular menses.

Who Can Take the Pill?

The majority of women can take oral contraceptives. Women who use oral contraceptives must be sufficiently motivated to take the pill day after day and must be free of certain health problems. Oral contraceptives are particularly attractive to women who strongly wish to avoid pregnancy and would be adverse to abortion in the case of contraceptive failure. They are an excellent form of contraception for women who have active sex lives, as well as for women who suffer from dysmenorrhea or premenstrual tension.

If a woman wishes to use birth-control pills, she must first undergo an interview and an examination, either by her physician or in a family-planning clinic. The purpose of the interview is to reveal past medical and family history of any condition that might be a contraindication for the use of oral contraceptives. If there are contraindications, the physician should suggest another, more appropriate, method of contraception. However, if the medical history is benign, the physician performs a complete physical examination, including blood pressure, to rule out hypertension, a pelvic examination to exclude uterine abnormalities such as fibroid tumors, and a breast exam to determine any form of breast tumors. All are contraindications to the pill. A urine specimen should be obtained for analysis of sugar and protein levels to rule out diabetes or any kidney condition.

If a woman is placed on birth-control pills, she should see her physician at least twice a year. At this biannual visit, blood pressure should be checked, breasts examined, and urine analysis performed. A Pap smear should be taken once a year.

Absolute Contraindications to the Pill

Women who have any of the following conditions *must not* take oral contraceptives:

Thrombophlebitis. The formation of a blood clot within a vein, which then breaks loose and travels to another part of the body (such as the lung or the brain), with the potential of causing extreme damage and even death.

Cerebral Vascular Disease or Accident. A history of stroke, aneurysm, or any other form of intracranial bleeding.

Cardiovascular Disease. Abnormalities in the vascular system, such as a history of *myocardial infarction* (heart attack) or congenital heart abnormalities.

Markedly Impaired Liver Function. Liver damage subsequent to conditions such as severe hepatitis or cirrhosis.

Malignancy of the Reproductive System. Suspected or treated cancer of the breast or uterus.

Pregnancy. The hormones in the oral contraceptives can cause congenital malformation in the fetus.

Other Conditions that Usually Prohibit the Pill

Women who have the following conditions *should not* take oral contraceptives:

Hypertension. Women with severe high blood pressure who are on antihypertensives should not take oral contraceptives. Women with mild hypertension can take the pill, but they should be placed on a low-estrogen pill. These women must be carefully monitored and should be seen every three months for blood-pressure checks.

Diabetes. Oral contraceptives can interfere with carbohydrate metabolism. Therefore, women with diabetes who require daily insulin administration should not use oral contraceptives. Prediabetic women and women in whom the diabetes can be controlled by diet alone can take birth-control pills. These women should be placed on a low-dose estrogen pill and must be closely followed by their physicians with annual or semiannual glucose-tolerance tests.

Fibroid Tumors. The growth of fibroid tumors can be stimulated by estrogen. If a woman with fibroids insists on oral contraceptives, she should be placed on the lowest-dose estrogen or on the minipill.

Conditions that Limit the Pill

Oral contraceptives are potent drugs which cause profound effects throughout the body. When deciding on the value of birth-control pills, a woman must weigh the advantages against the problems in order to make an intelligent and informed decision. There are a number of conditions that appear to be affected by oral contraceptives, and women with these conditions must be aware of the possible adverse effects of the pill. These conditions are epilepsy, migraine headaches, and significant psychological disorders, such as severe depression. Women with these conditions should be on a low-estrogen dose and should be aware that if the condition becomes worse, oral contraceptives should be terminated. Women suffering from severe asthma should probably not take oral contraceptives, since any water retention may adversely affect the lungs. Women who are over thirty-five and heavy smokers should use an alternative form of contraception, because of a significant increase in cardiovascular problems. Women with varicose veins can take oral contraceptives, but they should be particularly alert to any occurrence of leg pain indicative of blood-clotting disorders. Women who have sickle cell anemia or who are breast-feeding should also refrain from the pill. Sickle cell trait is not, however, a contraindication.

Age and Oral Contraceptives

The years between about sixteen and thirty-five are the most fertile time of a woman's life. During these years, the birth-control pill is a most attractive form of contraception because of its great effectiveness. Because women who have not had children usually have a harder time adjusting to an IUD, oral contraceptives are particularly acceptable to younger women. Women who have a number of sexual partners usually would rather depend on the great protection afforded by birth-control pills rather than worry about less effective techniques such as barrier methods. Finally, women at this age have, as a group, a lower incidence of those medical problems which contraindicate the use of oral contraceptives.

Women under eighteen who are sexually active can take birth-control pills, since the risk of the pills is probably less than the risk of an abortion. As with older women, a teenager experiencing only intermittent sex, perhaps once every few months, might be better off with some other contraceptive technique. If a teenager is having very irregular periods, early use of oral contraceptives is not strongly recommended.

There has been some concern that early use of oral contraceptives stunts growth, but this is *not* true. Estrogen must be given in *very* high doses—amounts that far exceed the amount in birth-control pills—for a long period of time immediately following puberty to have even a 50 percent chance of limiting growth. A teenager who assumes the adult responsibility of sexual intercourse must also realize her responsibility to protect herself from unwanted pregnancy. Oral contraceptives should be available to her.

After the age of forty, the risks involved with oral contraceptives, particularly the risks of myocardial infarction (heart attack), must be carefully weighed against the risk of pregnancy and the acceptability of other forms of contraception. For women over forty, the excess risk of developing a fatal heart attack is 27.6 per 100,000 women on the pill; this is particularly aggravated by smoking. However, the risk of death is 124.1 fatalities per 100,000 pregnancies in women between 40 and 44. Pregnancy is still more of a risk than the pill, but since fertility is lower in this age group, other contraceptive techniques should be closely examined. If a woman over forty elects to use oral contraceptives, she should take a pill containing less than 50 micrograms of estrogen and must be carefully followed by her physician.

How to Take the Pill

Once a woman and her physician determine she is a candidate for oral contraception, she can take the pills on the following schedule:

Combined Oral Contraceptives. A woman counts the very first sign of menstrual bleeding as day 1 of her cycle. On day 5, she starts taking the combined estrogen-progesterone pills for twenty-one days. If she has a twenty-eight-day pill packet, she takes a placebo for seven days. After these seven placebo or pill-less days, no matter when withdrawal bleeding has initiated, she will restart her pills. In other words, if a woman starts taking the combined birth-control pills on a Sunday, she takes her last effective pill twenty-one days later on a Saturday. She then takes either a placebo for seven days or no pill for seven days. She starts her new packet of pills on Sunday again. From that day forward, she always starts a new packet every twenty-eight days on Sunday. The pill packets are usually designed so the pills are matched with the days of the week. In this way, it is easy to determine if a pill has been taken or forgotten.

Sequentials. The instructions for the proper administration of the sequential oral contraceptives are omitted, since these drugs have been removed from the market.

Minipills. As with the combined birth-control pills, a woman originally starts the minipill on day 5 of her cycle. However, the minipills are taken constantly, day after day, with no interruption in the medication.

Most women on oral contraceptives try to incorporate taking the pill into their daily schedule to minimize the chance of missing a pill and in any way diminishing protection. An attempt should be made to take the pill at the same time every day to keep a steady level of drug in the body. A number of women find that the side effects are fewer if the pills are taken after the evening meal or right before bedtime. A woman should have an extra packet of oral contraceptives at her place of work or in the purse she uses every day just in case she forgets to take the pill at home.

What If a Pill Is Forgotten?

If a pill is forgotten, a woman should take that pill as soon as she remembers it and the next pill at its regular time, even if it means taking two pills during the same twenty-four-hour period. If a woman forgets to take the oral contraceptives two days in a row, she should take two pills as soon as she remembers and two pills the following day. She should also employ some additional form of contraception, such as a spermicidal foam or condom, for the remaining part of the cycle. If the pills are forgotten for three or more days, no further pills should be taken from that packet. In that case, a woman should stay off the pills for seven days and then start a new packet. During this time, and for the next cycle on the pills, there is a chance that ovulation will occur, and additional contraception must be employed. A second school of thought lets a woman who has missed three consecutive pills continue taking the pill by starting the new packet of pills immediately. This may, however, cause some irregular bleeding.

If a woman forgets two or more pills during a cycle and her period is delayed, she should have a pregnancy test prior to initiating a new pill packet. If any *minipills* are forgotten, a woman must immediately double up on the pill. Since there is a high failure rate with the minipill, an additional form of contraception should be used for three to four weeks even if a single pill is missed.

How Long Can a Woman Stay on the Pill?

A woman can use oral contraceptives for as long as she wishes. There are at the present time no contraindications for taking the pill for ten or even twenty years. A woman must see her physician at least annually, and biannually after age thirty-five, when she is on birth-control pills. However, the prolonged administration of pills is directly dependent on the absence of any adverse reaction or the occurrence of any of the conditions previously described as absolute contraindications to the pill.

In the past, it was routine for a woman to stop the pills every two or three years to let the body "recycle." A woman stopped taking the pills until she experienced three menstrual cycles and then would start them again, leaving herself unprotected for a period of up to six months. It was theorized that such a routine recycling acted as a check of the normal interaction of the pituitary and the ovary. This theory is given little credence today. A woman need *not* stop the pills to recycle.

Vitamins, Iron, and the Pill

There is an increased need for vitamins B_1, B_6, B_{11}, B_{12}, and vitamin C when oral contraceptives are used. Of these vitamins, the need for vitamin B_6 seems to be the greatest. The birth-control pill creates a pseudopregnancy; it is, therefore, easy to understand why a woman needs extra vitamin intake. The requirement for iron might, however, be slightly reduced; women on oral contraceptives tend to bleed less, and thus lose less iron. There is also an increase in iron absorption when a woman is taking the pill. It is suggested that women take at least one multiple vitamin daily, preferably a vitamin with a high concentration of vitamin B_6. Several such pills are now available (for example, the Feminins tablets). Instead of a multiple vitamin, an extra vitamin-B complex, possibly in combination with vitamin C, can be taken, especially for women who feel tired and run down. The extra intake of vitamin B_6 might also help prevent acne and depression.

The Pros and Cons of Oral Contraceptives

The combined oral contraceptives are usually effective in the prevention of pregnancy from the taking of the first pill. Dur-

ing the first month, there is a minimal chance of escape ovulation, and some backup form of contraception such as a condom or spermicide should be used. The failure rate of the combined birth-control pills is estimated at 0.1 pregnancy per 100 woman-years of use if the oral contraceptives are taken according to schedule. However, since human error cannot be eliminated and pills can be forgotten, the actual failure rate is from 2 to 5 pregnancies per 100 woman-years. Any woman who consistently has difficulty remembering to take her birth-control pills on schedule should examine her attitude toward the pills and contraception in general.

Freedom from the fear of pregnancy is the greatest benefit of the oral contraceptives to many women. Sexual intercourse may be enjoyed spontaneously, without the need for concern or for any preparation. Still, oral contraceptives have advantages other than effective birth control. Combination pills help regulate a woman's menstrual period, ease painful menstruation (dysmenorrhea), and decrease excessive bleeding from 50 to 75 percent. They prevent the cyclic buildup of hormonal peaks, which reduces the amount of uterine lining and subsequent menstrual flow. This helps women with anemia. The pill is valuable for women who tend to develop ovarian cysts, because it prevents formation of the Graafian follicle where the cysts can develop.

The pill is *not* intended to provide protection from venereal diseases. New regulations by the FDA require this warning information to be on all prescriptions for the pill in the United States. Additional information about possible side effects is also required.

The sequential birth-control pills have a theoretical failure rate of one to two pregnancies per hundred woman-years of use, even when taken faithfully. The minipill has a theoretical failure rate of one to four pregnancies per hundred woman-years when taken every day. The chances of escape ovulation are high if even a single minipill is forgotten. The majority of women who become pregnant on the minipill do so during the first six months. Some secondary form of contraception should be employed during this period to provide additional protection.

There are about twenty-five to thirty different brands of oral contraceptives currently available. The pill, especially the new low-estrogen type, is perhaps most popular in northern Europe. In the Netherlands, for example, nearly 35 percent of women use the pill in their birth-control programs. In the United States and Great Britain, the pill is taken by about 20 percent of women. The use of combination pills has been grow-

ing steadily, while, fortunately, the less effective and more dangerous sequentials have been removed from the market.

Side Effects of Oral Contraceptives

The rise and fall of estrogen and progesterone experienced with a normal menstrual cycle are replaced by steady levels of these hormones furnished by the combined birth-control pills. These artificial (pill-produced) steady levels of estrogen and progesterone give the pill its contraceptive effectiveness, but they are also responsible for its side effects. The side effects can be attributed to estrogen excess, progesterone excess, and, conversely, estrogen deficiency and progesterone deficiency. Some of the synthetic progestins have a degree of androgenic activity and can also be a source of pill-related side effects.

Minor "Estrogen Excess" Side Effects

Probably the most common side effects related to estrogen excess are nausea and vomiting, which usually occur only at first and subside after a while. Some women find these gastrointestinal side effects are minimized by taking the pill either following the evening meal or at bedtime. Dizziness is reported by about 2 of every 100 women. Headaches can occur at the beginning of the cycle, but if they persist from cycle to cycle, an alternate form of contraception should be found. Water retention is reflected in a number of possible symptoms—edema of the legs accompanied by leg cramps or cyclic breast enlargement and difficulty with the fit of contact lenses, caused by water retention swelling the entire eye. Water retention is usually mild and can be controlled by carefully watching salt intake and drinking adequate amounts of water to dilute sodium in the system. If the symptoms of water retention are more severe, diuretics might be taken for the last few days of the cycle prior to withdrawal bleeding.

An increase in breast size due to an increase in "female fat" deposition is also caused by estrogen excess. This condition is often considered a side benefit. *Leukorrhea,* a clear, nonodorous vaginal secretion, can also be an estrogen-related side effect, and while it may be a minor annoyance, it presents no medical problem.

One of the rare side effects related to estrogen excess is the appearance of freckles on the brow, across the bridge of the nose, and under the eyes; this is *cholasma,* the so-called mask of pregnancy. Cholasma most often appears after exposure to strong sunlight. Cholasma, while completely benign, is under-

standably disturbing from a cosmetic viewpoint. It usually is an indication that the birth-control pills should be replaced by some other form of contraception.

If any of the estrogen-excess side effects become difficult to tolerate, a woman should change to a pill with lower estrogen content or consider the minipill, which is estrogen-free.

Minor "Progesterone Excess" Side Effects

One of the most commonly reported side effects, occurring in almost 13 percent of oral contraceptive users, is depression. This change in mood is attributed to "progesterone excess." Levels of some vitamins are lowered by the use of oral contraceptives, and a dietary supplement containing vitamin B$_6$ may alleviate any pill-related depression. Progesterone excess sometimes causes an increased appetite, which can result in weight gain. Fatigue and tiredness can be the result of progesterone excess and can be partly eliminated by supplementary vitamins, particularly B$_6$. Progesterone excess, particularly in combination with estrogen deficiency, can alter the vaginal milieu and cause *monilia vaginitis*. If this condition persists even after local administration of antiyeast medication, a change to birth-control pills with lower progesterone or higher estrogen might be necessary.

A few women complain of decreased libido. If this occurs, change to another pill, perhaps one with a different type of progesterone, like norgestrel, which has a more androgenic or male-hormone effect. If this does not increase the libido, change to a pill with a higher estrogen content.

Oiliness of the skin or acne are usually caused by pills having a progesterone with stronger androgenic effects, particularly in combination with low estrogen (Lo-ovral, for one). These problems can usually be alleviated simply by changing to another brand with a less androgenic progesterone and a higher estrogen content.

Progesterone excess in combination with estrogen deficiency can cause irregular or no uterine bleeding. This is more common in women with a history of irregular bleeding, and occurs when the lining of the uterus does not build up sufficiently to be sloughed off during the seven days the pills are not taken. Pill-induced amenorrhea is not a serious condition per se, as it only indicates that the uterine lining is at rest. This can be beneficial, particularly for women who suffer from severe menstrual cramps. If a woman is concerned about absent or irregular bleeding, she should change to a pill with a higher estrogen content or a different progesterone. If amenorrhea occurs after the first pill cycle, particularly with the minipill, a woman should have a pregnancy test performed. Amenorrhea after three months on the pills, especially if no pills have been forgotten, is very seldom a sign of pregnancy. Regular menstrual bleeding usually starts again spontaneously once the pills have been discontinued. If the amenorrhea persists, the physician administers either a progesterone or an estrogen to trigger the cyclic hormone changes.

Minor Side Effects Related to Estrogen Deficiency

Side effects related to estrogen deficiency are most commonly found among users of the minipill. Estrogen deficiency can result in inadequate endometrial buildup. Spotting and breakthrough bleeding are common phenomena. Because of this, the minipill cannot be recommended to women who have histories of irregular bleeding.

Other symptoms of estrogen deficiency are fatigue, loss of libido, and acne. If any of these symptoms occurs, a woman should increase intake of vitamins, particularly B6. If this does not help, she should change to a pill with more estrogen.

Minor Side Effects Related to Progestin Deficiency

If the level of progesterone provided by the pill is insufficient, the development of the endometrium can be overstimulated, which can result in profuse bleeding that is often irregular in character and not cyclic. These symptoms are best treated by changing to another brand of pill which contains more progesterone in relationship to the estrogen.

Breakthrough Bleeding

Breakthrough bleeding is the term used to describe the occurrence of either vaginal bleeding or spotting at any time during the oral contraceptive cycle, other than the time of withdrawal or cyclic bleeding. This condition is a minor, but frequent, side effect of oral contraceptives. It is usually encountered during the first three cycles and may be caused by both estrogen and progesterone deficiency. A woman need not be concerned about *mild* vaginal spotting for the first few cycles, but if this persists after three cycles, she should inform her physician.

If a woman experiences true breakthrough bleeding, she should take two pills a day either until the bleeding stops or, preferably, until the end of the cycle. If bleeding persists at two pills per day, a third pill may be taken without worry. If breakthrough spotting or bleeding persists for more than three cycles, a pill with higher estrogen and progesterone should be considered.

Serious Side Effects Related to Oral Contraceptives

The serious side effects related to oral contraceptives are those that so profoundly disturb the normal functioning of a woman's body that they can lead to permanent damage or even death.

Thromboembolic Disorders. Thromboembolic disorders are the result of the abnormal formation of a blood clot within either a superficial (near the skin surface) or a deep vein. The increased incidence of thromboembolic disorders among women using contraceptives has received widespread publicity. Oral contraceptives increase the chances of developing some type of thromboembolic disorder by five to ten times. However, these statistics must be taken in perspective. Normally, each year 200 of 100,000 women of childbearing age develop *superficial thrombosis* (phlebitis) in the leg; among women taking oral contraceptives this number is increased to 300. The risk of *deep-vein thrombosis*, which is much more serious and potentially life threatening, is increased from 20 to 110 per 100,000 women per year. The risk of *thrombotic strokes (cerebral thrombosis)* is increased from 10 to 40 per 100,000 women per year. The presence of a number of pre-existent health problems such as hypertension, vascular problems, diabetes, and obesity appears to predispose women taking oral contraceptives to the development of clotting disorders. Smoking is a particularly potent factor in predisposing pill users to cerebral thrombosis. The clotting abnormalities appear to be related to the estrogen component, because the incidence of deep-vein thrombosis is reduced by 25 percent when estrogen is reduced to 50 micrograms. Thus, again and again the indications for low estrogen—below 50 micrograms—content in birth-control pills become stronger. Women are also advised to increase their fluid intake to help keep a good fluid balance. The effects on blood clotting exist only while the pills are being taken. Once a woman stops taking the oral contraceptives, the hormones rapidly metabolize and the increased risk disappears. Women scheduled for surgery should not take the pills for at least ten to fourteen days prior to the operative procedure. This reduces the chance of abnormal postoperative blood clotting.

The symptoms of early superficial phlebitis are tender and swollen leg veins. For deep thrombophlebitis, there is usually pain deep in the back of the legs. As the condition becomes more advanced, the leg swells.

The symptoms of cerebral thrombophlebitis are severe one-sided headaches and disturbance of vision. If any of these symptoms occurs, a woman should immediately stop taking the pill and contact her physician. Superficial phlebitis can usually be treated by local heat applications and aspirin. Deep-vein phlebitis and cerebral phlebitis require hospitalization and closely supervised anticoagulation treatment.

Heart Attack. The use of oral contraceptives increases a woman's chances for heart attack (myocardial infarction), particularly as her age increases, and even more so if she smokes. The incidence of fatal heart attack among nonusers between thirty and thirty-nine years old is less than 2 per 100,000 per year. This increases among users to 5.4 per 100,000 per year. Between ages forty to forty-four, risk of fatal heart attack among nonusers is approximately 3 per 100,000 per year and among users the risk is 20 per 100,000 per year. Although the risk of heart attack increases as age increases, particularly above forty, it must be remembered that these are the women who would be most at risk from the strain of pregnancy and/or delivery. The risk of the pill must be weighed against these risks. Still, if a woman over forty wishes to take the pill, she should take a very-low-estrogen pill.

Hypertension. Mild elevations in both *sytolic* and *diastolic* blood pressure are seen in women who have taken the birth-control pills over a period of years. In general, these elevations are quite small and do not elevate the blood pressure beyond normal levels. However, in 5 percent of women who take the pill for five years, the development of hypertension with blood pressure reading beyond 140/90 has been observed. Unfortunately, there is no way to predict in advance who will develop hypertension and who will not. In some women, the development of hypertension has been linked to some underlying medical problem, such as chronic kidney disease or the absence of a kidney, which would normally predispose a patient to hypertension.

The hypertensive effects in women who do not have any underlying disease processes are reversible, and blood pressure usually returns to normal once the pills are discontinued. It is essential to have blood pressure checked every six months, since hypertension is asymptomatic in its early stages. If a woman's physician fails to check her blood pressure, she should firmly request that readings be taken and perhaps consider another doctor. Women on oral contraceptives should limit their intake of salt, and, if they notice water retention, diuretics might be taken; these two measures can have antihypertensive effects.

Gallbladder Diseases. Gallstones occur about twice as frequently among users of birth-control pills. The hormones may cause the formation of gallstones by decreasing the amount of bile and increasing the cholesterol concentration in the bile. There also appears to be an increased incidence of *cholecystitis* (gallbladder infection) among pill users. Although these conditions may require surgery, they are rarely fatal.

Liver Tumors. Adenomas of the liver (liver tumors) are extremely rare. Forty-two cases have been reported in the last six years, and a statistical correlation between this condition and oral contraceptives has been established. There has been a further correlation between the types of estrogen used—a greater number of tumors occurred in women taking *mestranol* as opposed to *ethinyl estradiol.* Although the majority of these tumors have been benign, death from intraabdominal bleeding has been reported. The tumors are diagnosed by the discovery of abdominal masses. Women with such masses should see their physicians.

Pregnancy and the Pill

There is mounting evidence that if either progestins alone, such as in the minipill, or progestin-estrogen combinations, such as in the combined birth-control pills, are taken during the early part of pregnancy, congenital malformations may occur in the developing fetus. If a woman becomes pregnant while taking oral contraceptives, she should stop taking the pills the moment pregnancy is *confirmed.* There is no way to determine prior to birth whether the fetus has been severely affected by the pill, so early termination of pregnancy may be considered. The effects of the pill on the developing fetus can last even when conception has occurred after the pill has been stopped. There was an increased incidence of severe malformations among the spontaneously aborted fetuses of women who became pregnant soon after they had stopped taking high doses of oral contraceptives (estrogen above 50 mcg.). Although there is no such evidence indicting the low-dose oral contraceptives, a woman who wishes to conceive should stop taking the pills for at least three months prior to conception. This gives the body a chance to resume normal cyclic menstruation. Another form of contraception should be used in the interval.

Cancer and the Pill

There is no evidence that a woman who takes oral contraceptives increases her chances of developing breast cancer. In fact, the incidence of benign breast diseases, such as fibrocystic disease and chronic cystic mastitis, is less among pill users. Since the pill helps protect a woman against these benign breast diseases which are thought to predispose a woman to the development of breast cancer, it might protect her against breast cancer, although this has not been proven.

There is, similarly, no evidence that a woman who takes oral contraceptives increases her chances of developing cervical cancer. However, the portrait of the woman who runs the highest risk of cervical cancer (a woman who is sexually active at a young age, has a number of sexual partners, and has a child early in life) is probably the very woman who will opt for contraception via birth-control pills. One study showed that women who used the diaphragm rather than the pill for contraception had a lower incidence of cervical cancer, but this was attributed to the protective properties of the diaphragm rather than the direct effect of the pill.

There is some preliminary evidence that oral contraceptives increase the risk of developing endometrial cancer. In the spring of 1976, twenty-one cases of endometrial cancer were reported in women under the age of forty who used oral contraceptives. Thirteen of these women used the sequential birth-control pills, which have since been withdrawn from the market. Although the incidence of cancer is very low, women who experience irregular bleeding that is neither controlled by increasing the dosage of the pill nor subsides after the first three cycles should have an endometrial biopsy.

Summary

There is no perfect form of contraception. It seems that as the effectiveness of the contraceptive increases, the risk inherent in its use also increases. However, the benefit-risk ratio is very favorable for oral contraceptives. Besides their extreme effectiveness, oral contraceptives relieve severe dysmenorrhea, decrease the amount of blood lost during menstruation by 50 percent, and alleviate premenstrual tension. Women with chronic cystic mastitis and fibrocystic breast disease receive some symptomatic relief from taking oral contraceptives. Oral contraceptives produce a decreased incidence in ovarian cysts, duodenal ulcers, sebaceous cysts, and acne. There is even a 25 percent decrease in ear wax production!

There are risks involved in oral contraceptives, but they are not as great as the risks involved in pregnancy. Women should be aware that the pill can have serious side effects. The risk involved in oral contraception is magnified for women who smoke. They should protect themselves by notifying physicians of the appearance of any symptoms. It has been said there are no safe drugs, only safe physicians. This could be changed to: There are no safe pills, only informed women.

The pill has changed the life-style of almost an entire generation of women. It has given them a new freedom of expression in their sexual, academic, and financial lives. Perhaps most importantly, it has given them the expectation that a reliable method of birth control is their right. The pill may not be the ultimate method of contraception, but if that ultimate method is ever discovered, it will be based on the expectations raised by the pill.

THE "MORNING-AFTER" PILL

The so-called morning-after pill should not be considered a routine method of contraception but used only as an emergency measure. It is used in extreme cases such as rape and contraceptive failure. The theory behind the morning-after pill is that extremely high doses of estrogen over a period of days prevent implantation of a fertilized egg. The administration of this hormone must be started within seventy-two hours of unprotected intercourse. The dose schedule is 25 milligrams of diethylstilbesterol twice a day for five days, or 5 milligrams of ethinyl estradiol (administered in ten tablets of 0.5 mg.) for five days. Some physicians administer a type of estrogen at a dose of 1.25 milligrams three times a day for five days. These very high amounts of estrogen often produce severe side effects: constant nausea, vomiting, and water retention. If the morning-after pills fail to interrupt the pregnancy, abortion is usually indicated. The high dose of estrogen has been found to cause abnormalities in the fetus and diethylstilbesterol has been found to cause vaginal cancer in the daughters and genital abnormalities in the sons of treated women.

It must be emphasized that the morning-after pill should only be used for emergency situations and not as a routine contraception. The effects of its long-term and continued usage have not been estimated. Recent studies indicate that an IUD inserted immediately after intercourse has been effective morning-after treatment for unprotected intercourse and may be considered an alternative to the morning-after pill.

PROGESTERONE INJECTIONS FOR CONTRACEPTION

An injectable progesterone contraceptive, Depo-Provera, is being used by nearly a million women around the world. It works by inhibiting ovulation, making the cervical mucus impenetrable to the sperm and the lining of the uterus unreceptive to a fertilized egg. It has an apparent effectiveness rate of about 99 percent.

The administration of Depo-Provera consists of a simple shot of 150 milligrams of injectable progesterone once every three months. Though the contraceptive works well, there are several side effects, including irregular bleeding, amenorrhea, and weight gain. The irregular bleeding usually straightens itself out after a few months. If there is no change in the amenorrhea, the injections may have to be discontinued. The average time for conception after discontinuing Depo-Provera has been about a year, although menstruation begins in about three months. Animal studies in the United States showed Depo-Provera may lead to breast cancer in beagle dogs. As beagles do not metabolize hormones in the same manner as humans, the studies do not necessarily prove that there would be similar side effects in women. Depo-Provera might soon be released by the Food and Drug Administration for contraceptive use in the United States.

BREAST-FEEDING AS A FORM OF CONTRACEPTION

If a woman fully breast-feeds her newborn child, she is usually protected from pregnancy for two to four months after delivery. However, as soon as she shows any sign of menstruation, even minimal vaginal spotting, or starts giving her child a supplementary bottle, she must seek some other form of contraception. Oral contraceptives are contraindicated in a breast-feeding woman because the synthetic hormones could be passed to the infant via the milk. An IUD, a diaphragm, or contraceptive jellies are all acceptable alternatives.

DOUCHING FOR CONTRACEPTION

Many people still believe that a quick douche after intercourse prevents pregnancy. In fact, sperm swim so fast, they can reach the uterus and the fallopian tubes within three to five minutes after coitus, or often before you get to the bathroom. Douching, therefore, has absolutely no effect as a contraceptive. Too frequent douching may wash away the normal defensive bacteria of the vagina. It may even push the sperm into the uterus. Postcoital douching may be of some undetermined benefit in reducing the chance of contracting venereal disease, but it has no value as a contraceptive.

One of the prevailing myths among teenagers in the United States is that Coca-Cola is a particularly effective douche. Girls who do not get pregnant after a Coke douche are simply lucky; the Coke is about as effective taken vaginally as it would be taken orally.

THE FUTURE OF CONTRACEPTION

There is a continuing search for safe, effective, and reversible forms of contraception. The major thrust of this research has been aimed at women. There has been research focused on the inhibition of sperm production in the male, but it seems easier to interrupt the mechanism involved in the production of a single egg a month, compared to blocking the millions of sperm which are produced in a man every day.

Silastic Implants

There has been research in a number of foreign countries into the contraceptive effectiveness of progesterone released slowly from a silastic device implanted under the skin of the arm. These silastic devices are "injected" under the skin with special instruments and usually have to be replaced every year, although some devices release progesterone for a period of three years. The major side effect is extremely irregular bleeding. There have been reports of breakthrough bleeding, weight gain, and, on occasion, irritation from the site of the injected silastic capsule.

Vaginal Rings

Doughnut-shaped vaginal rings that slowly release progesterone have been developed. These steroid-releasing devices are placed in the vagina for three weeks, then removed for one week to allow cyclic bleeding. They are then replaced. It is believed that these devices act like the minipill in that they do not inhibit ovulation but prevent fertilization and implantation. Devices are also being tested that are left in the vagina for more than three weeks.

The advantage of such a device over the pill is that it requires insertion only once every month, eliminating the need for daily medication. The major disadvantage is that it is a foreign body within the vagina and might predispose the user to vaginal infections.

Menstrual Induction

A woman with an active and unprotected sex life would, on the average, become pregnant every three to four months. Even without contraception, a woman would not get pregnant every cycle. Women who try to become pregnant find that it is almost impossible to pick the exact month in which they will conceive. A delayed menses is often one of the first signs of pregnancy. Vaginal suppositories comprised of *prostaglandin analogs* are being studied for the induction of uterine contractions and menses in the nonpregnant woman, and contractions causing a very early abortion in the, pregnant patient. More than two hundred women with confirmed pregnancies of under seven weeks have received these prostaglandin suppositories and successfully aborted in Sweden.

In this country, similar research is being performed with the prostaglandin suppository on pregnant women who are no more than one to two weeks late. The suppository is inserted into the vagina and usually within two to four hours the woman experiences cramps. There will be cramping and vaginal bleeding for the next five to ten days with occasional severe cramping associated with the passage of large clots, similar to a delayed heavy period. Most women who have undergone this procedure have been pleased with the method since it avoids any surgical manipulation. This technique is still in the research stage and will not be generally available for at least two to three years.

New Oral Contraceptives

Recent drug research has yielded a promising new agent, *Danazol.* By inhibiting the release of LH and FSH from the pituitary gland, Danazol suppresses stimulation of ovulation. Danazol has been effective in the treatment of endocrine disorders, as well as pelvic endometriosis and chronic cystic breast disease. Since it has a further advantage of containing no estrogen, work is being done to determine its use as a birth-control pill. Additional research is needed before any affirmative statement can be made about Danazol as an oral contraceptive.

The contraceptive effectiveness of an *antiprogesterone drug* is being investigated. The progesterone produced after ovulation is necessary for the maintenance of pregnancy once an egg is fertilized. Any drug that inhibited progesterone production would also prevent pregnancy. This antiprogesterone would not have to be taken throughout the cycle, only during the immediate postovulation days. Such an antiprogesterone has been developed and has been tested in 160 women in Haiti, but the pregnancy rate on it is still too high. The concept, however, is valid, and more work is being done.

Vaccination for Contraception

Vaccines have been used to protect the body against a variety of diseases from measles to polio. Perhaps a vaccine could be developed that would interfere with normal conception. When a person is vaccinated against any disease, a small amount of material resembling the disease is injected into the body— briefly, the person is given a very, very mild case of the disease. The body's natural defenses rally to destroy the injected material by producing antibodies. These antibodies then continue to circulate in the blood, giving prolonged protection against future invasion by a similar germ. In some diseases the protection is lifelong. With other diseases, the antibodies need renewing and booster shots are needed at periodic intervals.

For years, it has been hoped that the ability of the body to produce antibodies against foreign substances could be used for contraceptive purposes. It is well known that prostitutes are usually extremely infertile. They produce antibodies against sperm, and it is believed that their overexposure to sperm is the basis for this condition. A woman's production of antibodies to her partner's sperm is one of the causes of infertility. Attempts have been made to isolate and synthesize these sperm antibodies, but there has been little success in this area.

Another approach in the search for a contraceptive vaccine is far more subtle and involves stimulating the body to produce antibodies against *hormones* involved in conception. In other words, the body is asked to raise antibodies against a natural substance rather than against a foreign invader. Vaccinations against the gonadotropins LH and FSH have been studied in both female and male animals. In female animals, antibody inactivation of LH and FSH prevented ovulation and also severely affected the menstural cycle, while decreasing the production of female hormones. In male animals, antibodies raised against LH caused testicular atrophy, and a severe drop in testosterone caused a decreased libido. This change was so exaggerated that these male animals were rejected by the other inhabitants of the animal colony.

It was concluded that disruption of the normal process of reproduction by antifertility vaccines is more feasible in women, since women can be immunized to placental hormones or proteins. Thus pregnancy might be prevented without interfering with the normal female hormones, ovulation, or menstruation. In men, there are few substances that can be inhibited with antibodies without disturbing vital hormone production as well as other organs.

Complex proteins which appear to play a necessary role in the maintenance of pregnancy have been isolated from the placenta. Antibodies have been produced against these proteins in rabbits and sheep. These antibodies have produced abortion in pregnant monkeys.

There is a very particular type of HCG (human chorionic gonadotrophin), called *beta-subunit HCG*. This is only found during pregnancy, and the maintenance of pregnancy might be prevented by a vaccine against beta-subunit HCG. Antibodies that destroy the biologic activity of beta-subunit HCG have been raised in laboratory animals and, when injected into other animals, these antibodies have caused interruption of a pregnancy by preventing, if conception occurred, the formation of the placenta. Researchers in India and Sweden have vaccinated women volunteers with the beta-subunit HCG antibodies. This single vaccination appears to have prevented the maintenance of pregnancy. The vaccine seems to be without other significant side effects, but the women seem to be irreversibly immune and unable to conceive for the rest of their lives.

There are enzymes normally present on the surface of the sperm. One of these enzymes, *lactic dehydrogenase* (LDH-X), has been isolated from the surface of mouse sperm and found to cause a cross-reaction with the similar enzyme in several species, including humans. Female mice and rabbits who were injected with the purified lactic dehydrogenase developed antibodies against this sperm enzyme, with a consequent reduction in fertility of up to 80 percent, *and the effects were reversible*. Studies of this type of active immunization are being carried out in monkeys, but the antifertility effects of the injected enzyme must be improved. The mouse lactic dehydrogenase was also injected into male rabbits, and fertility was decreased in direct relation to the amount of antibody in the blood, without any effects on libido. Again, the antifertility effect of the vaccination was reversible. A number of other sperm enzymes are also being investigated for their antifertility effects.

The Male Pill

Contraceptive research has not been limited to methods of female fertility control; there have been a number of studies into the efficacy of agents which will inhibit sperm production in the male or render the sperm incapable of fertilizing the ovum. High doses of female hormones such as estrogen may decrease sperm production, but would have a number of side effects such as decrease in libido and the development of female secondary sex characteristics. Administration of high doses of estrogen is a primary step in a male-to-female transsexual operation.

The antifertility effect of a new drug, Danazol, on men has shown some promise. This potent drug, which inhibits the gonadotrophins (LH, FSH), has recently been released by the Food and Drug Administration under the name of Danocrine for the treatment of pelvic endometriosis. Danazol is also being tested in women as an oral contraceptive. When Danazol alone was given to a group of male volunteers, the reduction in sperm count was not consistent and the men complained of decreased libido. In later trials, 600-milligram doses of Danazol daily were given in association with a monthly intramuscular injection of testosterone. This combined therapy resulted in a striking drop in sperm count—to infertile levels—within four to eight weeks. More than fifty men have been treated with Danazol and testosterone with no apparent side effects and no decrease in libido or sexual potency. The antifertility effects of this combined treatment are reversible, and sperm count returns to fertile levels eight to ten weeks after discontinuation of the Danazol. Widespread and long-term studies are needed to determine the full antifertility effects of Danazol in the male.

Even if a male pill is developed, there is some doubt that women would actually trust the man to take it. A male pill would be acceptable in an established relationship where both partners assume responsibility for contraception, but there may be little acceptance among people practicing casual sex.

Heat as a Male Contraceptive

One approach to birth control has been to increase the temperature of the testes. In both humans and animals, sperm must be stored at a temperature a few degrees lower than body temperature to maintain their fertility. This is why the testicles are outside the body, with their own specialized circulatory system. The effect of heat on the inhibition of sperm is consistent throughout the animal kingdom; no animal has hair or fur on the testicles. If the temperature of the testicles is raised a few degrees, the fertility of the sperm drops. The contraceptive effects of hot baths have been tested by the Japanese. Other researchers have developed a "testicle warmer" to be worn constantly. Although these somewhat bizarre methods appear effective, they have very little general appeal.

WHICH CONTRACEPTIVE METHOD IS BEST FOR ME?

It has been demonstrated that there is a safe method of contraception for every woman, although the same method cannot be used by every woman throughout her fertile age. If a teenager decides she is ready for sex, she should also be ready to assume the responsibility of obtaining contraception; a doctor or family-planning clinic can help her choose the method best suited to her needs. Recent studies conducted in Great Britain and the United States have shown that birth control pills containing less than fifty micrograms of estrogen when used by healthy, informed women are relatively risk free. No late ill effect of these low estrogen birth control pills has been found, and it is believed that this type of oral contraceptive is particularly suited to young women who have not borne children and in whom pregnancy would be a catastrophe. Young women are much more fertile and they need an extremely effective method of contraception. An intrauterine device might also be advised although some women who have not carried children seem to have more difficulties with this method. However, the pill can still safely be used by motivated women after their teens. There has been a reported higher incidence of cardio-vascular side effects among pill users who smoke. The difference between smokers and nonsmokers, though, is not significant until the age of 35. Women who don't smoke could continue taking the pill until age 40, but should then use another method. The barrier methods—diaphragm, foam, creams or jellies—are all effective for women at any age; however, the effectiveness greatly depends on a woman's motivation to use them and on her understanding of her own body. Finally, the condom, easily available over the counter, should always be kept in mind as an effective alternative.

chapter 10

VOLUNTARY STERILIZATION

In the wake of society's ongoing concern over birth control, an age-old procedure, improved by modern techniques, still provides a great number of women and men with a safe and reliable method of contraception. That procedure is sterilization, a viable and voluntary alternative to other contraceptive methods.

Voluntary sterilization has been the victim of some very unfair attacks and myths. Many people associate it with castration and/or any one of a number of cruel punishments. Still others think it desexes a person.

In fact, voluntary sterilization is one of the greatest aids to the world community. It helps rich countries and Third World nations alike. It's no wonder that it has become the world's leading method of final and definitive contraception.

The United States arrived late at full acceptance of voluntary sterilization. Just ten years ago, only a few hospitals in the country allowed women to undergo the procedure voluntarily. Even then, women had to have four or five children and submit to a hospital committee before gaining approval for the operation. This was the subject of many lawsuits in the late 1960s.

When New York State passed its Abortion Law in 1970, it was a major breakthrough for the advocates of voluntary sterilization. That law, supported by recent Supreme Court rulings, effectively gave women control over their own bodies. No longer could doctors or society dictate to women or rule their bodies. For the first time in history, a woman could choose what to do with her body—to have a child or not. Of course, this ethical and legal concept naturally extended to the area of sterilization.

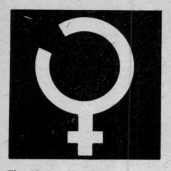 

Fig. 10-1: The female and male sterilization symbols. The female is to the left and the male to the right. These are the classic sexual symbols, with a portion removed from the circle. Some men who have undergone vasectomy wear pins bearing the male sterilization symbol; these are called vasectomy pins.

Today, people all around the nation and world can volunteer for sterilization. Some hospitals still require a woman to have her husband's consent, which seems unjust, because, after all, a man doesn't need his wife's consent to have a vasectomy.

BENEFITS OF STERILIZATION

Voluntary sterilization protects not only against unwanted pregnancies, but also against "accidents" as well. Accidents happen to everyone. A woman can forget to take her pill. A diaphragm can be inserted improperly. An IUD can lose its chemical effectiveness. A man can have a condom slide off at just the wrong moment. These are not uncommon events; they are altogether human. While these contraceptive methods are relatively effective, it is interesting to note that the failure for each is composed largely of such accidents. These are prevented by sterilization.

The virtual certainty of pregnancy prevention brings many side benefits. It relieves the anxiety of unwanted pregnancy, while allowing a couple their choice of family size. It allows the retarded to marry and lead normal lives. It prevents the transmission of hereditary abnormalities. It also relieves the family and society of a financial burden.

Happily, sterilization in no way effects hormonal change in the body, nor does it interfere with sexual pleasure. In fact, most women find sex more pleasurable when the anxieties surrounding unwanted conception are relieved.

Side Effects

Many people still think sterilization causes horrendous side effects—voices become lower or higher, hair growth increases or decreases, and so forth. The gist of these myths is that after sterilization, a woman becomes more like a man and a man becomes more like a woman.

These myths are patently ridiculous. In fact, by the late 1960s, more than 95 percent of those who had undergone sterilization pronounced themselves happy with the results. There are however physical and psychological side effects following both male and female surgical sterilization (See below).

FEMALE STERILIZATION

Sterilization for a woman is called *tubal ligation*. It is a procedure in which the continuity of the fallopian tubes is interrupted. There are many new and emerging techniques, but this surgery is basically separated into two categories: (1) sterilization through the abdomen; and (2) sterilization through the vagina. In both, the tubes are either cut, tied, or clamped so that the egg will not meet a sperm and pass into the uterus. There is, of course, no pregnancy if the egg does not meet the sperm.

Sterilization does not interfere with sexual intercourse. Menstruation and all other functions continue normally.

Postpartum Sterilization (Sterilization after Childbirth)

An ideal time to perform female sterilization is immediately after childbirth, usually within one or two days. At that time, the uterus is enlarged, making it much easier to find the fallopian tubes. The woman is usually placed under a general or spinal anesthetic. An incision approximately one and a half inches long is made immediately underneath or inside the navel. One finger can usually sweep over the fundus (top) of the uterus and reach the fallopian tubes, or the surgeon can use a small instrument to pick up the tubes. With the tubes in direct vision, the sterilization can be performed very easily.

By having the so-called *postpartum* tubal sterilization done, a woman does not need a second hospitalization; she can recuperate from the delivery and the surgery at the same time. She

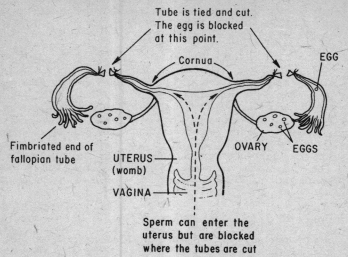

Tube is tied and cut.
The egg is blocked
at this point.

Cornua

EGG

Fimbriated end of
fallopian tube

OVARY   EGGS

UTERUS
(womb)

VAGINA

Sperm can enter the
uterus but are blocked
where the tubes are cut

Fig. 10-2: Locations in which tubal ligations have been performed. Ovulation can occur, but the egg is blocked where the tube has been tied and cut. The egg, therefore, dies and is reabsorbed in the tube. The sperm can freely swim into the uterus, but cannot reach the egg, since the sperm are blocked where the tube has been tied and cut.

The fimbriated ends of the fallopian tubes are also shown. A *fimbriaectomy* is a form of sterilization in which the fimbriated ends on both sides are removed. A *cornual resection* of the tubes is a complete removal of the fallopian tubes from the cornua area of the uterus (indicated by arrow).

also does not have to worry about leaving the child alone if she should be readmitted for a tubal ligation.

The abdominal approach is also applied when sterilization is performed at the time of Caesarean birth. As that area is opened during the bearing, it is a good time to perform tubal ligation.

It should be kept in mind that a woman *must be certain* this will be her last childbirth before undergoing sterilization. A woman carrying an unwanted pregnancy should not hastily choose to have her tubes ligated.

Tubal Ligation during Laparotomy

In 1834, Dr. Von Blundell, the first physician to write about tubal sterilization, suggested total resection of the fallopian tubes, but thought that simple division of the tubes might prevent pregnancy. A Dr. Lundgren performed the first tubal ligation in the United States in 1881. Since then, a variety of techniques has been described. Tubal ligation was often performed by just placing a suture around a loop of the tube without cutting a part of the tube. This method proved to be unsuccessful, since the tie often slipped off and the woman became fertile again.

The Pomeroy technique of tubal ligation was developed to insure a higher success in permanent sterilization. This technique involves tying the fallopian tube, plus cutting out a small section of the tube, thereby ensuring sterilization even if the tie slips off. Almost all tubal ligations during laparotomy (an operation in which a section of the abdominal cavity is exposed through an abdominal incision) are done utilizing the Pomeroy technique.

Other basic methods of sterilization include the fimbriectomy, the removal of the fimbriated ends of the fallopian tubes. These ends catch the egg, so their removal allows the egg to go unfertilized. Fimbriectomy is performed through an abdominal incision.

Also performed abdominally is a cornual resection of the uterus. The entire cornual area (the upper corners of the uterus) is excised. This, however, is an extensive and rather unnecessary operation. The Pomeroy technique seems to be the most efficient operation, with an almost 100 percent success rate. Tubal sterilization by exploratory laparotomy is performed in vast numbers, but its popularity has decreased in the past few years because it requires a postoperative hospitalization of five to seven days.

Voluntary Sterilization by Minilaparotomy

A mini-lap is an operation through a very small incision. This technique is less complicated and faster than a regular laparotomy (abdominal operation). It is done under general, spinal, or local anesthesia. The operation takes twenty to thirty minutes and is, basically, a simplification of a laparotomy. This procedure is often done for postpartum sterilization. The mini-lap is done the world over and is, in several countries, the preferred mode of sterilization. More importantly, it can be performed on an outpatient basis—if the patient tolerates the procedure, she can go home the same day. In the United States, a woman usually stays in the hospital for a few days, but in other countries, it is a same-day procedure.

Very similar to the laparotomy, an incision only one-third the size of a normal laparotomy incision is made just above the pubic hairline. The one-inch incision allows the doctor to insert small instruments and bring the tubes into direct vision. He can then tie the tube and excise a small segment in a modification of the Pomeroy technique. The tubal ligation can also be done by placing a special clip on the tube. This method is relatively new but makes reversibility more possible.

The complication rate with this technique seems extremely low, although if a woman is very obese, the procedure becomes more difficult. For example, in 2,800 procedures performed recently by 112 surgeons at fifty different hospitals in Thailand, complications ranged from only 0.4 to one percent.

Sterilization Via the Band-Aid Procedure (Laparoscopy)

Laparoscopy is presently the preferred technique in this country. The *laparoscope* is a periscope-type instrument that is inserted through an incision in the navel. It makes readily visible all parts of the abdomen—most importantly, the uterus, the ovaries, and the tubes. This slender, tubular instrument has many advantages. Primarily, it has a fiber optic light source which allows the physician to visualize the internal organs. Fiberoptics (a cold, nonburning source of light) have improved almost all *endoscopic,* or internal, instruments. Infections can be spotted through the laparoscope, tube endings can be checked for infertility problems, and fibroid tumors can be detected on the uterus.

For a sterilization using the laparoscope, a woman is placed under a local or general anesthetic. She is then placed in the Trendelenburg position (a tilted position in which the head is lowered and the legs are elevated). A small incision is made in the navel. In order to get a better visual field and push the bowels toward the diaphragm during the operation, carbon dioxide (CO_2) is first injected into the abdominal cavity. The laparoscope is then inserted and the light source attached. The physician first closely observes the bowels, and maybe the appendix. His attention is then focused on the uterus, the tubes, and the ovaries.

The sterilization can be performed through the laparoscope itself by insertion of an abdominal forceps through the instrument. More often a second incision is made near the pubic hairline and the abdominal forceps is inserted through that incision. From here, a variety of techniques can be effected; the most common is tubal cauterization. During this procedure, the fallopian tubes are picked up by the abdominal forceps and are

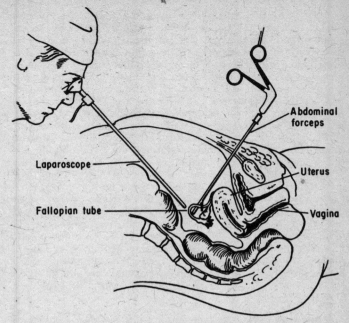

Fig. 10–3: A tubal ligation performed through a laparoscopy (the Band-Aid operation). If a tubal sterilization is performed, abdominal forceps can be inserted through a small hole in the lower abdomen (as shown in figure). The forceps can also be inserted through the laparoscope.

then cauterized (burned), and a piece of the tube is removed. This is quite effective, but there is a possibility of burning the bowels. It should, therefore, only be done by physicians who are familiar with the procedure.

Recently there has been some experimentation with clips and rings. A device called the *tantalum wick hemoclip* can be inserted through the laparoscope and attached to the tubes. The portion of the tube between the clips is then removed.

Also, the *silicone ring* (fallopian ring) is experiencing recent success. The "ring" is squeezed down on the tubes during laparoscopy, cutting off canalization of the tubes. An advantage to this technique is that reversibility is more feasible, since only a small portion of the tubes has been damaged.

After the actual sterilization, the physician checks through the laparoscope to see that no bleeding has occurred. The instrument is then pulled out, the CO_2 is expelled, and one or two sutures are placed underneath the skin. A small Band-Aid is placed over the incision. It takes only about thirty to fifty minutes, and the patient who has been under a local anesthesia can go home the same day; the patient who has general anesthesia can usually be discharged the following day.

There are contraindications to laparoscopic sterilization. Prime considerations are previous appendectomy or other previous abdominal surgery causing adhesions. Cardiac disease might make the operation dangerous, since the abdomen is distended with the CO_2, causing pressure on the lungs. Obesity is another factor. In the case of an overweight woman, it is almost impossible to insert the laparoscope correctly. One final caution: Make certain the physician is trained and experienced in laparoscopy. The laparascope is a delicate instrument, and one with which not all doctors are familiar. A physician can easily perforate the bowels and burn organs if he is not expert. If a large portion of the tubes are damaged by coagulation, there could be a decreased blood supply to the ovaries resulting in abdominal pain and future irregular bleeding.

Culdoscopic Tubal Sterilization

Another means of female sterilization is via a *colpotomy*, an operation in which the abdominal cavity is entered through a small incision in the vagina. The *culdoscope* is a periscope which is inserted through the vaginal wall rather than the abdomen (see Fig. 16–7). The woman is placed in the knee-chest position, which is a position in which she sits on her knees, hands forward, resting her chest on a table (see Fig. 16–6). The operation is always performed using only local anesthesia. A speculum is inserted into the vagina and pulled backward to increase the physician's ability to see the area. The cervix is then held with a tenaculum (special forceps) and a small incision is made behind the cervix, through which the culdoscope is inserted. A fiberoptic light source attached to the culdoscope enables the physician to see the pelvic organs. After visualization, the tubes are picked up through the culdoscope by a small instrument. The fallopian tubes are ligated, most likely with the use of a special hemoclip, which is squeezed around the tubes. A portion is then excised between two clips.

The infection rate has been high after this type of operation. Yet if a doctor is familiar with colposcopy this poses no real problem. Actually, this operation has no really deterrent factors, as there is no need for gas insufflation in the abdominal cavity. In skilled hands, this is a twenty-minute operation and a good method. The woman can be discharged the same day. The operation is, however, associated with considerable discomfort because of the position in which the woman must be and because only local anesthesia is used. In this country, culdoscopy is used only in rare cases for sterilization.

Hysteroscopic Sterilization

The final internal instrument to be discussed is the *hysteroscope*. The hysteroscope is another periscopic-type tool passed through the vagina and the cervix on its way to visualizing the uterine cavity. It has been considered valuable for inspecting and diagnosing cancer of the uterus.

The major difficulty with the hysterocope is that the uterine cavity has to be distended to get a clear view. Different types of hysteroscopes have been developed. The first type had a balloon on the tip, which was blown up inside the uterus to expand the cavity. The more recent ones use Dextran (a highly viscous solution) or CO_2 to distend the uterine cavity to give a better view. When the cavity is distended, it can be carefully inspected through the hysteroscope and the opening of the tubes can be seen. A fine operative instrument can then be placed through the hysteroscope. Biopsies from the uterus can be obtained and various types of tubal sterilizations can be performed.

Recently, means of closing the fallopian tubes through the hysteroscope have been investigated. As yet there is no definitive technique, but cauterization of the cornual area of the fallopian tubes is being attempted, as is the placement of various types of plugs into the tubes to prevent sperm migration.

A method is being examined in which a solution is injected directly into the tubes through the hysteroscope. Research is being done on just this kind of solution, which would block off the tubes permanently, or at least for a long period of time. If hysteroscopic sterilization one day becomes readily available and the technique is improved, this would be a highly recommended method, since the sterilization could be done on an outpatient basis and would result in only minimal pain and discomfort.

A few researchers are exploring the possibility of inserting "plugs" into the fallopian tubes via the hysteroscope. These plugs would block the tubes while they were there, but could be removed if pregnancy was desired. A new form of *reversible*

Hysteroscopy

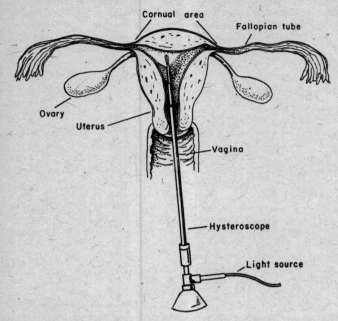

Fig. 10–4: Hysteroscopy is a procedure in which a hysteroscope (a periscope-type instrument) is inserted into the uterine cavity to enable the physician to look into the uterus. The hysteroscope is inserted through the vagina and the cervix into the uterus without any need for an abdominal incision.

sterilization will be born if this technique proves safe and feasible. It is now still in a developmental stage.

The methods discussed, with the exception of hysteroscopy, are all highly effective. The pregnancy rate after tubal ligation is less than one percent, and those were cases in which the tubes were incorrectly burned or the physician was inexperienced.

Are Tubal Ligations Reversible?

Simply, reversibility is the process of recanalizing the fallopian tubes so that a woman is again fertile. Factors such as remarriage, death of a child, and improved financial conditions all make reversibility a desired prerequisite. Reversibility might also eliminate some of the religious and cultural objections to sterilization.

Devices such as clips and silastic rings seem to be the hope of the future. Surgical reconstruction of the tubes has the highest rate of success, but only when performed by very skilled physicians familiar with these procedures. However, the pregnancy rate after these operations is usually as low as 10 to 20 percent.

Many factors affect surgical reconstruction, all of which can alter a woman's chance for reversibility. The major factor is how close the excised portion of the tube was to the uterus. As it gets closer, the chances for reconstruction get higher. The type of sterilization is also important. A fimbriectomy has a very low chance of reversibility because the fimbriated ends of the tubes are impossible to reconstruct. As was stated before, it is these fimbriated ends which catch the egg and determine fertility.

If a woman decides to attempt reversibility, she should be aware that surgical reconstruction isn't nearly as simple an operation as a tubal ligation, and the chances of conception are very slim. Sterilization should only be considered as a final method of contraception.

Hysterectomy—The Most Effective Sterilization?

Several physicians advocate hysterectomy as a means of final sterilization. Women occasionally experience irregular bleeding after a tubal ligation; this might be due to the operation interfering with the blood supply to the ovaries. To avoid this, many gynecologists recommend hysterectomy as sterilization because it avoids later complications. For women with uterine abnormalities, irregular bleeding, or vaginal prolapse who have completed their families, hysterectomies might possibly be considered as a means of sterilization. This most drastic form of sterilization should be limited to rare, clearly indicated instances.

When Should Sterilization Be Considered?

All factors considered, one basic element remains: Only a woman who has completed her childbearing, or a woman for whom pregnancy and childbearing would be dangerous, should undergo sterilization. Women in their early twenties with unwanted pregnancies shouldn't hastily decide to have their tubes tied because they are temporarily angry at the entire male population. Likewise, young women with one or two children would be wise to use a form of birth control until they are older and certain they have completed their families. There are few emotional side effects to sterilization in the case of the thirty-five-year-old career woman, whereas there are many when dealing with the occasional young woman who never wants to see another man in her life. When the anger ebbs and she returns three years later with a prospective husband, she faces the uncertain prospect of reversibility. A woman should not only think twice, but perhaps three times before she consents to sterilization.

Which Type of Sterilization Should a Woman Choose?

The simplest form of tubal sterilization is the Band-Aid procedure—tubal sterilization via laparoscopy. This procedure requires only one or two days of hospitalization, and the incision can usually be made inside the navel so that no scar is visible. Whether a silastic ring or a hemoclip is used is left to the discretion of the physician. A laparoscopy cannot be performed if you have had previous extensive abdominal surgery or if you are very obese. A laparotomy is then suggested.

What Does Tubal Sterilization Cost?

Among private physicians, fees vary from doctor to doctor. If you have good health insurance, it might pay a portion of this fee. It would be wise to discuss the fee with the doctor or his secretary before the surgery. The hospital fee is usually covered by health insurance. If you go to clinics, the operation is often completely covered. Patients with Medicaid usually get the entire procedure covered through the Medicaid. However, check locally, since this also varies from place to place.

MALE STERILIZATION

Vasectomy, or sterilization of the male, is not *castration.* Castration is a removal of the testes, and the connotations surrounding it in former days prevented the growth of popularity of vasectomy, which is a completely different procedure. Anything that remotely resembled tampering with the male organs was in the past avoided. As the unwarranted fears relating to vasectomy were dispelled, it affected more men on a worldwide basis. In spite of the fact that vasectomy is much less complex than tubal ligation, tubal ligation was for years the preferred method of sterilization. Recently, however, the popularity of vasectomy has increased rapidly.

In Asia, for example, vasectomies have exceeded tubal ligations in number. Between 1968 and 1972, six million vasectomies were performed in India. The rates are equally staggering in Pakistan, Nepal, and Bangladesh. In fact, the numbers have been increasing in many Third World countries, most notably in Latin America.

The concept of vasectomy was initiated in 1885 by Felix Guyon of France, who concluded that blocking off the *vas deferens* (the two tubes which carry semen) caused an atrophy of the prostate. At the beginning of this century, vasectomy was performed for eugenic reasons on criminals, the mentally ill, and those with hereditary diseases. It became popular in Asia in the 1950s, as it tried to replace ineffectual birth-control practices.

Even in the United States and Europe, vasectomy has seeped into the consciousness of the male population. As oral contraceptives received adverse publicity, and as feminism stirred feelings of male responsibility, the figures took on a startling change. In 1969, a quarter of a million men in the United States

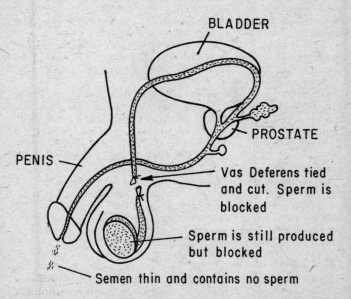

BLADDER

PROSTATE

PENIS

Vas Deferens tied and cut. Sperm is blocked

Sperm is still produced but blocked

Semen thin and contains no sperm

Fig. 10-5: A vasectomy. The vas deferens (the tube which leads the sperm from the testes to the prostate gland) has been tied and cut. This blocks the sperm, which continue to be produced in the testes.

had vasectomies. In 1970, it was three quarters of a million, a two hundred percent jump!

Procedure of Vasectomy

The operation is simple enough and, in most cases, is done by a urologist in his office. As there are many different techniques, a specialist may perform a specific type of sterilization.

In most cases, the patient is given a local anesthetic, injected into the skin of his washed scrotum. Although an occasionally squeamish man may ask for a general anesthetic, it is not recommended. The pain is minimal and he can usually be released minutes after the surgery.

After the scrotum is numb, a small incision is made and the *vas deferens* are pulled out. Clips are placed on the two ends and a small piece is excised. Depending on the skill of the physician, a suture may be used instead of a clip. For those so trained, *electrocautery* or *electrocoagulation* of the vas can be performed.

A small gauze bandage is then placed on the scrotal incision and held by an athletic supporter, or *scrotal suspensory*. The patient need stay off his feet only the first day.

The follow-up to this simple operation is as important as the surgery itself. The patient should not engage in sexual intercourse for at least a week. The pressure can prevent the vas from healing.

Secondly, the patient must know that he is not sterile for at least six weeks. All the residual sperm and products of ejaculation must be expelled before complete sterilization is effected. The stored sperm may take from one to several months to leave the body. Postoperative semen tests are recommended. These tests normally begin at the sixth week and end when two consecutive sperm counts are found negative.

Again, there are contraindications to sterilization, although they are much less severe for the man than for the woman. Local infections and blood disorders are the primary ones, but even previous hernia surgery can be a hindrance to the operation, depending on its severity.

Side Effects of Vasectomy

Those who undergo vasectomies should be warned of possible postoperative side effects. Most, such as discomfort and swelling, are common and go away in a week or so. Certain infections and hematomas can develop, and are treated accordingly. These are, luckily, rare.

Epididymitis (swelling and tenderness near the testes) has occurred in less than one percent of all vasectomies. It is treated with heat and/or a suspensory.

Sperm granuloma, an inflammatory response to the leakage of sperm, is another post-op problem. Again, it is usually not severe enough to be harmful, but if it does cause problems, the sperm can be drained surgically. *Granuloma* occurs in 0.1 to 3.0 percent of all vasectomies.

Reversibility

Again we approach the subject of reversibility, and again the prospect is not favorable. There are three major methods of reversal of vasectomy being researched. Only one is past the point of experimentation. This process is called *vas anastomosis* (also *vasovasotomy*). This is a surgical reconstruction of the vas. The vasovasotomy is a lengthy surgery which must be performed by a specially skilled surgeon. To date, it has been fairly successful, but not many physicians are familiar with this difficult operation.

There are two other methods of reversal which are still in the experimentation stage: (1) storage of the semen, and (2) vas-occlusive devices. Neither of these methods is yet accepted. The vas-occlusive (blocking) clips and silicone rings have been used only on monkeys. As for semen storage, this is not really reversibility; it is artificial insemination. A man about to decide whether he should be sterilized should know that vasovasotomy is his only chance of reversal. The word *chance* should be stressed.

Physical Factors

As vasectomy becomes more prominent the world over, certain physiological questions have been asked.

First is the question of the alteration in the male hormone count. The *spermatogenesis* (production of sperm) continues unchanged soon after the operation. There is no FSH or LH change whatsoever. There is, however, an increase in testosterone, which is produced in the testicles. If anything, this is a positive factor, as it is thought to increase desire.

Another controversy is the issue of sperm antibodies. It is true that one third to one half of all vasectomied men develop antibodies to sperm. This is an immunity established within the body which inhibits sperm activity. The condition is known in fertile men, but is more common in infertile ones.

Does Vasectomy Lead To Heart Disease?

The sperm antibody which follows vasectomy may be involved in the development of atherosclerosis. In a very well-controlled and well-conducted study by Drs. Nancy Alexander and Thomas Clarkson ten monkeys were fed a high cholesterol diet for six months. Five of the monkeys were then vasectomized and all were maintained on the high cholesterol for another six months. At the end of this time a significant increase in atherosclerosis was shown in the vasectomized monkeys as compared to the similarly treated control group. Although the number of animals in this initial test sample was small and the amount of cholesterol employed about twice as high as that in the average American diet, the results were consistent and significant. This study has been expanded in an effort to confirm and explain these results. At the present time it might be advisable for a man with a heart condition, history of high blood cholesterol, or atherosclerosis to reconsider vasectomy very carefully until the final results of long-term testing are available. If a man is already vasectomized, it might be advisable for him to avoid excess dietary cholesterol.

Psychological Factors

There is a psychological factor that remains in many men—fear. The fact that a doctor takes steel instruments, scissors, and hypodermic needles to his genitals can overwhelm many a timorous man. Yet a healthy man should be able to allay any fears with proper counseling. After all, there is certainly a bright side to being sterile.

First, in the hands of a skilled surgeon, the failure rate almost does not exist. The pregnancy rate is 0 to 0.15 percent. The recanalization of the vas is as unlikely as honesty in politics. It is, in fact, this release from anxiety which enhances the sex lives of a majority of vasectomied men.

In the United States alone, sterile men have a twenty percent higher frequency rate of sexual intercourse. Without the bother of birth control, the possible financial burden, and the increase of testosterone, the sterile man has become more sexually active.

The only noticeable sexual change is that the semen is somewhat thinner. This is because the semen is coming only from the gland and the prostate. Indeed, when a man decides whether or not he should undergo a vasectomy, the emotional and financial relief should far outweigh some remotely possible physical change. However, men with serious neuroses or sexual maladjustments are not advised to submit themselves to the surgery. The psychological ramifications can be much more harmful than the physiological ones.

Recommendation

Vasectomy should not be performed so that a man can be more promiscuous. It should be an act of respect. Still, in Western culture, pride often stands in the way. Some men fearful of losing their masculinity would rather have their wives undergo the more complicated surgery than have a vasectomy in ten minutes. This is chauvinistic. For a couple healthy in mind and attitude, the vasectomy seems to be the preferred method of sterilization.

What Is the Cost of Vasectomy?

Done by a private physician, the complete cost (with interview, operation, and sperm count after the procedure) should be about $150 to $200. These prices are, of course, individual. Medicaid or private health-insurance companies might cover part or all of these expenses.

Further Information

If you want more information about voluntary sterilization and vasectomies in particular, contact your nearest Planned Parenthood affiliate (you can find it in your telephone directory) or one of the regional offices listed below:

GREAT LAKES (Illinois, Indiana, Kentucky, Michigan, Ohio, and Wisconsin): 1001 Washington Boulevard Building, 234 State Street, Suite 802, Detroit, Michigan 48226 (313)962-4390

MID-ATLANTIC (Delaware, District of Columbia, Maryland, New Jersey, and Pennsylvania): Medical Towers Bldg., 255 South 17th Street, Suite 2005, Philadelphia, Pa. 19103, (215)732-4744

MIDWEST (Colorado, Iowa, Kansas, Minnesota, Missouri, Montana, Nebraska, North Dakota, South Dakota, Utah, and Wyoming): 406 West 34th Street, Room 725, Kansas City, Missouri 64111 (816)JE1-2243

NORTHEAST (Connecticut, Maine, Massachusetts, New Hampshire, New York, Rhode Island, and Vermont): 810 Seventh Avenue, New York, New York 10019 (212)541-7800

SOUTHEAST (Alabama, Florida, Georgia, Mississippi, North Carolina, South Carolina, Tennessee, Virginia, and West Virginia): 3030 Peachtree Road N.W., Rooms 301–303, Atlanta, Georgia 30305 (404)233–7117

SOUTHWEST (Arkansas, Louisiana, New Mexico, Oklahoma, and Texas): 4928 Burnet Road, Room 204, Austin, Texas 78756 (512)452-6417

WEST (Alaska, Arizona, California, Hawaii, Idaho, Nevada, Oregon, Utah, and Washington): 785 Market Street, Room 1017, San Francisco, California 94103 (415)777-1217

The United States national voluntary agency for sterilization information is:

Association for Voluntary Sterilization
708 Third Avenue
New York, N. Y. 10017 (212)986-3880

The use of saline gained widespread acceptance in the 1940s, until reports from Japan and England showed a high incidence of infection, uterine hemorrhaging, and occasionally brain hemorrhaging. Saline is still used today, but in limited, safe doses and only under strict supervision. It has, in many places, been replaced by the prostaglandins.

Following the Second World War, Swedish researchers succeeded in isolating a substance called prostaglandin from the prostate gland and the semen. This substance causes uterine contractions, and in 1970, reports from Sweden and Uganda confirmed that it could be used successfully to induce *midtrimester abortion*. Unfortunately, this type of abortion was accompanied by nausea, vomiting, and diarrhea. The drug was administered in many different manners until it was found that intraamniotic injection alleviated severity of the side effects and provoked uterine contractions strong enough to cause expulsion.

THE FIRST SIGNS OF PREGNANCY

If conception occurs, the pituitary secretes a hormone called HCG (human chorionic gonadotrophin), which stimulates the corpus luteum, or yellow body, in the ovary to produce progesterone. Progesterone, in turn, prepares the uterus to receive the fertilized egg. Four weeks after conception, or six weeks after the last period, most HCG production is replaced by the placenta, an organ whose sole purpose is to provide nourishment to the fetus. HCG is excreted in the urine and levels of HCG in the urine can be measured in the laboratory. This laboratory measurement of urinary HCG is the most commonly employed pregnancy test and takes from four to eight hours to complete. These tests can be performed in a doctor's office with a diagnostic kit, but the levels of HCG in the urine must be very high for a positive reaction; the laboratory test is more sensitive. A positive reaction in either of these tests means that you are pregnant, but the opposite is not true. It is possible to have a negative pregnancy test, particularly in the first three to five weeks after conception, yet still be pregnant. Pregnancy tests should be repeated every week until there is either a positive sign of pregnancy or the most positive sign of nonpregnancy—menstruation.

A urinary pregnancy test is usually not positive until two weeks after the first missed period, six weeks from the last menstrual period, and four weeks from the time of conception.

In order to have the ability to detect pregnancy *with accuracy* soon after conception, researchers at Cornell University Medical Center in New York have developed an ultrasensitive *receptor assay* for HCG which gives a positive reading as early as two weeks after conception, even before the first missed period. The levels of HCG in the blood are tested with this technique, which is available in a number of centers throughout the country. There are also over-the-counter kits for pregnancy testing in the home which detect levels of HCG in urine. These techniques make the early detection of pregnancy more practical.

One of the first visible signs of pregnancy is enlargement of the breasts and deepening in color of the areola surrounding the nipple. A physician can check the uterus for signs of softening, but uterine enlargement is usually not detectable until six or seven weeks after a missed period. Nausea, a bloated feeling, and breast tenderness are often the first signs noted by a patient. Persistent elevation of the Basal Body Temperature is another indication of pregnancy. If all these signs are monitored and pregnancy is detected early enough, abortion can be relatively simple. The earlier the abortion is performed, the fewer are the complications that can be anticipated.

MENSTRUAL EXTRACTION, OR MINIABORTION

The quickest, easiest, and safest method of abortion is the so-called *menstrual extraction* developed by a California physician in an effort to minimize the psychological trauma of abortion. The procedure was initially performed on women who had missed a period, yet showed negative pregnancy tests. It was felt, though, that if a woman did not know she was pregnant, the abortion procedure would have a better chance of psychological acceptance. Thus the name—menstrual extraction, which is the simple removal of the endometrium which would normally be expelled during menstruation. Some feminist leaders even advocated replacing the normal form of six-day menstruation with this operative procedure, which lasts only a few minutes. Extensive studies, though, have indicated that this procedure should not be performed on nonpregnant women, since there are dangers of infections and excessive bleeding. Because of this, the term *menstrual extraction* is now considered a misnomer and the technique is called a *miniabortion*. It is the recommended procedure only if a pregnancy test is positive and a woman is less than 7 weeks from her last menstruation.

A miniabortion is performed either in a clinic or in a doctor's office. The procedure is not without discomfort and a tense person is advised to take either a tranquilizer or a mild painkiller thirty minutes prior to the procedure (the doctor should always be advised as to the pharmacological agent that has been taken). The woman is placed on an examining table with her legs in the stirrups, a position similar to that used in the normal pelvic examination. A manual internal examination is performed to determine the size and position of the uterus. A speculum is then inserted into the vagina to provide the physician with good visualization of the cervix. The vagina is swabbed with an antiseptic solution. A local anesthetic of Novocaine is injected with a very fine needle at three points on the cervix—the top and on either side. The cervix is then held with a special type of forceps, called a tenaculum. A thin, flexible, plastic tube five to seven millimeters in diameter is inserted through the cervix into the uterus. With most patients, the cervix does not have to be dilated to permit insertion of the plastic tube; this minimizes cervical damage. The plastic tube is attached to a suction apparatus. Through mild suction, the lining of the uterine wall, complete with the products of conception, is gently removed within one or two minutes. On occasion, the tube is removed and cleared, then reinserted to make certain that removal is complete. Since the procedure can be associated with strong uterine cramps, nausea, and a feeling of sweating and faintness, the woman should not be moved from the examining table for fifteen to thirty minutes. It is advisable for a woman undergoing this procedure to be accompanied by a friend or relative to help her return home safely.

There are many advantages to this procedure. It is fast, relatively simple, can be performed without the need for general anesthesia, and the cost of a hospital stay is eliminated. A woman should not have intercourse or use a tampon for three to four weeks after the procedure to avoid complication or infection. Bleeding after the procedure should stop within one to two weeks. If it continues, you should return to your doctor for evaluation. Normal menstruation usually occurs four to eight weeks after the procedure. Non-surgical menstrual induction is presently under investigation in a number of medical centers (See p. 240).

FIRST-TRIMESTER SUCTION ABORTION

Today, a suction abortion, or curettage, is the technique of choice for interruption of pregnancy between the seventh to the twelfth week after the last menstrual period.

The art of suction abortions has progressed significantly in recent years. When suction or vacuum abortions were first developed, many of the pumps did not exert sufficient power, and in several instances complications occurred. Since the liberalization of abortion laws around the world, more attention has been given to the development of safe abortion apparatus, and the procedure has become more sophisticated. Still, complications do occasionally occur, and it is important to go to an experienced, competent physician to minimize these risks. If you want an abortion but are unsure where to go, a Planned Parenthood clinic or referral center in the city nearest you should give you reliable information.

Suction abortion can be performed up to the twelfth week of amenorrhea, or the tenth week after conception. After that time, the fetus is too large and severe bleeding may occur if a suction abortion is attempted. A good chance also exists that the physician may tear the cervix to accommodate such a large fetus.

Suction abortion can be performed either under local or general anesthesia. Most abortion clinics prefer local anesthesia because the patient can go home much sooner after the procedure. Hospital abortions are usually performed under general anesthesia, since the hospitals feel that this procedure, although it is more expensive, should be available to women who do not wish to be conscious during the abortion. Even at hospitals, though, one will usually be admitted in the morning and go home the same evening. A patient placed under a general anesthetic will experience no pain during the abortion.

Technique of First-Trimester Suction Abortion

The technique of suction abortion is outlined as follows: If the patient is undergoing local anesthesia, she will usually receive an intramuscular injection of one of the various painkillers such as codeine or Demerol. The patient is then placed on the operating table with her legs in the stirrups. An internal examination is performed to determine the size and the position of the uterus. The vagina is then washed with an antiseptic solution and a local anesthetic is injected into the cervix to numb the nerves. If a patient is having this procedure performed under general anesthesia, she initially receives an intramuscular injection of Atropine one hour prior to the procedure. This decreases the mucous secretion of the lungs in preparation for the later administration of general anesthesia. An intravenous infusion is then started. The anesthesia is usually initiated with intravenous injection of sodium pentathol through the intravenous infusion. The sodium pentathol puts the patient to sleep and then a general inhalation anesthetic,

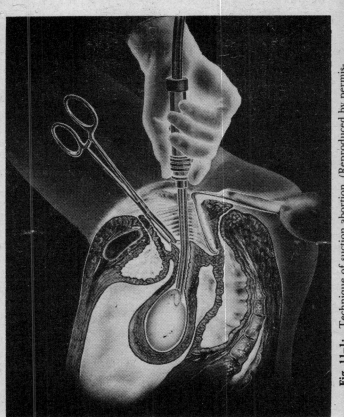

Fig. 11–1: Technique of suction abortion. (Reproduced by permission of the Berkeley Bio-Engineering, Inc., San Leandro, California.)

such as nitrous oxide, is administered through a mask during the operation. Once the patient is completely asleep, she is examined and her vagina is washed with an antiseptic. From this point, the procedure for patients under local and general anesthesia is identical.

The cervix is held by a tenaculum and then dilated slowly by the insertion of a progression of cervical dilators, each one somewhat larger than the last. The cervix is stretched until the opening allows the insertion of a suction tip *(vacurette)*. These tips have diameters ranging from 8 to 12 millimeters and, as a rule, a patient is aborted with a tip that is one size larger than the week of gestation; that is, if a patient is eight weeks from her last menstrual period, the physician will employ a nine-millimeter suction tip. As the vacurette tip is inserted into the uterus, it is attached to a suction apparatus via a flexible tube. This vacuum aspirator can either be an electrical or a mechanical pump, and it indicates the amount of vacuum suction it produces (see picture). The suction should go up to at least 60 centimeters of water pressure to evacuate completely the products of conception. The suction from the pump gently loosens the fetal tissue from the uterine wall and aspirates it through the suction to contract the uterus, thus decreasing the blood loss. With local anesthesia in a clinic, an injection of *ergotrate* is used to contract the uterus; this can cause nausea and vomiting.

If the abortion is performed under general anesthesia in a hospital, the patient is usually fully awake and ready to go home four to five hours following the operation. With a local-anesthesia abortion, the patient can go home after about two hours, but may feel a little faint and should be accompanied by a friend or relative.

Suction abortion under local anesthesia is not without discomfort, so it might be advisable to take a tranquilizer beforehand, if the clinic or the doctor permits it. The pain usually subsides during the first hour following the procedure.

A woman experiences contractions the first few days after the abortion as the uterus returns to normal. Bleeding usually occurs for up to two weeks following the procedure. In order to minimize the pain, a woman should take it easy the first few days after the abortion to give the uterus a rest and to decrease bleeding. If the bleeding is heavy or if a temperature develops after the operation, the clinic or doctor should be contacted immediately.

Blood type should be checked before any suction abortion. If a woman is more than six weeks pregnant and her blood type is Rh-negative, she should have an injection of Rhogam, an anti-

Rh-positive agent which prevents a woman from being immunized in future pregnancies (this is usually not necessary after a miniabortion). If the fetus has Rh-positive blood, and some of its blood gets into an Rh-negative bloodstream, an allergic reaction results causing subsequent pregnancies perhaps to abort spontaneously or result in death of the fetus. Rhogam prevents this from occurring.

A woman should be aware that the cervix will take three to four weeks to close up following a suction abortion. Because it is dilated, the uterus is particularly susceptible to infection, so during this period women should refrain from inserting tampons into the vagina or engaging in intercourse. Any object pushed into the vagina at this time might push bacteria from the vulva into the uterus. She may shower, but not bathe.

Since ovulation might occur two to three weeks after an abortion, birth control should be planned immediately. If the pill is the chosen method of birth control, the cycle should begin a few days after the abortion. If a woman opts for an IUD, it can be inserted while she is still anesthetized from the abortion. Regular menstrual periods usually occur four to eight weeks following an abortion.

ABORTION IN THE GRAY ZONE

The so-called gray zone is that period of time between the twelfth and the sixteenth week after the last menstrual period. Abortions are generally not performed at this time. During this interval, the fetus is too large for a suction abortion and there is too little amniotic fluid (the fluid which fills the sac surrounding the fetus) to allow an intraamniotic injection for a midtrimester abortion. This means that women who discover that they are pregnant after three months, or for some reason put off their decision to have an abortion until that time, must wait an additional month until they enter the time of the midtrimester, when abortion is feasible. Psychologically, this can be an extremely long month.

Recent research, however, has developed what appears to be a relatively simple, apparently safe method of "gray zone" abortion. These abortions are accomplished by means of *vaginal suppositories* of prostaglandin E2, a drug which causes uterine contractions and abortion. This method has been tried in over one thousand women with excellent results.

The half-life of prostaglandin in the circulation is less than thirty seconds, which means the body inactivates the drug in about half a minute. Therefore, vaginal suppositories are ideal for administration, because the prostaglandin is released slowly when the suppository is placed in the vagina. The suppositories are held in the vagina by a diaphragm that is altered by having a portion of the center removed. A physician may then determine when the abortion has occurred. Without the diaphragm, the prostaglandin tends to leak out, requiring more repeated suppository insertions, perhaps every two hours. With the diaphragm, suppositories must still be inserted repeatedly, but only every three or four hours. Expulsion of the products of conception usually occurs within ten to fifteen hours after insertion of the first suppository. Side effects such as nausea and diarrhea can be somewhat alleviated with prophylactic drugs.

Another form of prostaglandin has been developed which can induce abortion in the "gray zone"—a synthetic prostaglandin called 15(S)-15-methyl prostaglandin F2 alpha. This drug is injected intramuscularly every two to three hours and results in expulsion of the products of conception in about fourteen hours. This analog seems to relax the cervix as it stimulates the uterus, thus reducing the pain associated with abortion.

These two forms of "gray zone" abortions—vaginal administration of prostaglandin E2 suppositories and intramuscular injections of 15(S)-15-methyl prostaglandin F2 alpha are very effective in the midtrimester and have been approved for that use by the FDA. Often, traditional midtrimester abortions with intraamniotic instillation of saline cause excessive bleeding or are difficult to perform. Research continues into the development of the prostaglandin for abortion induction. These methods for gray zone abortions have not yet been approved by the Food and Drug Administration; it appears that they eventually will be. They will perhaps replace those presently used for midtrimester abortions.

Finally, researchers are working on a silastic device (a silicon material compatible with biological tissues, often used in plastic surgery) impregnated with 15(S)-15-methyl prostaglandin F2 alpha. This device can be inserted into the vagina and slowly releases the drug into the system, eliminating the need for replacement of the suppository. In the future, it might even be possible to perform first-trimester abortions using a prostaglandin device, thus eliminating entirely the need for suction abortion.

There is usually some bleeding and mild cramping for one or two weeks following the gray zone abortion. The same instructions as for midtrimester abortions should be followed after this procedure.

MIDTRIMESTER ABORTION

Midtrimester abortion, or the interruption of pregnancy from the sixteenth to the twenty-fourth week of gestation, is the most difficult and complicated of all the abortion techniques. Although pregnancy may be legally interrupted up to the twenty-fourth week from the last menstrual period, many hospitals and clinics will not perform the procedure after the twentieth week unless the woman's health is in danger or there are indications of a malformed fetus. These restrictions are observed in some institutions in order to avoid any possibility of delivering a fetus with signs of life, a circumstance which proves very disturbing to both the woman having the abortion and the professional staff attending her. Women should be aware of the difficulties related to midtrimester abortion. Because of the difficulties, if a woman is considering pregnancy interruption, she should have it interrupted as soon as it is known she is pregnant.

Pregnancy can be interrupted between the sixteenth and the twenty-fourth week of gestation by intraamniotic instillation of either saline or prostaglandin, or by hysterotomy.

Intraamniotic Instillation

An intraamniotic instillation of either saline or prostaglandin causes abortion by stimulating the uterus to contractions similar to those of labor, and the products of conception are expelled, mimicking a natural miscarriage. Abortions of this type are considered major procedures and should only be performed in hospitals on an inpatient basis so that the woman can be carefully watched throughout the entire procedure. In this way, if any complications occur, they can be immediately and adequately handled by a competent professional staff. A woman undergoing this type of abortion must expect a hospital stay of one and a half to three days in an uncomplicated procedure.

A woman must fast for at least six hours prior to her admission to the hospital. On admission, a blood specimen is obtained for typing and cross-matching, so that blood replacement is immediately available if the woman has bleeding complications. An intravenous infusion is then started.

The woman is then taken to either an operating or treatment room and is asked to lie on her back on the treatment table. The procedure is initiated by a careful washing of the lower abdominal region with an antiseptic solution; there is no need for shaving of the abdomen. A sterile drape is placed over the lower part of the body and the area from the pubis to just below the naval is left exposed. The physician performs the operation wearing a mask and sterile operating gloves to eliminate the risk of infection. The physician palpates the abdomen to determine the position of the uterus and the appropriate area for the injection. A local anesthetic such as Novocaine is injected into the area where the needle will be inserted. Once this area is anesthetized, the procedure, an *amniocentesis*, is performed. In general, *amniocentesis* is the puncturing through the abdominal wall of the amniotic sac, the sac of fluid which surrounds the fetus, by a fine needle and the aspiration or withdrawal of some of the amniotic fluid. This procedure is performed for a variety of reasons, such as determining the genetic makeup of the infant for chromosomal studies, determining fetal abnormalities and fetal lung maturity at term, and finally for the initiation of abortion by intraamniotic instillation of drugs.

If saline is used to induce the abortion, an 18-gauge, 3½-inch-long spinal needle is inserted through the abdominal wall and into the amniotic sac. Between 50 and 200 cubic centimeters of amniotic fluid are withdrawn via a syringe attached to the needle. Approximately 200 cubic centimeters, or approximately seven fluid ounces, of a 20 percent saline solution are slowly injected through the needle by a syringe into the amniotic fluid.

If, on the other hand, prostaglandin is used, only a very small amount of amniotic fluid is withdrawn. This is simply to determine the correct positioning of the needle. Eight milliliters, containing forty milligrams of prostaglandin F2 alpha are slowly injected into the amniotic sac. The needle is then removed and the site of the amniocentesis covered with a sterile dressing. If it is done by an experienced physician, amniocentesis is a rapid and relatively painless procedure.

The woman's blood pressure and pulse rate are then measured. If the readings are within normal limits, she is returned to her room and requested to remain in bed for one hour. After this time, the woman may be allowed to walk around for as long as she wishes. A clear liquid diet is provided until the expulsion of the fetus. For the first few hours after the amniocentesis, a woman should experience only a minimal amount of pain. As time passes, abdominal cramps of increasing strength develop, similar to cramps experienced with the onset of menstrual flow. The cramps, or contractions of the uterus, cause a softening of the cervical muscle in preparation for the dilation required for the expulsion of the products of conception. As cervical dilation occurs, the pain associated with cramps increases to a peak. This happens immediately prior to the expulsion of the fetus,

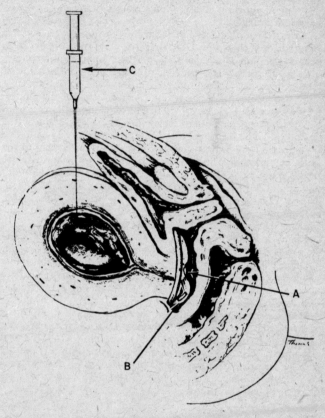

Fig. 11-2: Midtrimester abortions are usually performed by intraamniotic instillation of either a hypertonic saline solution or prostaglandin. During amniocentesis, the needle is inserted through the abdominal wall into the uterus and amniotic fluid is aspirated with a syringe, as shown in C. The hypertonic saline or the prostaglandin is then injected and the needle withdrawn.

Vaginal suppositories, as shown in B, containing prostaglandins have been administered for induction of midtrimester abortion and a number of various techniques are under investigation. Some investigators also insert a diaphragm, as shown in A, to prevent the leakage of the suppositories.

and the cervix is the most stretched at this point. In women who have not previously delivered a child, the pain associated with this type of abortion is somewhat stronger than in women who have had children.

During the early part of the abortion, a woman may receive a tranquilizer such as Valium to help relax her over the abortion period. As pain and cramping increase, something stronger, such as Demerol, is required. However, if an injection of Demerol is administered too early, it stops the uterine contractions and prolongs the abortion. Demerol should not, therefore, be given before the cervix begins to dilate. As contractions become stronger, a woman feels more comfortable in a sitting position than in a supine position. As the woman begins to feel strong rectal pressure, often an indication that passage of the fetus is imminent, she may be asked to sit on a bed pan (to facilitate the passage of the abortus) and asked to use voluntary abdominal exertion. When the abortion takes place, the patient usually remains in her hospital bed and is aided by the nursing staff. Only rarely is she transferred to an operating or delivery room.

The time from the intraamniotic instillation of either saline or prostaglandin to abortion varies from patient to patient. Women who have previously borne children abort somewhat faster than women who have not. A relaxed woman appears to abort more rapidly than a tense woman. The abortion time is approximately eighteen to twenty hours.

If the placenta is not expelled spontaneously as the fetus is aborted, the gynecologist must remove it. It usually comes out by itself an hour or two after abortion, but if it doesn't, removal is simple and often accomplished manually or with the aid of a sponge forceps. After passage of the placenta, the uterus contracts and the bleeding stops. In extremely rare cases, the placenta is hard to remove, and a D&C is required.

Oxytocin Administration during Midtrimester Abortion

One of the main factors influencing the time it takes to complete an abortion is the length of time it takes for the cervix to dilate and permit passage of the fetus and placenta. In order to speed up the dilation of the cervix, *laminaria digitala* (dried seaweed steam) is inserted into the cervix. The laminaria absorbs body fluid, causing it to expand slowly and to create a very gradual dilation of the cervix. Another method of decreasing abortion time is to increase uterine activity. This is achieved by the intravenous infusion of oxytocin.

This hormone must be administered carefully in a saline solution, like Ringer's lactate, because oxytocin can work as an antidiuretic, preventing the excretion of water from the body and causing water retention. There have been cases where the water in the body has reached toxic levels and has diluted the bodily sodium concentration. This leads to seizures and even death. When oxytocin is given, careful attention should be paid to urine output. If there is a decrease in urination, diuretics should be given, oxytocin should be stopped, and electrolytes should be checked for sodium levels.

If oxytocin is given with intraamniotic instillation of prostaglandin, it may cause overly violent contractions which rupture the cervix. However, if the oxytocin is not administered for six hours following amniocentesis, there are few problems. After instillation of saline solution, there should be a two-hour interval before administration of oxytocin.

What to Expect following a Midtrimester Intraamniotic Abortion

The patient may leave the hospital six to ten hours after the abortion. For two weeks following a midtrimester abortion, there will be bleeding and the passing of a few large clots. The patient should try to remain relatively inactive. Because the cervix is dilated, no foreign objects should be introduced into the vagina or infection may be pushed into the uterus. This means no tampons and no sexual intercourse. A woman may shower, but not bathe during this time. After four weeks, the patient should have a follow-up examination. If the uterus has healed and the cervix has closed, normal sex life may resume.

Birth control should begin as soon as possible. If a woman elects to use the pill, she should begin taking it a few days after the abortion.

If heavy bleeding or a sign of infection occurs after a woman has left the hospital, she should immediately contact the clinic or doctor who did the abortion. If neither can be reached, she should go immediately to the nearest hospital emergency room. Women should expect a very heavy flow during the first menstrual period following abortion.

Since midtrimester abortion is actually induced labor, the endocrine mechanism of the body is fooled into producing milk. Women should expect milk secretion for several weeks after abortion. Nothing can be done about this, but a tight breast binder or bra helps decrease tenderness. Breast movement stimulates milk production, as does applied heat.

If a midtrimester abortion is performed by an experienced physician in a good hospital, the procedure resembles a miscarriage and no physical harm should result to the uterus. The ability to conceive and have children will not be affected. In fact, it might even be easier to conceive since the cervix has been opened.

Hysterotomy

Hysterotomy is an operative abortion, a procedure almost identical to a Caesarean section, in which the products of conception are surgically removed. This is considered a major operative procedure requiring a hospital stay of six to eight days. After a hysterotomy, a woman will have a scar on her abdomen. More importantly, she will also have a scar in her uterus. In the future, she will have to be delivered by Caesarean section. Because of this, hysterotomy is seldom employed.

The operation is usually performed under general anesthesia, but can be done with spinal anesthesia. When the woman is asleep, the abdomen is shaved and sterilized. The patient is draped sterilely and an abdominal incision is made, either transverse (from side to side) or up and down. When the abdomen is open, an incision is made in the lower part of the uterus. The amniotic sac containing the products of conception is carefully freed from the inner uterine wall and removed via the incision. The uterus and the abdomen are then surgically closed.

The patient is given a postoperative intravenous infusion for two days. She is then slowly given clear liquids. Finally, during the last part of the hospital stay, she is allowed to have solid foods. If the woman's recovery is uncomplicated, she is usually discharged on the seventh postoperative day.

A patient undergoing a hysterotomy must expect a longer period of recuperation than if her pregnancy is terminated by intraamniotic instillation of either saline or prostaglandin. Complete healing does not occur for four to six weeks following surgery, and during this period, a woman should not have intercourse, lift any heavy objects, or even return to work.

Hysterotomy is associated with the highest complication rate of any type of abortion and should only be performed in a very limited number of indicated cases, such as in cases of uterine abnormalities.

Mental Health and Late Abortions

Besides the medical complications, late or midtrimester abortions have also been associated with more pronounced psychological difficulties. The late abortion is usually a rather painful procedure—it is actually a drug-induced miscarriage—but psychological trauma is often a greater problem for women who undergo this type of abortion. Many hospitals recognize this and have set up counseling centers to deal with the depression which often accompanies midtrimester abortions. Because the fetus is so far advanced, many women have religious conflicts. Unmarried women may allow a pregnancy to continue too long in the hope of marrying the child's father and are emotionally devastated when he refuses. Still others refuse to face the possibility that they are pregnant, sometimes indicating a weak grip on reality and the potential to break down.

The psychological depression that can occur after late abortion may be very severe, sometimes suicidal. Some women are so depressed that they require hospitalization. This should be recognized by the family and parents, who should help any woman as much as possible after any abortion. Women should know that this depression will disappear and if the abortion was performed in a recognized clinic or a good hospital, there should be no difficulty in conceiving and carrying a child in the future. It is important to note that many women emerge from an abortion experience unscarred and with a healthy attitude toward contraception.

If you need psychological counseling and don't know where to get it, your nearest Planned Parenthood center should be able to help. There should be a Planned Parenthood office in your state, but if you don't know how to contact it, call the main office in New York City at (212)541-7800. Counseling and referral for abortion can also be obtained in many cities from the Clergy Consultation Service, an organization of women and men of all religions who recognize the difficulty a woman experiences when she has an unwanted pregnancy. This organization is also able to refer you to the best abortion facility or the best counseling. Their main office is also in New York City, and they can be reached at (212)254-6230.

CHOOSING THE METHOD OF ABORTION

When a woman is pregnant and does not wish to maintain the pregnancy, it is important for her to decide on interruption as early as possible. The miniabortion and the early, first-trimester curettage are the least complicated procedures, in both the medical and psychological senses. As a general rule, the later an abortion is performed, the higher the complication rate. Statistics collected from 1972 to 1975 in the United States indicated that the death rate associated with suction abortion was 1.6 per

100,000 abortions; the death rate related to intraamniotic instillation of saline was 22.9 per 100,000 abortions; and the death rate for hysterotomies was 45.0 per 100,000. Prostaglandin was approved by the Food and Drug Administration in 1973, and initial studies indicate that it is even safer than saline. Labor and full-term delivery are associated with a death rate of approximately 20 per 100,000; thus it is evident that early abortion is even safer than full-term delivery.

When performed by experienced physicians, intraamniotic instillation of prostaglandin is the safest form of abortion from the sixteenth to the twentieth weeks of gestation. However, because of the possibility of the fetus being aborted with some signs of life in an abortion performed after twenty weeks, the majority of physicians induce abortion with saline in these later gestations.

Recent research indicates that intraamniotic instillation of saline results in damage to the placenta and fetal death, as well as causing an expansion in the volume of the uterus. It is hypothesized that instillation leads to the release of prostaglandin; it is the prostaglandins which cause uterine contractions, which result in the expulsion of the products of conception.

ABORTION IN THE FUTURE

In the future, with more sex education and counseling, women will better understand their bodies and be better able to detect the signs of pregnancy early. It is hoped that pregnancy testing facilities or home pregnancy kits for detection of early pregnancies will be readily available to every woman to determine if she is pregnant without fear of recrimination. If a pregnancy is confirmed and cannot be maintained, it should be interrupted in the earliest stage, when there is the greatest margin of safety and a lesser chance of permanent damage to the body.

Research is being conducted with the administration of different types of prostaglandins for the induction of very early first-trimester abortions. It may be that, in time, prostaglandins will replace many types of mechanical abortions or suction techniques. Prostaglandin causes uterine activity, which results in the expulsion of the products of conception. In the future, this type of prostaglandin may even be used to induce a period if a woman is a few days late.

chapter 12

INFERTILITY

Infertility—the inability of a couple to conceive—is, for many people, a completely irrelevant concern, since most young couples are preoccupied with preventing conception and many even live in constant fear of unwanted pregnancy. In fact, the most remote thought in a young woman's mind is that she might be barren. Probably as a result of our upbringing and cultural conditioning, we tend to expect our bodies to perform on demand, and for this reason, many couples become hysterical if they do not conceive within the first months of trying.

Our social attitudes and values are undergoing profound changes at present. Many women now postpone childbearing until their late twenties, early thirties, or even later years, waiting until they have fulfilled career ambitions as well as other personal goals. Because of this, more and more women are coming to realize that it is increasingly difficult to get pregnant as they get older. This is caused by many factors, not the least of which is the fact that women and men can develop various medical conditions in the intervening years which make conception more difficult and which may even cause sterility.

The realization that a couple might be sterile often comes as a shock and can cause tremendous psychological distress. This is particularly true of couples who have postponed childbearing in order to achieve certain career goals and a degree of financial security. When such couples are faced with the realization that they might remain childless, their dreams can be completely shattered.

The word *infertility* has a nightmarish ring of finality. The thought of it cuts straight to our genetic core, for it is our biological heritage, to say nothing of our societal expectation, to reproduce. That is how our species survives and progresses. Yet, far from being a permanent condition, infertility is often the result of a relatively minor psychological, physical, or chemical problem. It is a condition which can be reversed. Rather than being a permanent curse, infertility is often a matter of poor timing, nervousness, or hormonal imbalance. In this chapter, infertility is defined as the inability of a couple to conceive after *one year* of coitus without contraception. About ten percent of all married couples fit this description.

Partly as a response to the great number of unwanted pregnancies in our society, many people believe it is easy to conceive. Actually, it is rather difficult to conceive. Women are fertile for only two to three days each month, while sperm survives in the uterus for only two to three days. Therefore, conception usually occurs only during a period of three to five days each month. If the timing is off, it can take months for a woman to become pregnant. Patience is often a successful self-help fertility program, but if patience fails after one year, it is time to consult a fertility specialist.

CAUSES OF INFERTILITY

The process of fertilization is so complicated that any minor disorder can prevent it. First, an egg must be released from the woman's ovaries. This egg must be able to move freely into the fallopian tube, which in turn must be normal and unobstructed all the way into the uterus. While this occurs, hormonal changes should open the mouth of the cervix during ovulation to make a channel for the sperm. The sperm, assuming the man is able to produce healthy, motile (fast-swimming) sperm, must then reach the egg alive and penetrate it. Then the fertilized egg must move into the uterus and embed itself in the uterine wall, at which time it should be under the influence of the correct hormonal conditions.

This complex process can break down from a wide variety of causes originating in either the woman or the man, or both (as, for example, when the woman develops an allergic reaction to the man's sperm).

Female infertility can be caused by emotional stress, radical weight changes, thyroid dysfunction, vaginitis, mycoplasma (microorganisms in the cervix or the vagina), amenorrhea (cessation of menstruation), ovarian cysts, endometriosis, pelvic tumors, cervical stenosis (narrowing of the cervix), or synechia (scar tissue in the uterus).

Male infertility can result from excessive drinking, stress, lack of exercise, hormonal disturbance, or varicose veins in the testes. Most male infertility stems from permanent damage done by mumps, venereal disease, or physical trauma to the genitalia.

These causes are discussed at greater length later, but there is one additional problem that deserves mention here: the fear of infertility. Sometimes a couple assumes that they are infertile because they have been unable to conceive after several months of trying. This assumption becomes an emotional stress that, in itself, is enough to prevent normal conception. Such couples often conceive soon after seeing a fertility specialist, even if he prescribes no treatment.

Finally, many women believe that a tilted uterus prevents pregnancy. This is a myth. Recent studies have shown that the angle of the uterus has no influence on fertility. Some doctors still perform surgery to move the uterus forward by tightening the uterine ligaments, but any subsequent improved fertility is to be attributed to psychological rather than physiological factors. This procedure is now performed only if the uterus is tilted back so far that the veins are obstructed, causing abdominal pain.

WHAT TO DO BEFORE CONSULTING A SPECIALIST

Since conception is such a complicated process, there is no reason to suspect a fertility problem until at least a year of intercourse without the use of contraceptive measures has elapsed. In the case of women taking the pill, a longer period may be necessary from the time she stops taking the pill, since it may take a few months for normal ovulation to resume.

On the other hand, older couples might consider seeing a specialist after about six months of unsuccessful attempts at conception, since the mechanism of ovulation in the woman deteriorates with age and the amount and motility of sperm begins to decrease in men as early as the mid-twenties. Thus the older a couple is, the more difficult it becomes to conceive, and the greater the likelihood of infertility for such couples.

During this trial period, intercourse should be carefully timed to fall within the few fertile days each month when the woman is most likely to conceive. These days usually fall about fourteen days prior to the onset of the next menstrual period, no matter what the length of the menstrual cycle. Because of this, the couple should have intercourse daily from between seventeen to eleven days prior to the onset of the woman's next menstrual period. Chances of conceiving before ovulation are greater than after ovulation.

After coitus, the man should withdraw his penis from the woman's vagina so that the sperm will not dilute on the shaft of the penis. Pillows placed beneath the woman's buttocks give the sperm a much-appreciated downhill swim. Any jelly or Vaseline used during intercourse may harm sperm, so saliva is recommended if a lubricant is necessary.

Emotional stress can disrupt both male and female hormonal balance, so periods of relaxation, like vacations, are good times to conceive. The man should be careful not to drink too much or become exhausted from too much sightseeing. He might even want to take vitamin supplements.

A good example of stress-related infertility is the case of a woman who held a hectic professional position—one that made her extremely nervous. This, coupled with her anxiety concerning her inability to conceive, was making her infertile. Her physician, who found nothing abnormal during a physical examination, suggested she take a glass or two of wine each evening to help her relax, and one evening at a party, she had intercourse standing up in the garden and conceived.

If, after relaxing, eating properly, cutting down on excess drinking, taking regular exercise, timing intercourse, and following the optimum coital procedure for conception, a couple has not conceived after one year, it is then time to seek professional help. It is important to find a fertility specialist, not just any gynecologist. Even though most gynecologists claim to have some expertise in treating infertility, this does not qualify them as fertility specialists. The head of the department of obstetrics and gynecology at any major medical center should be able to refer a couple to a competent fertility specialist.

FREQUENCY OF SEX

During the investigation of the frequency of sex, it is important to understand the relationship between the partners and the amount of sex experienced. It is important to know that orgasm has no influence on the ability of a woman to conceive. Orgasm is merely satisfying and pleasurable for the partners, but conception can occur even without it, as, for example, during artificial insemination, where there is no sexual pleasure at all. During the investigation of a couple's sex habits, it is not so much a question of how often they have sex as it is the understanding of having sex on the right days. In this area, the physician should help a woman calculate the days when she is most likely to be fertile, since this time of maximum fertility amounts to only a few days each month. There are different beliefs as to how often intercourse should take place during the woman's fertile days. Some physicians believe that couples should have intercourse only once every other day in order to build up the semen and break down the acid-base difference between the sperm and the mucous plug. On the other hand, if sperm are too old, they tire easily and have less motility. Therefore, it is probably advisable during a woman's fertile days for a couple to have intercourse every day. It is also important, during those days, that the man is well rested, takes vitamins, and does not drink too much.

DIAGNOSING FERTILITY PROBLEMS

Infertility Workup

The first step in determining the cause of infertility is a comprehensive medical history and a physiological examination. You should be absolutely candid with your doctor. Remember, it is his responsibility to keep your medical history confidential, even from your husband. Your doctor should know about any previous pregnancies, miscarriages, or abortions (especially illegal ones) which you may have had, because these indicate that you do ovulate, at least occasionally, and this information could also point to possible fallopian complications resulting from infection or scar tissue. If you have conceived before but your partner has not, the problem could be his, not yours.

A menstrual history is vital to a proper understanding of the nature of infertility. If regular periods occur every twenty-eight days, ovulation is highly probable, so the problem must be elsewhere. Irregular menstrual bleeding, sometimes spanning eight weeks between periods, might indicate a problem such as Stein-Leventhal syndrome, in which the ovaries are enlarged and have a thicker capsule, making ovulation difficult or impossible.

An erratic menstrual history may also indicate hormonal imbalance, especially when accompanied by increased hair growth on the face and arms. This can often be solved with hormone injections or fertility drugs.

The release of hormones is radically affected by anxiety. Two key hormones, the releasing hormones FSH-RH and LH-RH, are produced in the hypothalamus area of the brain and stimulate the production of FSH and LH, both of which are released by the pituitary gland. Anxiety affects the hypothalamus and, in turn, affects the release of these hormones, resulting in sterility. For example, a group of women college students who were under a great deal of stress were found not to release these hormones at all, and therefore developed amenorrhea. However, as soon as they went home to their parents for a vacation and were relaxed, they released these hormones again, and normal menstruation resumed. FSH and LH are responsible for stimulating the ovaries to produce estrogen and progesterone, and without them, abnormal menstrual periods result. It is important to include any psychological or emotional stress in your history so your doctor can consider these factors in his diagnosis.

At this point, it is worth noting that approximately 25 percent of all infertility problems are caused by male infertility. This is due either to the fact that the man does not produce enough sperm or that his sperm are abnormal in size or shape. For example, some men produce sperm with two heads, two tails, and various other abnormalities. Often a man produces enough sperm, but if their motility (i.e., swimming speed) is too slow, this can cause sterility in the man, even if his sperm are normal in shape and size.

Since such a high percentage of infertility is caused by male infertility, it is important for a man to undergo a complete physical examination, including a sperm analysis, in order to determine if a couple's infertility problem is related to any physical abnormalities in his reproductive system. In this way, if the problem lies with the man, the wife can be spared the time, inconvenience, discomfort, and expense of extensive tests when, in fact, it is her partner who is infertile.

Of course, certain diseases in a woman's past may have caused damage to the ovaries or fallopian tubes. Venereal diseases are particularly dangerous, so a woman should not be shy about reporting them to her doctor. He is there to help cure infertility problems, not to pass any kind of moral judgment.

If there is any thyroid dysfunction in your family, you should be tested. Actually, you should have this done anyway. Thyroid function is very closely associated with ovulation, and many infertile women who complain of fatigue show a low level of thyroid function in blood tests. A thyroid pill often cures both the fatigue and the infertility.

The loss or gain of as little as five pounds can also throw off a woman's menstrual cycle. Therefore, if you have been dieting or if you have recently gained weight, be sure to include this information in your medical history. A return to normal weight generally causes your menstrual cycle to return to its normal pattern.

Any physical examination prior to diagnosing the cause of infertility should be thorough. Your eyes should be normal, your neck should be without thyroid gland enlargements, your heart and lungs should be functioning normally, and your blood pressure should be normal. Any problems in these areas could mean trouble, from thyroid dysfunction to kidney problems. For instance, if your blood pressure is high, you could be suffering from chronic hypertension. This is sometimes caused by kidney abnormalities, which in turn often cause infertility. A urine sample can isolate many of these problems, and at the same time, it can be checked for possible diabetes.

A pelvic examination often reveals startling problems, such as a total congenital absence of the uterus or fallopian tubes. A speculum inspection of the cervix should be performed to be sure that it is open. The hymen should also be examined to make certain that it is not intact. A bimanual examination, with two fingers in the vagina and the other hand on the abdomen, reveals any uterine tumors. You must relax completely for this examination to be successful, although this is often more easily said than done.

Basal Body Temperature

One essential indicator which the doctor will want to evaluate is your basal body temperature (BBT). This is usually taken orally, although some physicians prefer it be taken rectally. BBT takes a month to measure, so you should have taken your BBT for one month before visiting your doctor. This not only saves time, it also gives your doctor the advantage of additional data for his initial diagnosis of your fertility problem.

BBT is obtained by taking your temperature every morning,

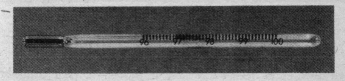

Fig. 12–1: Ovulation Thermometer. This is a special type of thermometer, since it is only able to measure temperatures between 96° and 100°F.

beginning on the first day of your period, as soon as you awaken and before you get out of bed. It is important that the basal body temperature be taken before you smoke a cigarette, brush your teeth, drink coffee, make love, or do anything else, since the slightest activity affects BBT. After a month of plotting your BBT on a graph, you know exactly when, or if, you ovulated.

Immediately after menstruation, the ovaries are stimulated by the hormone FSH to produce an egg. During the growth period of the egg, the BBT remains relatively low and stable, but at the time of ovulation, there is a small *decrease* in the BBT, followed by a sharp increase (see Fig. 5–2).

As the egg makes its way into the uterus, the scar tissue in the ovaries, where the egg was expelled, turns into the so-called yellow body, or corpus luteum. This yellow body starts to produce progesterone, which reduces the contractions of the uterus and tubes, thereby simplifying conception. This increase in progesterone also increases body temperature, which remains high until immediately prior to menstruation. If your BBT shows an early drop at this point, you probably have a luteal problem, caused by insufficient production of progesterone. While it is possible to conceive with this condition, the contractions of the uterus might increase, squeezing the egg out of the womb and resulting in miscarriage. Treatment is therefore recommended if you have a luteal problem.

If the BBT does not decrease before the anticipated time of your next menstrual period, you might be pregnant. BBT is the cheapest and easiest pregnancy test. If you have reason to believe you are pregnant, continue charting your BBT for another two weeks just to be sure, at which time a pregnancy test can be done.

The Cervical Factor

The cervix is more than a passive barrier to be negotiated by the sperm; it is an active organ whose functioning is essential to conception. Studies show that cervical problems are responsible for between 30 and 50 percent of all female infertility.

The cervix changes shape throughout the menstrual cycle. For instance, it opens and shortens to let blood pass from the uterus during the menstrual period. It is during this phase that vaginal infections can be sucked into the tubes by the pumplike contractions of the uterus, resulting in *salpingitis* (inflammation of the fallopian tubes), or even into the abdominal cavity, resulting in *peritonitis* (inflammation of the peritoneum, the smooth,

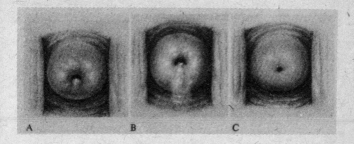

Fig. 12-2: A close-up view of changes in the cervix throughout the menstrual cycle. (A) A few days after menstruation has ceased, the cervical canal is closed and the cervix points backwards. (B) The cervix, during ovulation, moves forward, and the cervical canal opens to approximately 3 mm in diameter to facilitate sperm transport. The cervical mucus is clear, watery, and slimy, which makes sperm adhere more easily to the cervix. (C) The cervical opening closes again during the luteal phase and will again point somewhat backward. The cervical mucus has almost disappeared. (Reproduced by permission from *Progress in Infertility;* 1968; Little, Brown and Company, Inc.; Boston, Massachusetts.)

transparent membrane that lines the abdominal cavity). After menstruation, the cervix usually points backward and closes to an opening of only about one millimeter.

At the time of ovulation, the cervix usually opens to about three millimeters. It softens and points forward in order to catch the sperm. The cervical secretions become thinner, like saliva, to aid the sperm's passage through the fine channels of the mucous plug at the mouth of the cervix. Many women describe this change as "becoming wetter." This wetness also increases sexual sensations, remotely resembling the mechanisms of *estrus* ("in heat") in other species. After ovulation, the mucus thickens. Women who practice the rhythm method of birth control call this their "dry" or "safe" period. What is vital to understand here is that all of these changes are governed by estrogen levels.

Your doctor can ascertain a great deal from mucus samples. The mucus should stretch up to ten centimeters and be long and slimy. This enables the mucus to draw the sperm into the cervix and lead it on into the uterus and tubes. If there is no change in the amount of mucus and its ability to stretch (also called *Spinbarkeit*), there may be no ovulation.

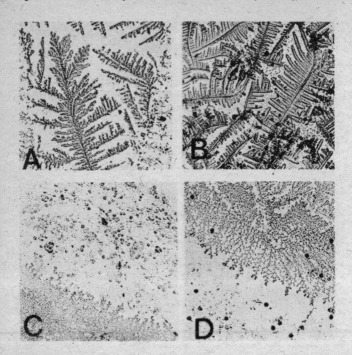

Fig. 12–3: Fern pattern of the cervical mucus. This illustration shows how the dried mucus, as it appears under a microscope, changes throughout the menstrual cycle. (A) The fern pattern a few days after menstruation. (B) A well-developed fern pattern at the time of ovulation. Note how the mucus crystallizes, forming small, fine channels in which the sperm can travel. (C) The fern pattern is broken up in the mid-luteal phase, days 20–24 of the menstrual cycle. Sperm cannot pass through this mucus. (D) Poorly developed fern pattern in a patient with a vaginal infection, which could be contributing to her infertility problem. (Reproduced by permission from *Progress in Infertility;* 1968; Little, Brown and Company, Inc.; Boston, Massachusetts.)

The Postcoital Test

Dr. Papanicolaou, who discovered the Pap-smear test for cancer, found that cervical mucus, when dried, forms distinctive patterns which change as the mucus changes. When a woman is fertile, these patterns, during ovulation, resemble in shape a fern or palm leaves, opening channels through which the sperm can swim freely. This pattern is important in evaluating the estrogen and hormone levels. When the mucus thickens, after ovulation, the "leaves" appear to bunch up and the channels are closed off, acting like miniature diaphragms to prevent the entrance of sperm.

A visit to the doctor as soon as possible after intercourse, preferably within two to three hours, enables him to extract samples of sperm and mucus to determine whether the sperm is able to move through the fern patterns. This test is also valuable for finding out if the sperm can survive in the mucus, since many women are allergic to sperm, and this reaction causes the sperm to die in the mucous plug.

The Influence of Vaginal Infections on Fertility

The effect of vaginitis on fertility is hard to evaluate, but there is little doubt that increased discharge lowers sperm concentrations by diluting semen. Trichomonas in the vagina is likely to cause an increased pH in the vagina, and this elevation of the pH could interfere with sperm survival. Whether the elevated pH permitted the vaginal infection to develop or whether it is secondary to the discharge produced is uncertain. Vaginal moniliasis does not increase the vaginal pH. However, clinical vaginitis of both types may diminish fertility because the resulting discharge impedes sperm migration and dilutes the sperm concentration. It is, therefore, important to understand that infertility can be caused by infections of the vagina, and the physician should examine you for both monilia and trichomonas, as well as for cervicitis. If any of these conditions are present, they should be treated, as they could be the only factors causing infertility.

Mycoplasma

Mycoplasma is a condition wherein microorganisms are found in the cervix and vagina. Some studies have recently shown that this condition *could* influence fertility by decreasing sperm motility and/or survival; however, other studies deny the importance of these findings. Treatment with tetracycline (250 milligrams, taken four times a day for ten days) should be sufficient to kill the infection. It might also kill other infections present, and therefore increase fertility. However, when a woman is treated with a broad-spectrum antibiotic such as tetracycline, the balance in the vagina between yeast and bacteria is often altered, thereby causing a yeast infection, which, in turn, causes infertility. Therefore, if you are treated with antibiotics, you should always be treated at the same time with an antiyeast medication such as myocostatin suppositories or any other antiyeast cream or jelly, to maintain the proper balance between yeast and bacteria in the vagina.

Tubal Insufflation (The Rubin Test)

The Rubin Test, in which the fallopian tubes are inflated with carbon dioxide, can determine if at least one of the tubes is open. Unfortunately, this test cannot distinguish between bilateral and unilateral blockage, nor can it determine the existence of a partial blockage of one or both of the fallopian tubes. For this reason, the Rubin Test is considered to be obsolete by many modern fertility specialists. On the other hand, the advantage of the Rubin Test is that it can be performed in the doctor's office, but other tests must be performed concurrently in order for it to have any credibility. During this procedure, if the fallopian tubes are clear, gas (carbon dioxide) escapes into the abdomen, and there is no high pressure. The escaping gas can be heard with a stethoscope, and when the woman sits up, she feels a pain in her shoulders, because the gas has irritated the thoracic diaphragm, thereby stimulating the phrenic nerve.

Hysterosalpingogram

Rather than resort to the Rubin Test, most modern gynecologists and fertility specialists prefer the *hysterosalpingogram,* an X-ray of the uterus and the fallopian tubes. In modern hospitals and clinics, where extensive infertility studies are performed, X-ray facilities have been set up specifically for this test.

First, the patient lies on a gynecological table. A special forceps (a tenaculum) holds the cervix, while a tubelike instrument connects a syringe to the cervix. A water-soluble dye is then injected with the syringe into the uterine cavity, flushing through the tubes. This dye, as it shows up on an X-ray film or a fluoroscope, reveals any abnormalities of the uterus or the tubes. Often the dye flushes out obstructions in the tubes, and if no other problems are influencing the woman's infertility, the pregnancy rate increases 40 to 50 percent within four months of this test. The hysterosalpingogram can be painful, so a Valium or an aspirin tablet might be taken beforehand. Aside from identifying obstructions, a hysterosalpingogram can also indi-

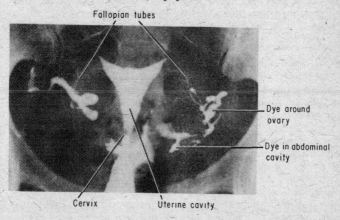

Normal Hysterosalpingogram

Fallopian tubes

Dye around ovary

Dye in abdominal cavity

Cervix

Uterine cavity

Fig. 12–4: X-ray picture of a *hysterosalpingogram,* which shows a normal uterine cavity and normal and open fallopian tubes. The dye flows freely out through the tubes on both sides and surrounds the ovaries.

cate cervical stenosis and/or synechia (scar tissue inside the uterus).

Endometrial Biopsy

In an endometrial biopsy a small spoon is placed through the vagina and cervix into the uterus to take a specimen from the endometrium (see Fig. 16–2). As has been described before, the lining of the uterus, or endometrium, changes and becomes thicker toward the end of the menstrual cycle, making it ready for implantation of the egg. During the menstrual period, the endometrium is expelled due to contractions of the uterus. A biopsy from the uterine lining determines if ovulation has occurred. The best time for the biopsy is the first day of menstruation, because when the uterus starts contracting, the cervix opens and it is easier to insert the biopsy instrument. This test is painful, but less so if it is performed during the time of menstrual bleeding. A good pathologist grades the biopsy by studying the vascularity and structure of the tissue, thereby determining if ovulation has occurred and if implantation was possible. Endometrial biopsy is still considered a good test, and it should be a part of an infertility workup.

Laparoscopy

If, after a hysterosalpingogram or a Rubin Test, your doctor suspects pelvic adhesions, he should perform a laparoscopy (waiting three to four months after the hysterosalpingogram to see if conception occurs in the interim). This is a fairly simple procedure, usually performed in a hospital under general anesthesia because it causes severe pain when the abdomen is distended with four liters of carbon dioxide. A periscope is inserted through the navel to give the doctor a complete view of the pelvic organs. The periscope is the same instrument used for tubal cauterization or ligation during voluntary sterilization (see illustration in Chapter 10, Voluntary Sterilization).

Small adhesions and obstructions are treated through the laparoscopy. Sometimes a problem requires more extensive surgery, such as a *laparotomy* with a *tuboplasty* (see Tuboplasty, below), and the patient should be prepared for this eventuality so that the doctor can proceed while she is still under anesthesia. Laparoscopy is also used to evaluate pelvic tumors or endometriotic masses. Several women have become pregnant after this operation, even when no cause of infertility was found. This could be due either to psychological factors or to the fact that the operation perhaps stimulated the ovaries to normal functioning.

Culposcopy

As in a laparoscopy, a periscope is inserted into the abdomen during colpotomy. Instead of being inserted through the navel, the periscope is introduced through the vagina for this procedure (see Fig. 16–7). Today, culposcopy has been largely replaced by laparoscopy, because a culposcopy can push into adhesions and cause even further damage. At the same time, the procedure is uncomfortable for the patient, since she must be in a knee-chest position under local anesthesia (see Fig. 16–6). Most physicians today have abandoned the culposcopy.

Tuboplasty

If laparoscopy reveals abnormalities such as adhesions or tubal occlusions of the fimbriated ends, an exploratory laparotomy (an operation in which the abdomen is surgically opened) must be performed to correct the condition. Occlusion, or blockage of the tubes, is often caused by gonorrheal infections. Other severe pelvic infections, such as those following a septic abortion or infections after delivery, also cause this closure. During the laparotomy, a dye is usually injected into the uterus so the physician can see if the tubes are open. If there are pelvic adhesions, a careful dissection and surgery must be performed, perhaps using an operative microscope, and the doctor has to be very careful in freeing the adhesions of the ovary and tubes. The rougher the physician is during this procedure, the more is the chance of subsequent adhesions.

If tubal surgery is performed, this is called *tuboplasty*. Tuboplasty calls for delicate surgery with fine instruments. If there are adhesions on the outer part of the tubes, they should be gently freed and the fimbriated ends opened and folded up like a flower. For conception to occur, the tubes and ovaries should be able to move freely in relation to each other. Freed adhesions could recur, and an attempt should be made to prevent this. It has also been found that if steroid hormones are injected into the abdominal cavity and the patient is treated with steroids, antibiotics, and tranquilizers after the operation, chances of recurrent adhesions are less.

If there is severe tubal occlusion, several modifications of tuboplasty can be done. However, it has been found that the more successful the doctor is in restoring the natural anatomy of the tubes, the higher are the chances for conception to occur afterward.

If the obstruction in the fallopian tube is closer to the uterus, one can bring the tubes closer to the uterus by reimplanting the tubes into the uterus.

If the fimbriated end is amputated due to severe adhesions or damage after infection, the chance of conception is small. Therefore, the most important task of tuboplasty is to restore the fimbriated ends of the tubes, free adhesions, and prevent the recurrence of adhesions by administering steroids, tranquilizers, and antibiotics immediately following the procedure. The ovaries and fallopian tubes are highly fragile organs, so the chance of conception after this procedure is often as low as 30 percent, depending on the extent of damage the infection has done to the pelvic organs.

Cervical Stenosis

Cervical stenosis is a narrowing of the cervix, leading to painful menstruation (dysmenorrhea). In some cases, this has been linked to a psychosomatic condition in which the fear of bleeding causes a woman to tighten her cervix to such a degree that sperm cannot enter. This condition is usually corrected with a dilatation and curettage (D&C). Following childbirth, it corrects itself.

Synechia

Synechia are scars inside the uterus. These scars usually result from scraping the uterine walls too aggressively during abortion or for control of bleeding after delivery. Today, with modern abortion techniques, synechia are becoming less frequent.

If a D&C is not successful in freeing adhesions from synechia, a laparotomy may be necessary. After synechia are freed, IUDs effectively prevent new adhesions from forming. Birth-control pills or estrogen and progesterone therapy aid in building up the lining of the uterus.

Immunological Factors—Can a Woman Be Allergic to Her Husband's Sperm?

The human body can be allergic to anything, especially to any foreign body. To a woman, nothing could be more foreign than sperm. The simplest way to evaluate whether a woman is allergic to her partner's sperm is to perform the postcoital test, as previously described. If an allergic reaction is found, there is no known cure for this cause of infertility, but if the allergy-causing factor (i.e., the sperm) is removed, the reaction subsides somewhat. A man whose partner is allergic to his sperm should refrain from ejaculating into the vagina for several months, perhaps by using a condom, and thereafter he should use the condom at all times except during the woman's most fertile days of the month. This has resulted in many pregnancies. If the condom technique doesn't work, artificial insemination with a donor sperm may be necessary.

Endometriosis as a Cause of Infertility

Pelvic endometriosis is a condition in which endometriotic masses are spread in the pelvis. The exact cause of endometriosis is not known, but it usually develops in highly strung women who have severe menstrual cramps. The menstrual blood is pushed out through the tubes to the pelvic cavity during menstruation, where it stays like normal tissue and is under the influence of the hormones which stimulate its growth. Endometriosis can grow all over the pelvic organs and block the tubes and ovaries, thereby causing infertility. Usually if tumors of this nature are found, the patient should undergo laparoscopy or exploratory laparotomy to determine the location of the tumors.

The usual treatment involves surgical removal of the endometriosis. However, this usually grows back and can, therefore, cause persistent infertility. Recently a new synthetic hormone called Danazol was developed, which blocks the release of LH and FSH, thereby causing amenorrhea. This hormone has proven effective in melting away all endometriosis and in many cases has restored normal fertility. This new hormone has helped many women who, after six months of treatment with Danazol, returned to normal fertility and successfully conceived. Danazol has recently been released by the Food and Drug Administration for general use. The usual dosage is 400 to 800 milligrams daily for six months, which is usually sufficient for the majority of women who have endometriosis. Of course, some women need a more prolonged period of treatment with Danazol in order to obtain the desired result.

TREATMENT OF FEMALE INFERTILITY

Infertility Caused by Pelvic Tumors or Adhesions

If the factor causing infertility in the female is tumors in the pelvis, the woman should be evaluated for an exact diagnosis. A laparoscopy, using a periscope inserted through the navel, enables the physician to examine the pelvic organs. If there are adhesions or growths around the tubes or ovaries, tuboplasty should be performed. Ovarian tumors should be very carefully evaluated and removed if they are causing infertility.

Infertility Caused by Congenital Abnormalities

If infertility is linked to unusual physical conditions such as double vaginas, uteri, or the absence of the uterus altogether, there is usually little, if anything, your doctor can do to remedy the situation. In the case of double uteri, pregnancy is possible, but the miscarriage rate is high, and premature deliveries are common. If the problem is merely a septum (a dividing wall or membrane) in the middle of the uterus, it can be removed surgically (by the Strassman operation) and the uterus can be reconstructed to reduce the chance of miscarriage. Other forms of uterine abnormalities will not be discussed here, since they are relatively rare and treatment for them is complex.

Evaluation of Amenorrhea

Amenorrhea (the absence of menstrual bleeding) is caused by any number of factors, but it always results in infertility. When a woman does not menstruate, it is because the lining of the uterus has not built up normally since the hormonal changes essential for ovulation have not occurred.

Amenorrhea can be caused by prolonged use of birth-control pills. After a certain time, the pill takes over the hormone functions of the body and, because it maintains a steady level of estrogen and progesterone, there is no stimulation to cause the buildup of the uterine lining. Once a woman stops taking the pill, it may take several months before menstruation resumes. If, after several months, menstruation does not resume, estrogen treatment followed by the administration of progesterone may bring it back.

Emotional stress can also be responsible for amenorrhea, as it affects the hypothalamus, which controls the release of FSH and LH from the pituitary gland. When this release does not occur, a woman will not bleed. This condition is sometimes called *anorexia nervosa*. Women who suffer from this condition often refuse to eat, thereby becoming increasingly thinner. This throws their hormonal balance even further off. Eventually such women break down physically and must be hospitalized. Treatment for anorexia nervosa must be of a psychological nature, and it may be a prolonged process. When the woman's weight, along with her eating habits, returns to normal, the rest of her body processes usually follow suit, and menstruation recurs.

A pituitary tumor can also cause amenorrhea. This will show up on a skull X-ray and must be removed surgically.

Hormone assays should be made to insure that the ovaries and the adrenal glands are not overproducing the male hormone androgen. Overproduction of this hormone can also cause menstruation to stop. If an infertility problem stems from the adrenal glands, there is probably overstimulation of or a tumor in the adrenal glands. This condition requires surgery. If, on the other hand, activity in the adrenal glands seems to be normal but the level of androgen is high and thus prevents ovulation, there is a rare possibility that a masculinizing ovarian tumor is responsible. The ovaries may have several types of tumors, some producing female hormones, others producing male hormones. The recent development of sensitive methods for checking testosterone level in the blood aids in this diagnosis.

Sometimes the ovarian capsule becomes thickened. As the thickening grows, it becomes increasingly difficult for ovulation to occur and cysts form. This is called Stein-Leventhal syndrome, or polycystic ovaries, and causes irregular or absent bleeding. The problem is treated surgically by removing a wedge of the ovary so it returns to normal size. Pregnancy occurs more easily after this procedure. The new fertility hormones have also proven effective in the treatment of Stein-Leventhal syndrome.

Alkaline Douches as a Treatment for Infertility

An alkaline environment is extremely important to sperm survival, motility, and ability to penetrate the cervical mucus. For this reason, it might be beneficial for a woman to take an alkaline douche prior to intercourse during ovulation. One tablespoon of sodium bicarbonate (baking soda) added to one quart of warm water will suffice for this purpose. Precoital use of this solution might be particularly beneficial for women whose cervical mucus is less than normally alkaline. After use of an alkaline douche prior to intercourse, postcoital tests often reveal an improvement over the previous condition by showing a greater percentage of actively motile sperm in the cervical mucus. Some physicians even recommend adding a small amount of glucose to the alkaline-douche solution, since this helps create an environment in which sperm have an increased chance for survival.

Fertility Drugs

If you are not ovulating (BBT is the easiest way to determine this), then your doctor may prescribe fertility drugs. One of the most successful of these drugs, and the most benign, is *clomiphene citrate* (Clomid). This drug has made many barren women fertile. No one knows exactly how it works, but it probably teams up with the estrogen already present in the body to stimulate and release eggs from the ovaries. One tablet a day should be taken from the fifth day of the menstrual period. If this proves unsuccessful, the dosage can be raised to four or five tablets daily. Clomid does not generally cause multiple births, but it can.

Some doctors follow Clomid with an injection of HCG (human chorionic gonadotropin). Your doctor should treat you with progesterone tablets or suppositories to decrease uterine contractions that can squeeze out the egg. Clomid may also improve the luteal phase merely by normalizing ovulation.

The fertility drug which sometimes causes the much-publicized multiple births is *Pergonal*. This drug is only indicated in rare cases and is generally prescribed for women who do not respond to Clomid. Pergonal is a mixture of LH and FSH collected from the urine of older women. The reason the urine of older women is used is that the secretion of these hormones from the pituitary gland is much higher after menopause. Most Pergonal is produced in Italy, where it is often collected from the urine of elderly nuns.

Pergonal is administered by injection. Your doctor then checks urine, blood, or cervical mucus for estrogen. When the estrogen reaches a certain level, an injection of HCG is administered. This should cause ovulation, but since the levels of FSH and LH are unusually high, several eggs might be released at the same time, causing multiple birth. A specialist experienced with Pergonal knows how to watch the hormone levels carefully, thus decreasing the chance of multiple birth. Still, Pergonal, which is very expensive, should be a last resort.

MALE INFERTILITY WORKUP

The production of sperm is a delicately balanced process, one that can be toppled by anything from too little exercise to too much alcohol. If sperm analysis reveals that the sperm is not sufficiently motile, that is, that it does not move fast enough, vitamin B complex or perhaps extra caffeine may be all that is required.

More often the cause of infertility is related to a hormonal imbalance. The man should have his thyroid function and pituitary production of gonadotropin checked to be sure they are fulfilling their roles in the production of sperm. A urologist can best evaluate both these functions, as well as abnormalities such as diabetes and hypertension as they relate to infertility. Most hormonal imbalances are successfully treated with hormone drugs, whether the imbalances are caused by tension or by disease.

A partially understood cause of male infertility is varicose veins in the scrotum. Surgical removal of these varicose veins has been proven to increase tremendously the amount of normal sperm which a man produces. The prevailing theory is that the great number of veins in the scrotum raise its temperature to the point where the testes are adversely affected. Temperature control is essential to normal sperm production, and this is why in warm whether, the testicles hang low, away from body heat; but in cold weather, they draw up into the body. The temperature of the scrotum should be somewhat lower than normal body temperature.

A complete physical examination should determine the condition of the penis and the testicles. Many unexpected congenital abnormalities, such as the absence of the vas deferens (the tube which transports semen from the testes through the penis) may be discovered. Undescended testicles that have been squeezed and damaged at a young age can also be detected.

A sperm analysis must be done by a specialist. Semen is often collected at the laboratory (the man is asked to masturbate in a private room) so the sperm is fresh. For sperm to be considered healthy and capable of causing pregnancy, the ejaculate should be at least 4 cubic centimeters and should contain a minimum of 20 million sperm per cubic centimeter. The normal sperm count is about 90 million per cubic centimeter. At least 40 percent should have good motility and 60 percent should have no serious defects, such as double or abnormal head structures. The first sperm sample might appear to have a low count, since the man will probably experience anxiety the first time he goes to a urologist. The role which many men are raised to play often makes it difficult for them to admit to having reproductive problems—infertility is easily translated by cultural bias into weakness, or a less than manly condition. Thus, more than one visit might be necessary before the man feels sufficiently at ease with the doctor to render a normal sample.

Environmental factors such as excessively high temperatures, poor eating habits, severe fever, allergies, or the excessive consumption of alcohol or tobacco can also lower a man's sperm count.

In today's high-pressure world, with sexual roles under constant scrutiny, it is not unusual for a man to suffer from infertility. Though the causes are sometimes physical, the problem is usually of a psychological nature, and professional help should be sought. If the problem is physical, hormone treatment or surgery often remedy the condition.

TREATMENT OF MALE INFERTILITY

If a man's sperm count is found to be low, a specialist should evaluate the man's physical problems. For example, if the level of thyroid function is low, treatment with thyroid tablets often restores fertility. If the gonadotropin level is low, treatment with FSH and LH is indicated. Clomiphene citrate (Clomid), the fertility tablet for women, is also sometimes effective in treating male infertility by raising the sperm count to a normal level. A testicular biopsy is indicated to determine if the testes have normal sperm production. A few other conditions are

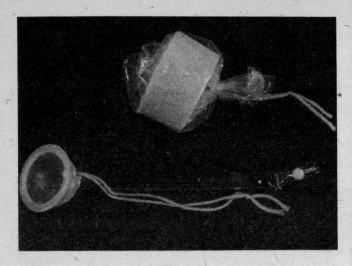

Fig. 12–5: This picture shows a vaginal sponge and a cervical cup, both used during artificial insemination. The vaginal sponge is covered with a plastic shield so it will not absorb the semen.

surgically or hormonally treated, but the majority of male infertility is caused by permanent damage, such as that resulting from mumps or accidents.

Men who undergo vasectomy should understand that this operation is generally not reversible and that their sterility is permanent, although isolated cases of restoring fertility through reconstruction of the vas deferens have been reported.

Unfortunately, the majority of male infertility problems cannot be treated. However, if a man is able to produce sperm, but the count and/or motility is low, the couple might consider artificial insemination.

ARTIFICIAL INSEMINATION

Twenty-five percent of all infertility problems, as previously stated, are attributable to the man. In the past, many couples have turned to adoption as an alternative to conception, but with the decrease in unwanted pregnancies due to modern birth-control techniques and legalized abortion, it is becoming increasingly difficult to find an adoptable child. Contemporary couples with infertility problems often solve their problem through artificial insemination.

The term *artificial* insemination is unfortunate. There is nothing really artificial about it. Perhaps *therapeutic* insemination would be a more accurate term. The procedure is timed to coincide with the woman's ovulation. If she has a regular twenty-eight-day menstrual cycle, insemination should be performed as many as three times between the tenth and the fourteenth days of the cycle. First, the doctor should check the fern pattern of the cervical mucus to ensure that the sperm will be able to penetrate it. Then the sperm should be checked, whether the husband's or a donor's is used. When brought to the doctor, the semen should be transported in a small bottle. The bottle should be kept warm (slightly below body temperature) or the sperm may die. Sperm are injected directly onto the cervix by the doctor in the hope they will move more quickly into the uterus and tubes. Insemination directly into the uterus is extremely painful and not particularly successful. A sponge is placed in the vagina to prevent the sperm from running out, and the woman's hips should be elevated slightly for fifteen to twenty minutes.

Alternatively, a cervical cup can be used. This apparatus fits over the cervix and has a tube running out through the vagina. The sperm is injected through the tube to the cervix. Uterine contractions create enough suction to hold the cup on the cervix, and a small valve prevents the sperm from escaping. The tubing is then folded into the vagina. Still, the woman should elevate her pelvis and remain on the table for fifteen to twenty minutes. After twenty-four hours, the woman removes the cup simply by pulling it out. There will be mucus and perhaps a little blood in the cup after removal, but this is normal.

The difficulty of artificial insemination is not in the procedure itself; rather, it lies in arriving at the decision to resort to this procedure. Most men find the idea threatening to their egos, especially if donor semen is used. Sometimes if the husband's sperm count is low but not necessarily useless, the doctor may mix the husband's sperm with the donor's. Although this might create an allergic reaction, just the possibility that the successful sperm was the husband's can work psychological wonders.

Many couples worry about who their donor will be, having read horror stories about blood donors recruited from Skid Row. Sperm donors are carefully screened and are matched as closely as possible to the prospective father. Hair color, eye color, race, and religion—all of these factors are taken into consideration when matching a sperm donor to the prospective father. Most sperm donors are medical students and generally an intelligent group of men.

One obvious advantage of artificial insemination over adoption is that the woman carries the child and the couple is involved in its birth. An understanding between the parents that no blame should be assessed for the original infertility is essential; it could just as easily have been the woman's problem as the man's. Sometimes professional counseling helps a couple understand that an artificially inseminated child is still their own child, a whole child, born of their love.

If the man is not infertile but has some inheritable disease—for instance, certain central nervous system diseases—or if he and the woman have incompatible Rh factors in their blood which may have already caused spontaneous abortion or stillbirths, the couple should consider artificial insemination with donor sperm. This greatly increases the possibility of a normal birth.

If artificial insemination is correctly performed by a specialist, conception should occur within a few months, although this is a generalization and not a firm rule. It may take years. The rate of success with artificial insemination is around 70 percent.

Is Artificial Insemination with the Husband's Sperm Worth the Effort?

Many people feel the entire procedure of artificial insemination is not worth the time and effort that it requires. Such couples often ask if it is not possible to achieve the same results at home with concentrated effort, by having intercourse during a woman's most fertile days and by using all optimum conditions for intercourse such as elevating the woman's buttocks by placing pillows under the pelvic area. It is true that this home method helps somewhat, especially when the man withdraws his penis from the woman's vagina shortly after ejaculation to prevent the dilution of the sperm on the shaft of the penis. However, if, after six months of trying at home, a couple still has not conceived, it is definitely a good idea to consult a doctor about artificial insemination.

Frozen Semen

In the past fifteen years, insemination with frozen semen has made progress. Today approximately one thousand babies

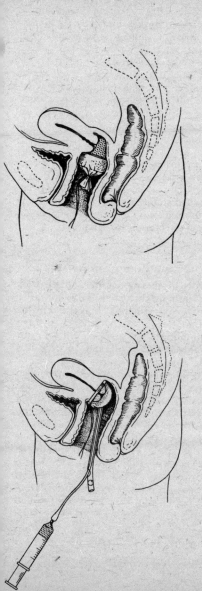

Fig. 12–6: This picture shows the cervical cup placed around the cervix and the semen being injected into the cup through plastic tubing. The little round plastic ball in the tubing pushes down to the cervical cup to prevent the leakage of sperm.

Fig. 12–7: Artificial insemination in which a vaginal sponge is placed high in the vagina to prevent the sperm, which are seen around the cervix, from leaking out.

have been born who were conceived with frozen, stored semen. Only about one percent of these have evidenced any abnormalities (as compared to six percent of the general population). The rate of successful impregnation with frozen sperm is only fifty percent. It is, however, a very practical method of donor insemination, since sperm banks have a large selection of donors, meeting almost all imaginable male genetic characteristics. The frozen sperm can easily be stored in the doctor's office for several days, and this makes insemination possible on weekends and in the evening. In this way, a working woman does not have to interrupt her office hours in order to visit her doctor's office.

The procedure for artificial insemination with frozen sperm is slightly different from that with fresh sperm, in that frozen sperm is actually allowed to thaw in the vagina. Motility is reduced more than 50 percent in some cases, so insemination is tried every month until impregnation occurs. The average length of time for a woman to become pregnant using this method is about eight months.

Should a Man Store His Semen Prior to Vasectomy?

Whether a man should store his sperm in a sperm bank prior to vasectomy has been increasingly discussed. Thus far, very few men have made use of this possibility. Even though this prospect appears attractive to some men, particularly to men who feel it might still be important to them, at some future time, to reproduce, it should be clearly pointed out that this procedure is still relatively new, and scientists do not know exactly how many years the sperm can be stored. It is known that sperm loses its motility, and the percentage of this loss is increased in direct proportion to the length of time during which the sperm remains frozen. As previously stated, the chance of conception with frozen sperm is only about 50 percent. Furthermore, there is no guarantee that a power failure might not occur one day, resulting in the destruction of all sperm stored in a given sperm bank. All of these factors should be taken into consideration before a man elects to undergo voluntary sterilization. In view of all this, it seems more reasonable to postpone vasectomy until a man has completely fulfilled his desire for reproduction.

Artificial Insemination with a Donor Uterus

In any discussion of artificial insemination, one usually considers the case of the fertile female partnered with the infertile

sion concerning artificial insemination of the husband's sperm into another woman who would act as surrogate mother, carrying the child until delivery and then surrendering it for adoption to the child's genetic father and his wife. This concept has even been explored in a recent movie, *The Babymaker;* however, in this case, the father impregnated the surrogate mother naturally. Such a procedure would undoubtedly cause a number of psychological problems, and family conflicts are certainly not suggested as a solution to fertility problems.

Nonetheless, one case has recently been publicized in which the husband was fertile and his wife infertile, and adoption was difficult. The husband placed an ad in a newspaper stating that he was married to an infertile woman and wanted to have a baby through artificial insemination with a woman whose background was similar to his wife's. There were more than 160 responses to this ad, and even though the man was willing to pay a good deal of money for this donor uterus, he found many women willing to carry the child just for payment of the doctor and hospital fees. The husband gave his sperm to a physician, and a woman submitted to artificial insemination. The woman delivered and the father adopted his child. The two parents never met. Although there are very few reports of this kind, artificial insemination with a donor uterus is considered another way to help the childless family and at the same time insure that some of the family's genes are transmitted to the child.

TEST-TUBE BABIES

"Test-tube baby" was the term used to describe Lucy Brown, the first live-born child to be conceived outside the mother's body in 1978. The term is a misnomer as it suggests the baby actually develops and grows outside the body. The proper term is *"in vitro* fertilization" since the mother's ovum (egg) is fertilized by the father's sperm *in vitro,* that is, in glass outside the woman's body. The full procedure is complex and requires the skills of several medical disciplines. The pioneering work in this field was done by Drs. Robert M. Edwards and Patrick Steptoe.

A woman whose infertility is based in tubal disorders such as damaged, blocked or missing fallopian tubes, who is healthy, with no ovulatory difficulties, and has a fertile partner, would be a candidate for *in vitro* fertilization.

When the fallopian tubes are blocked or missing, it is impossible for the normal pathway of conception to occur. What happens in nature must be replicated with great skill in the laboratory in an effort to bypass the tubes by artificially performing their vital functions. This is achieved in three basic steps.

Phase 1—Obtaining the Egg

The mother's egg or ovum must be obtained at the precise time of ovulation when it is about to be extruded from the ovary. At this time, the egg is mature and can be fertilized. The time of ovulation must be precisely determined by a battery of hormone tests. The operation to obtain the egg is called laparoscopy (See Chapter 16). Once the egg is collected, it is placed in a glass dish (therefore the term *in vitro*, in glass) containing blood serum and nutrients.

Phase 2—Fertilizing the Egg

Once the ripe egg has been obtained it must be fertilized. The husband's sperm is added to the dish containing the egg along with certain chemicals which permit the capacitation of the sperm, the ability of the sperm to fertilize the egg. The egg and sperm are placed in an incubator at body temperature in the hope that fertilization and cell division will occur. Great care must be taken to keep everything as free from contamination as possible. If the egg is fertilized, it will be ready for reimplantation within two and one-half days.

Phase 3—Reimplanting the Egg in the Uterus

The timing of the reimplantation of the fertilized egg must be again extremely precise. The zygote, two and one-half days after fertilization, is introduced into the uterine cavity by means of a slender tube passed through the cervix. If the zygote is at the right stage of development for implantation, and the mother's uterus is at the proper stage for reception, the fertilized egg will attach to the uterine wall and normal development will begin.

The Future of *In Vitro* Fertilization

The birth of Lucy Brown in England in 1978 proved that "test-tube" fertilization is possible and raised expectations in women for whom pregnancy had been impossible. However, a number of ethical problems have been raised. Will women in the future be able to hire surrogate mothers to carry their children? Whose baby would it be? These problems will only arise if *in vitro* fertilization becomes widespread. Since the technique requires exquisite skill and care, it will most likely be limited to the strictest indications.

chapter 13

UTERINE ABNORMALITIES

DEFINITION AND DESCRIPTION OF THE UTERUS

The uterus is a muscular organ whose sole function is to house the fetus during its growth and development. To this end, the interior of the uterus goes through monthly variations to prepare for conception.

The uterine wall is composed primarily of smooth muscle cells. These cells are lined by fibrous (connective) tissue and vascular tissue. The fibrous tissue supports the muscle cells, while the vascular tissue supplies blood and other energy-giving components to these cells through blood vessels.

As a muscular organ, the uterus has contractions or cramps continuing for the entire monthly cycle, even throughout pregnancy and delivery. Those cramps are much stronger at the time of menstruation, but they are evident throughout the month, even if they are not felt by the woman. The pain at menstruation is caused by the dilatation (opening) of the cervix. This dilatation permits the passage of the endometrium (the lining of the uterus), which is squeezed out of the uterus during menstruation.

CONGENITAL MALFORMATION

During the first three months of female fetal development, the beginning of the brain system, the intestines, and the urogenital systems are formed. The uterus (as well as the kidneys, the vagina, and the bladder) is developed from tissue originating on each side of the body, the so-called Müller's and Wolffian ducts. As these ducts fuse together in the midline, the uterus is

DEVELOPMENT OF FEMALE GENITAL ORGANS

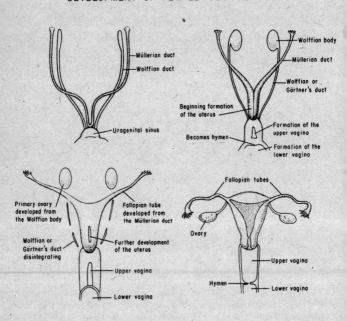

formed. The urogenitalia sinus, located in the lower part of the abdomen, joins with the newly formed uterus to create the vagina.

During this intrauterine life, an occasional developmental abnormality can occur. This is commonly precipitated by certain infections or viruses in the first three months of pregnancy or by any condition which might prevent the complete fusion of this tissue in the midline. In severe instances, a girl baby can be born with neither a vagina nor a uterus or with other severe malformations of the reproductive and urinary tracts. Sometimes the uterus will be only partially fused, and a child will be born with a double uterus. There are many variations of this, all of them dependent upon the degree to which this fusion has occurred.

Fig. 13–1: Development of Female Genital Organs. The genitalia start to develop during third to the fourth week of fetal life. Primitive cells fuse to become the Wolffian or Gaertner's duct about the fifth week after conception. The Müllerian duct starts to develop at about the sixth week of fetal life, about the same time as the urogenital sinus. *(See upper left drawing.)* The upper part of the Müllerian ducts develops into the fallopian tubes while the lower portion fuse together and form a uterus at about eight weeks after conception. *(See upper right drawing.)* The upper portion of the Wolffian duct develops into the Wolffian body which eventually becomes the ovary in a female (it would be a testicle in a male). The urogenital sinus likewise develops into the vagina.

The lower left drawing shows the stage of development approximately eleven to twelve weeks after fertilization. The development of the Fallopian tubes and the uterus has become clear. The Wolffian body has formed into a primary ovary, which will subsequently move downward. In the male fetus, this gonad moves all the way into the scrotum. The lower portion of the Wolffian or Gaertner's duct disintegrates in a female fetus. In a male, it develops into the *vas deferens* (the tubes carrying the sperm from the testes to the urethra).

The vagina lengthens and the vaginal opening becomes apparent. The hymen will be located between the developing of the upper and the lower vagina. If this normal progression is disturbed during the second to fourth month of fetal life, an abnormal uterus or vagina can result. Such disruption can be caused by drugs taken by the mother, or by various types of infections, as well as by radiation from X-rays. By the sixteenth week of fetal life, the female genitalia have their characteristic appearance, but development continues until birth. The lower right picture illustrates this final stage of development.

Such abnormalities often cause no symptoms and thus go largely undetected until they accidentally are discovered, either because a girl does not start menstruating or experiences trouble which leads to a complete gynecological examination. If malformations are suspected, they can be confirmed by special tests or procedures such as *hysterosalpingogram, laparoscopy,* or *hysteroscopy.*

Imperforated Hymen

During fetal development, the Müller's and the Wolffian ducts meet the urogenital sinus and form the hymen, a mucous membrane located approximately half an inch inside the opening of the vagina.

The hymen is closed to varying degrees in different women. In certain cases, there is very little hymen located on the wall of the vagina. In other cases, the hymen almost completely closes the vagina and makes penetration extremely difficult. If the hymen is completely closed (imperforated hymen), a problem would develop when the woman starts menstruation—the blood will collect behind the hymen period after period and cause severe pain, eventually requiring surgical intervention *(hymenectomy)*.

An intact hymen has long been considered a symbol, if not absolute proof, of virginity. In fact, it is not. Some hymens are so undeveloped that they are apparent only to a doctor as a *fragment* of tissue on the wall of the vagina. Intercourse can occur without breaking the hymen and so can conception.

If the hymen is so tight that intercourse is impossible, even after several attempts, you should see a doctor. He might have to perform a hymenectomy, a surgical procedure in which the hymen is cut open at several places and then sutured so that it remains open. After this procedure, a woman might have to use vaginal dilators if she does not have regular sex to keep the hymen open. This condition, however, in no way affects a woman's ability to become pregnant.

Absence of the Vagina or Uterus

Some women are born without a vagina or a uterus. Although this can occur separately, usually the absence of a vagina means the absence of a uterus, also. However, the ovaries are often intact, so normal development of sex characteristics occurs.

Women often do not realize this type of problem until they attempt intercourse and discover that there is no real opening, or until they consult a gynecologist about absence of menstruation.

This condition is not genetically derived; rather, it is a developmental abnormality occuring in the fetus often as the result of some disease or drugs taken by the mother during pregnancy.

If a woman has no vagina, which might be discovered through self-examination, the physician should test her chromosomes to determine if they are normal. He should also perform a laparoscopy (with a periscope inserted through the navel) to determine if the uterus and ovaries are present and normal. If the uterus and ovaries are both present, which is rare in these cases, a surgical vagina can be constructed with the same plastic surgery techniques used in male to female sex-change operations. In this operation, a tunnel is created, then covered with a skin graft obtained from the inside of the thigh.

The finished product has all the characteristics of a real vagina, from touch to smell. Since the skin graft is placed directly on nerve tissue, sensation is not impaired and frequency of orgasm is absolutely normal. This procedure can be performed even when the uterus and ovaries are missing, but in that instance, conception is not possible.

Double Vagina and Uterus

During the first three months of fetal intrauterine life, developing tissues from either side of the abdomen might not join properly. In some rare cases of female fetuses, two vaginas and two uteri may result. Quite often, each vagina is connected quite cleanly to one cervix, one uterus, and one fallopian tube, and the woman will exhibit no abnormal symptoms. A double vagina is usually divided by a membrane that is pushed to one side or the other by a penetrating penis, so it feels normal to both the man and the woman. Conception can occur in either uterus.

Problems occur, however, when the fetus begins to stretch the uterus. Since one sac of a double uterus cannot stretch as far as a normal uterus, premature birth or miscarriage is frequent. Surgery is not always necessary to remedy this condition, but if pregnancy occurs, the obstetrician should pay special attention to prevent complications.

What Problems Occur with Uterine Abnormalities

As seen in the illustration, there are various types of uterine malformations caused by incomplete fusion of the two parts of the uterus during the first three months of embryonic development. Any variation can occur, from a complete separation of the womb with a double uterus (uterine *didelphys*) or a double vagina to only a small uterine septum (a membranous partition within the uterus). Occasionally, only one side of the uterus develops, a condition known as *uterus unicornis*.

A woman with a double uterus can conceive. The only problem usually is miscarriage or premature delivery. Still, no corrective surgery is indicated.

If there is an incomplete septum in the middle of the uterus, pregnancy can also occur without problems, although there is a higher incidence of miscarriage. If a woman miscarries too often, a *hysterosalpingogram*, an X-ray of the uterus in which the septum or the abnormality can be clearly seen, should be ordered. If the septum is causing miscarriage, corrective surgery should be performed. This entails a Strassman's procedure, in

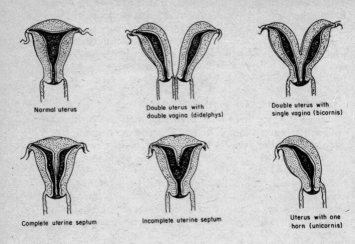

Normal uterus

Double uterus with
double vagina (didelphys)

Double uterus with
single vagina (bicornis)

Complete uterine septum

Incomplete uterine septum

Uterus with one
horn (unicornis)

Fig. 13–2: Some congenital uterine abnormalities. In the top row to
the left is a normal uterus. In the middle is both a double uterus, a
double cervix and two vaginas. To the right is a double uterus with
only one cervix and one vagina. In the lower row to the left is a uterus
with a complete uterine septum. In the middle, is an example of a
uterus with a small septum. To the right, is an example of a one-sided
uterus; the other side did develop in this particular case.

which the septum is removed and the uterus is repaired. After
this operation, women can usually carry children with no
further problems.

A woman with a unicornis (or "one horn") uterus usually
experiences no problem in conceiving if her cervix is open and
a normal fallopian tube and ovary are present.

Many women have variations of uterine abnormalities without ever knowing about them, since they experience normal
menstrual bleeding and childbearing. These conditions need to
be evaluated—by a physician or by X-ray—only if problems
occur.

Tilted Uterus

Normally the uterus is positioned forward, against the bladder. In infancy, the uterus lays backward a bit, but it shifts
forward as it develops. However, in about 20 percent of all

women, the developing ligaments holding the uterus forward loosen, and the uterus tilts back against the rectum. This syndrome is called *tilted uterus.*

Until recently, there was a widespread belief that a tilted uterus caused, among other things, infertility. Today, unless a tilted uterus causes pain or physical problems, it is usually left untreated. It is now considered to be a genetic condition, like freckles or a big nose.

There is a second type of tilted uterus that is not congenital, but is acquired usually from pelvic inflammation or endometriosis resulting in adhesions which pull the uterus backward. This is often painful and associated with infertility.

Acquired tilted uterus can also occur after childbirth, since delivery stretches the uterine ligaments and these ligaments subsequently relax after birth. With each delivery, the ligaments become weaker and looser, allowing the uterus to lean back more.

The most common symptom associated with tilted uterus is backache. This is probably a result of blood trapped in the uterus, causing the uterus to become enlarged and tender. This uterine tenderness inflames the nerves of the back and results in severe backache. This is called *pelvic congestive syndrome.*

Many women with tilted uteri also complain of pelvic pressure stemming from the pressure the uterus exerts on the rectum. Constipation generally follows, and there is abdominal pain often mistaken for inflamed ovaries. These symptoms increase prior to menstruation.

Treatment of Tilted Uterus

Treatment depends on the severity of the symptoms. When no symptoms are present, no treatment is necessary. If the symptoms are minor, some doctors simply prescribe an exercise regimen, stressing exercises in the knee-chest position to allow the uterus to fall forward and empty any congested blood.

Another alternative to surgery is the insertion of a *pessary,* a device which acts like a crutch to hold the uterus forward.

If your gynecologist suggests surgery, you should solicit a second opinion from another doctor. Surgery is sometimes required, but more often it is abused. The surgery is not dangerous; it is often merely unnecessary. The operation basically entails tightening the ligaments which pull the uterus forward.

FIBROID TUMORS OF THE UTERUS

The word *tumor* is shocking to everyone. If a doctor suddenly looks up after completing a pelvic examination and says, "You have a tumor of the uterus," most women will immediately begin planning their own funeral arrangements. It is a common fear, one that is possibly devastating to the psychological well-being of every patient.

It should be clear from the start that having a tumor *does not necessarily mean cancer*. A tumor is merely an enlargement or growth. That growth can be either benign or malignant. A benign tumor is noncancerous; only malignant tumors are cancerous. In the vast majority of cases (approximately 99 percent), a fibroid tumor is benign or noncancerous. This statistic should calm women's natural fears about fibroid tumors, but it should not divert attention away from other possibly serious ramifications of a fibroid tumor.

Definition and Origin of Fibroid Tumors

A fibroid tumor of the uterus, also called a *myoma* or a *leiomyoma*, is caused by abnormal growth of cells within the uterine wall (the *myometrium*). There are contrasting theories concerning the type of cells in the uterine wall that develop into fibroid tumors.

One theory is that fibroid tumors arise from primitive cells which normally develop into muscle cells, fibrous cells, or blood vessels. For some unknown reason, this normal development of primitive cells into special cell types has not occurred. Instead, these primitive cells develop into fibroid tumors. Since there is no known reason why these cells shouldn't develop along their normal lines into special types, this apparent malfunction could be genetic in origin. This theory tends to support the undeniable fact that fibroid tumors run in the family—if your mother had fibroid tumors, you have a higher risk of developing the same condition than a woman whose mother was free of fibroid tumors.

A second belief holds that the myomas come from the fibrous (connective) tissue cells in the uterine wall.

Other investigators have suggested that fibroid tumors originate in the fibrous tissue or muscle cells of the blood vessels in the uterine wall.

Finally, some scientists firmly believe that myomas are developed from the smooth muscle cells of the uterine wall, since the fibroid tumors have been found, on microscopic examination, to be composed of muscular tissue. This lends credence to the Latin words *myoma* and *leiomyoma*, both of which refer to muscle. If this is true, though, the layman's term—fibroid tumor—is technically inaccurate, since it is the muscle tissue, and not fibrous tissue, which causes the tumor.

The type of cells from which fibroid tumors develop is, however, more of scientific curiosity than clinical interest. What is important is the cause behind the growth of fibroid tumors, how to prevent or minimize their growth, and how to treat them in their various stages.

General Characteristics

Myomas are the most common tumors afflicting the female organs. It has been estimated that more than 20 percent of all adult women have fibroid tumors, although the vast majority of these women exhibit no symptoms of these tumors.

The incidence of fibroids is, inexplicably, five times greater in black women than in white women. Although it is not statistically verified, the incidence of fibroids tends to be higher in East European and Jewish women than in other white women. The youngest female known to have fibroid tumors was an eleven-year-old girl. Rarely do new tumors develop after menopause, and the majority of myomas found after the change of life actually developed before the menopause. If a new tumor does develop after menopause, there is more reason to believe it is malignant.

A woman can develop a single fibroid tumor, yet development of multiple tumors is far more common.

The size of fibroid tumors varies widely, from microscopic to enormous. The largest tumor ever reported weighed over one hundred pounds.

White in color, fibroid tumors are dense in structure. They are encapsulated and form whorllike masses.

Genetic Occurrence of Myomas

There are several misconceptions among women concerning the development and growth of fibroid tumors. Most of these misconceptions arise from fear and the subsequent ignorance it produces or from a misguided sense of morality.

It should be stated at the beginning that frequency or type of intercourse, or any past traumas or accidents, have absolutely nothing to do with the development of fibroid tumors.

The reason fibroids occur is most likely genetic. The significantly higher incidence of fibroids running through specific families backs up this genetic theory. As mentioned before, the more frequent occurrence of myomas in certain races also supports this belief. Since this genetic trace seems undeniable, it is vital that a woman in one of the racial or familial categories which have a greater tendency to myomas be aware of her situation. In this instance, a woman should be more alert and have a gynecological examination twice yearly to monitor the occurrence and/or growth of fibroids. Moreover, she should understand the phenomenon of myomas and not be frightened if a doctor tells her she has a fibroid tumor of the uterus.

Hormonal Stimulation of Fibroid Tumors

A woman is probably born with the seed of a fibroid tumor in her uterine wall. Although we don't know what exactly sets off the impulse for this seed to develop into a myoma, a growing body of evidence indicates that the female hormone estrogen may be the culprit. This is supported by the observation that these tumors almost always occur between the first menstruation and menopause—the only time when women produce estrogen hormones. Furthermore, when the production of estrogen is highest—during pregnancy—fibroid tumors grow more rapidly. Concomitantly, after pregnancy—when estrogen production diminishes—fibroid tumors usually regress to a certain extent. It has also been observed that there is a rapid enlargement of myomas in cases of estrogen-producing ovarian tumors.

Birth-control pills, particularly the kind with high estrogen content, have also been found to stimulate rapid growth of fibroid tumors. For this reason, many women taking oral contraceptives develop fibroids. Of course, these women might have developed fibroid tumors in any case, and the birth-control pill might only speed the onset of myomas. Women with increased genetic tendencies to fibroid tumors should, then, probably avoid use of oral contraceptives, particularly those with high estrogen content. Women who already have diagnosed tumors should definitely not use estrogen-containing birth-control pills. If you are taking an oral contraceptive and your physician discovers a myoma, even if it is very small, you should immediately discontinue the use of the pill and find another method of contraception.

It has recently been discovered that there is an association between high-fat diets leading to obesity and an increased level of estrogen production. It seems that obesity overstimulates the body's hormone production. This, in turn, leads to a greater stimulation of fibroid tumors, as well as an increased incidence of breast cancer (which is probably also dependent on estrogen levels). This indicates another important function of diet, but it also shows that if you are one of those women with a higher tendency to myomas, you should avoid becoming overweight.

Usually the growth of fibroids is slow. If, however, you have rapidly growing myomas and this fast growth cannot be connected to the overstimulation of hormones (such as by pregnancy or use of oral contraceptives), the fibroid tumor should be *very* carefully monitored. It is this type of tumor which is most often malignant.

Types and Descriptions of Fibroid Tumors

Fibroid tumors can be found in three general locations in the uterine wall, and the location of each fibroid determines the type of tumor in question and the treatment.

One type is the *intramural*, or *interstitial*, fibroid tumor, located in the middle of the muscular wall of the uterus. This type of tumor usually grows entirely in the wall, causes no pain, and poses no problem when it is small. If the intramural tumor is large, it will occasionally obstruct the fallopian tubes and/or the birth canal.

A fibroid can also be located in the subserosal area of the uterus, directly beneath the peritoneum (the outer lining of the uterus). This is the *subserous*, or *subperitoneal*, fibroid. These can grow anywhere on the outside of the uterus. Although they might cause some pain, they are usually not dangerous as long as they remain small. The subserous fibroids will occasionally achieve great size without causing any other symptoms, except perhaps a feeling of heaviness. If they are located in front of the uterus, they may press on the bladder and cause urinary discomfort, such as frequent or difficult urination. If they grow on the lower part of the uterus, the subserous tumors might also block the birth passage if they are large. This would make a natural delivery impossible. Sometimes large veins on the surface of subserous fibroids might rupture, causing severe internal hemorrhaging.

The subserous fibroids occasionally become *pedunculated*, meaning that they grow like a flower on the outside of the uterus, attached to the uterine wall by a stalklike protuberance. A pedunculated subserous myoma will also cause no problems unless it twists around its own stalk, thereby cutting down the blood supply to the tumor. This causes extreme pain and can only be treated by surgical removal of the pedunculated tumor.

A third type—the *submucous* fibroid—grows inside the uterine wall just beneath the endometrium (the lining of the uterus) and protrudes into the uterine cavity. Even though submucous myomas comprise only 5 percent of all fibroids, they are the type that instigate the most problems. Submucous fibroids will, when they enlarge, break the smooth lining of the

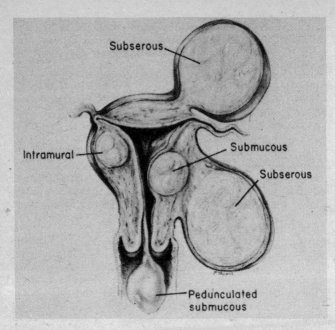

uterus, thereby causing heavy bleeding. This bleeding can, at times, become so severe a woman might bleed to death without medical attention. She might well require emergency surgery. A submucous fibroid can also disturb pregnancy. When the placenta, or afterbirth, starts to grow inside the uterus, it might grow into the area of the myoma. This area will not have the same blood supply as the normal part of the uterus. Consequently, the placenta will not adhere adequately to this area. This might result in bleeding and miscarriage.

Some submucous fibroids might also become pedunculated as they grow larger. The uterus then regards the fibroid as a foreign body, and it attempts to expel the fibroid by contractions. Even when the uterus succeeds in expelling the pedunculated fibroid through the cervix, the myoma will still be attached, via its blood-supplying stalk, to the uterine wall. This so-called self-aborting tumor tends to become ulcerated and infected and must be surgically removed.

If you have a fibroid, make sure you know what kind it is and where it is located. Remember, fibroids vary with each person—one woman will have a subserous fibroid while her

Fig. 13–3:   Three different types of fibroid tumors. On the left is an *intramural* fibroid, located *inside* the muscle wall of the uterus. As you can see, if this tumor grew to a large size, it could obstruct the passage to the fallopian tubes. On top of the uterus is a *subserous* fibroid. This tumor is *outside* the uterus and, although it is rather large as pictured here, it does not interfere with uterine function. A second *subserous* tumor can be seen in the lower right portion of the picture. Even at this relatively large size, this tumor would not generally cause any symptoms. However, in this location, on the lower aspect of the uterus, this tumor might be stimulated and grow due to the increased hormone level during pregnancy. It might grow to such an extent that it would obstruct the cervix and vagina and make natural delivery impossible. In the middle of the diagram, on the right side of the uterus, is a *submucous* fibroid, lying just underneath the endometrium (the lining of the uterus). This is protruding into the uterine cavity, pushing the endometrium in front of it. This breaks the smooth contour of the uterine cavity and can, therefore, cause bleeding. Protruding down through the cervix into the vagina, a *pedunculated* submucous can be seen. This pedunculated tumor started inside the uterus, but was expelled from the uterine canal by uterine cramps. It is still attached by its stalk to the inside of the uterine cavity and can, therefore, cause pain and bleeding. Each tumor is whorllike in substance, contrasted to the normal tissue of the uterine wall.

best friend or sister will have an intramural or submucous fibroid.

It is also important to know that it is not the number of fibroid tumors you have that is important. The vital fact is the size and location of the tumors.

The only type of smaller tumor you, as a patient, should be concerned about is the submucous fibroid. It is potentially the most dangerous type, since it may cause severe hemorrhaging.

Diagnosis of Fibroid Tumors

A fibroid tumor is usually diagnosed during a pelvic examination. A competent physician will most often be able to feel any abnormality in the size and shape of the uterus, particularly if the patient is relaxed during the examination. A thorough physician should, as soon as he feels even the slightest abnormality of the uterus indicating the development of a fibroid tumor, inform the patient of his diagnosis and the size and location of the fibroid.

Unfortunately, some doctors are not that good at determining the size and location of fibroid tumors. These doctors might unnecessarily frighten you by telling you that you have a large tumor that is very dangerous when, in fact, you have a small tumor that is quite harmless. No matter how much you like your doctor, if he suddenly springs this kind of diagnosis on you—a diagnosis that will scare most people—you should get a second opinion. This is especially true if you have been receiving regular examinations in which you were told you had no abnormalities.

To confirm a physician's diagnosis of a fibroid tumor, *sonography* (or *ultrasonography*) can be used. This is a newly developed technique which has become extremely popular in diagnosing both pelvic masses and the size of the fetus during pregnancy. Sonography has replaced X-ray for a variety of diagnoses, since ultrasound is completely harmless to the body. Essentially similar in principle to radar, sonography employs acoustical rather than electronic frequencies in making a diagnosis. Sonography projects a high-frequency sound into the body, and the impulses of the reflection of that sound measure the size and location of the tumor as it is shown on the sonar screen. If there is any doubt as to the location and size of your fibroid tumors, sonography might be the ideal tool to give you an exact description of your uterine tumors. Besides, it is completely painless and most hospitals have ready access to the equipment.

There might be occasional difficulty with sonography in determining whether a tumor on the side of the uterus is of ovarian or uterine origin. Ovarian tumors are far more dangerous than uterine masses. For this reason, it must be determined whether a mass is ovarian. To check this, a physician could perform a laparoscopy. This is a procedure usually done under a general anesthesia, though sometimes local anesthesia can be used. During this operation, a periscope-type instrument (a laparoscope) is inserted through the navel. By looking into the laparoscope, the doctor will have a direct view of the uterus, the fallopian tubes, and the ovaries. This allows an exact description of the size, shape, and origin of the tumor.

If there is a suspicion that you have a submucous fibroid, one of the best methods of diagnosing this condition is an X-ray of the uterus, called a hysterosalpingogram. With this type of X-ray, dye is injected into the uterus and a picture is taken. If a submucous fibroid tumor exists, it will distort the shape of the uterine cavity. This distortion will be readily seen on the X-ray.

A few doctors prefer to perform a D&C (dilatation and curettage) to determine the presence of a submucous fibroid tumor. During this procedure, the physician will explore the uterine cavity with a curette (a spoonlike instrument) in order to find out if the walls are smooth and regular. If the walls are irregular, a submucous tumor is most likely penetrating into the uterine cavity.

What Can You Do If You Have a Fibroid Tumor?

Most fibroid tumors cause very few problems, so if you show no symptoms whatsoever, the best thing you can do is relax and not worry about them.

However, if you have one or more fibroids with no symptoms, you should be seen by a good gynecologist two or three times a year to check the size of the fibroids. This is the only important action on your part, because you and your doctor can then determine what, if anything, is happening with the fibroid tumors.

If there is rapid growth of the fibroid tumors, it might cause suspicion. Rapid growth is one of the symptoms of malignant tumors, but is not an indisputable sign; tests may be necessary to find out if the tumor is, indeed, malignant. Sometimes you might even need an operation to remove the fibroid tumor for further analysis. This should determine whether the tumor is malignant. It should be pointed out, however, that this type of condition is extremely rare, happening in only one-half to one percent of all cases, and almost always when there is rapid growth of the fibroid tumors.

If your fibroid tumor causes hemorrhaging, you should have an examination under anesthesia and a D&C to determine the location of the fibroid. If the symptoms are severe, you should probably have an exploratory laparotomy, an operation in which the abdominal cavity and the uterus are explored.

Contraception and Fibroid Tumors

If you have a fibroid tumor, yet you experience no problems with it and can bear children, you really don't have to do anything about the condition except refrain from taking birth-control pills with high estrogen content.

You might, though, desire some form of contraception. Here a diaphragm may be the answer. Still, fibroid tumors sometimes disturb the vagina to such a degree that a diaphragm will not fit properly.

An IUD might be a perfect solution in this situation. Not only is there no hormone stimulation, the enlarged uterine cavity will make insertion of an IUD fairly easy. An IUD is not recommended when dealing with submucous fibroids, though, since it will probably cause more bleeding.

Of course, condoms and foam are other solutions to this problem and are widely used when fibroids disrupt normal contraceptive techniques.

As stated before, submucous fibroids often cause miscarriage. While certain cultures believe miscarriage is God's will and therefore a natural form of contraception, it is hardly the ideal method for today's woman. If you have a submucous fibroid where hemorrhaging and miscarriage occur, you should probably have the tumor removed. It is important to realize that a tumor can be taken out without removing the uterus.

Fertility and Fibroid Tumors

The vast majority of women with myomas have no difficulty whatsoever in conceiving. If, though, you do have any trouble conceiving, it might be due to obstruction of the reproductive passages by fibroid tumors. Surgery might be indicated in such an instance, but because myomas related to fertility are so rare, the physician should perform a thorough testing prior to any surgery.

The doctor should take an X-ray of the uterus (a hysterosalpingogram). If the X-ray shows that the fibroid tumors are obstructing the fallopian tubes, there might be cause to remove the fibroids. However, the physician should first make sure your ovaries are functioning normally and that you have a normal ovulation pattern. This is done by taking daily basal body temperature (BBT), which shows an increased temperature just after ovulation. The doctor can also take a biopsy from inside your uterus to make certain you do ovulate. Sadly, many women have operations to remove fibroid tumors only to find that it is an abnormal ovulation pattern which is preventing conception, not the fibroids.

The potential father is often overlooked. The doctor should examine his sperm to ensure his fertility before *you* undergo an operation to remove fibroids. Again, countless women have gone through such an operation only to find that the hopeful father does not have a healthy sperm count.

If these checks are made and it seems that the fibroid tumors are the cause of your infertility, it would probably be wise to have them removed.

Can Fibroid Tumors Be Removed without a Hysterectomy?

If the fibroid tumor is enlarged to an abnormal extent or causing symptoms, you will most likely need a *myomectomy,* an operation in which the fibroids, or myomas, are removed. This